*The*

# DIET HACK

## WHY 95% OF DIETS FAIL
## AND HOW YOU CAN SUCCEED!

### TIM STEELE, MSc

**The Diet Hack: Why 95% of Diets Fail and How You Can Succeed!**

Publishing services provided by 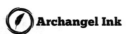 **Archangel Ink**

ISBN: 978-1-942761-93-8

# WHAT OTHERS ARE SAYING ABOUT
## *THE DIET HACK...*

Tim Steele's *The Diet Hack* is anything but a hack. He's done an excellent job reminding us that many rivers reach the sea, and the current state of diet tribalism is unnecessary and oftentimes unproductive. His book brings us back to the basics and provides a foundation people can use not only to lose weight, but to actually keep it off—which is the real challenge.

—Angelo Coppola, host and producer of the Latest in Paleo podcast and the Mostly Plant Diet™

Written in an entertaining and authentic tone, Tim Steele's newest book, *The Diet Hack*, explains how to stay healthy once and for all. Statistics confirm that less than half a percent of obese people who diet will ever reach a normal weight, so Steele entered an elite health circle when he not only lost nearly one hundred pounds but kept it off, shedding plenty of prescription drugs and health problems along the way. In this book, you'll find complex nutrition and health ideas presented in words that everyone can understand and apply; hard-core science is handily translated into real-life action plans. *The Diet Hack* is a solid forever diet plan written in such an honest way that it will have you vigorously nodding your head, occasionally busting out laughing, or even at times awkwardly smirking. Although enthusiastic nutrition experts and health nuts will find plenty of practical knowledge and fascinating facts to keep them busy, Steele writes for common people who wonder, deep in their hearts, if they can ever get and keep the weight off and how.

—Terri Fites, M.D., nutrition writer for Molly Green Magazine; hostess of The Homeschooling Doctor blog

Tim Steele writes *The Diet Hack* with the same fervor that he wrote the extremely popular *The Potato Hack*.

Written at a time, in the Western world when the standard diet is less than optimal for health, weight, or wellbeing, he has taken steps to identify why most diets ultimately fail, and what we can do to help ourselves.

He takes a lot of science and puts it together in a way that can be understood by most people with an interest in the subject, without bombarding the reader with heavy data.

If you are one of these people for whom diets don't work, other than in the short-term, then this could be the book for you to read. He brings together reasons why diets don't work for everyone and gives examples of how to approach it based on both science and experience. You'll learn how to make long-term changes to your lifestyle choices to help achieve long-term goals.

The section on gut health may be particularly interesting to those who are new to this concept.

—Mags Fegen, PhD, research coordinator for National Health Services (NHS Scotland)

Tim Steele has suffered from the medical consequences of the modern American diet. The reason why he is now lean is because he learned that most calorie restriction diets work for weight loss but fail to maintain a desired weight. *The Diet Hack* provides his simple guide to lifelong weight control. This is your last diet book.

—Dr. Art Ayers, Ph.D., former professor of cellular biology at Harvard University and host of Cooling Inflammation, a blog explaining the interaction of diet, inflammation, and disease mediated by gut microbiota

I've been a fan of Tim Steele ever since picking up his book *The Potato Hack*. Tim isn't tied to any specific dieting philosophy, and he simply digs deep into the current research to give out the best science-based advice.

If you want facts that aren't influenced by a hidden agenda, you will love Tim Steele's books.

—Rusty Moore, health writer, entrepreneur, host of Visual Impact Fitness blog

Tim takes a simple and unique approach to dieting, and good health in general, with a major focus on gut health being central to overall well-being. Tim coined a phrase in his first book, *The Potato Hack*, that I've used many times since reading it: "If you're not hungry enough to eat a plain, cold, boiled potato, then you're not hungry!" *The Diet Hack* removes the guesswork and will give you confidence that lasting success is well within reach.

—Andrew "SpudFit" Taylor, author and health coach at SpudFit.

# CONTENTS

# PREFACE

Here's a hard pill to swallow: most dieters will fail to achieve meaningful weight loss past the one-year mark, and 95% or more will have failed by their fifth year. Why do so many people fail at dieting? They don't. *People* are not the problem. The problem is that the deck is stacked against dieters, and hardly anyone really understands dieting. And losing weight is easier than keeping weight off.

There are several people we can blame: the Diet and Fitness Industry, the Pharmaceutical Industry, the Food Industry, the Medical Industry, the Supplement Industry, and several other "big boys" who don't care about your health as much as they care about your net worth. But *we're* to blame, too … for buying into their schemes and falling for hype that's obviously too good to be true.

I've learned their tricks. I know the dirty secrets. We *can* regain control of our health and weight if we understand how and why we lost control. I will show you how to focus on what matters and decipher what's just noise. I'll show you how *you* can beat the odds and keep your weight off for good. I'll even give you a brand-new diet that will prove to be more effective than most diet plans ever devised.

I promise: No tricks, no gimmicks, no crazy science. Just good food, a good life, and great health.

# INTRODUCTION

**TL;DR:** *Let me help you take the mystery out of weight gain, weight loss, and weight maintenance.*[1]

The Diet and Fitness Industry (aka "Big Diet") will hate this book. Because it's designed to take a huge bite out of their profits. There are thousands and thousands of diet and fitness books, apps, and programs designed to lure you in and tempt you to buy countless products. After reading this book, you'll never need them again. Just like Big Pharma wants to keep you sick, Big Medicine wants to keep you as a patient, Big Food wants to keep feeding you junk, and Big Tobacco wants to keep you hooked on nicotine. Big Diet? They don't really care that you lose weight or get fit. They just want you to buy billions of dollars' worth of diet and fitness products every year.

In this book, I will share *evidence-based* advice and *industry-insider* secrets that will allow you to craft a diet that works for you. After reading this book, you'll see why over 95% of dieting attempts fail to produce lasting weight loss, and you'll learn how *you* can succeed.

---

1    *TL;DR* is an internet term for a summary. It's used throughout diet and fitness forums to acknowledge that you wrote something waaaaay **t**oo **l**ong and you don't blame people if they **d**on't **r**ead it.

## Big Pharma, Big Diet, Big Medicine, Big Food, and Big Ol' Me

In 2009, my daily supplement regimen included Lopid, Colcrys, Zocor, Cozaar, and Synthroid.[2] My BMI was 35 ... obese. How could this have happened? I was dieting, drinking diet soda, eating low-fat potato chips and ice cream, skinless chicken breasts, whole wheat bread, and organic vegetables. I thought if I took the pills and ate like the (overweight) doctor told me, I'd soon get better. Wrong.

Everyone has a tipping point. The straw that finally broke this camel's back was an annual checkup that showed I'd gained another 10 pounds and my fasting blood glucose and hbA1C were firmly in the pre-diabetic range. I left that appointment with a prescription for Metformin and a sunken heart.

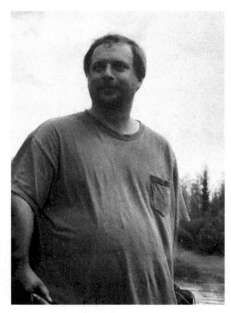

*Author, 2008*

2   Lopid is for high triglycerides, Colcrys is for gout pain, Zocor is used to lower high LDL cholesterol, Cozaar is a blood pressure medication, and Synthroid is used for hypothyroidism.

No freakin' way! I'd spent the last ten years watching my belly balloon as I did everything the doc told me. I thought, *If I'm like this at 43, what will I be like at 53? Will I even live to 63?*

Time to break out the big guns … Google, Bing, and Yahoo:

"Reversing T2D"

"Metabolic syndrome"

"Lowering blood glucose"

"How to get off high blood pressure meds"

"Low carb diets"

"How to *loose* weight"

I remembered doing Atkins back in the '90s with some success, so I started there. I ate lots of butter and steak for a couple weeks and lost a few pounds, but my gouty big toe had other plans. I joined an Atkins support group and realized I'd been doing it all wrong. After a couple more false starts, I came across the concept of Paleo dieting, eating as our ancestors did thousands of years ago.

Instead of lean chicken, I was eating two big fatty steaks for dinner along with piles of steamed veggies and some fruit. I stopped buying low-fat packaged food and just ate real, whole food … fat, skin, and all. Nuts, berries, and jerky were my new snacks. The enemies were potatoes, bread, rice, cheese, and any food unavailable 10,000 years ago.

After I'd lost a few pounds, I felt like exercising again. The Paleo diet is big on exercise and sleep. I went from not being able to do a single pull-up to doing twenty within a short time. I was in bed by 10 p.m. every night and slept in complete darkness.

It worked! Within six months, I'd lost over 40 pounds and was off most of my meds. But then my weight loss stalled, and my digestion suffered, so I regrouped and realized I was missing fiber from "non-Paleo" foods such as beans, rice, potatoes, and grain. I slowly started eating wholesome foods again, carbs be damned.

After another six months, I'd lost another 40 pounds and was at my goal weight, a weight I've maintained for almost ten years now. During this time, my thinking on what constitutes the best diet has evolved. I learned very quickly that the advice that helped *me* did not help *everyone*.

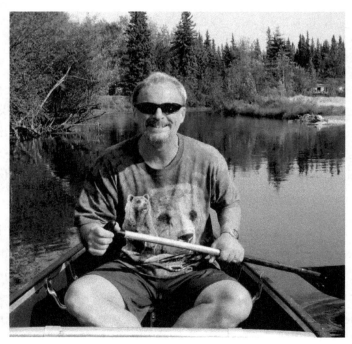

*Author, 2018*

For the past ten years, I've been studying different diet plans and watching the diet industry evolve. I've been active in dozens of weight loss boards, fitness forums, and Facebook groups; I've made thousands of comments on various blogs; and I've appeared in several podcasts. I presently host three popular health blogs (Vegetable Pharm, The Potato Hack Chronicle, and The Diet Hack), and I have a best-selling book, *The Potato Hack: Weight Loss Simplified*.

It's horrendously daunting to search for diet plans on the internet. You don't know what's real and what's a scam. We are continually bombarded on TV, radio, and browsers with ads for different diets. We are lured in by the sexy, slim bodies and promises of instant weight loss without hunger, instant abs without sweat, and effortless health with the right supplements.

I suffered through gout, fatty liver disease, gallstones, high blood pressure, high triglycerides, high cholesterol, pre-diabetes, and hypo-thyroidism. I found what worked for me. Now I'm writing this book to take the mystery out of diet and exercise and to help you find a plan that works for you. You'll learn how to create your *own* diet with elements from all the best plans available. Dieting is much more than simply eating the right foods. Some diet plans are really good, some are just plain awful. So, let's take a close look at what makes a good diet plan and how you can find one that suits you. By the time you're finished with this book, you'll know how to make the right diet work for the rest of your life.

# PART 1

# THE OBESITY EPIDEMIC

# INTRODUCTION TO PART 1

I'm not a doctor or a nutritionist. I spent the first 21 years of my adult life as an airman in the United States Air Force and the past 15 years working with electronics in a large hospital in Alaska. During this time, I earned a master's degree in biotechnology and started a biotech consulting company from my home, less than 200 miles away from the Arctic Circle. I learned a few things along the way: It's easier to fly at Mach 1 than it is to eat right. It's easier to harness 12,470 volts of electricity than it is to lose weight. It's easier to create immortal life[3] in a lab than it is to keep weight off.

Losing weight and keeping it off requires an attack from all sides. I'm happy when someone loses weight, but I'm more impressed when they keep it off. The goal of Part 1 is to show you why there is such an urgent need for dieting. I want to help you achieve long-term weight maintenance by focusing on several factors: diet, exercise, sleep, stress, diseases, medications, genetics, and gut health.

But first I want to show you where we are going wrong. From the food we eat to genes that control our destiny, if we don't understand why we got fat in the first place, how can we ever expect to fix the problems?

---

3 See my published paper: *Life begins at forty – hybridomas: ageing technology holds promise for future drug discoveries* (Steele, 2016).

# CHAPTER 1

## WHY WE GAIN WEIGHT

**TL;DR:** *Diet, exercise, sleep, stress, medical conditions, medications, environment, diseases, genetics, and gut health all play an intricate and interrelated role in our weight.*

You are most likely reading this because you need to lose weight, or you want to help someone else lose weight. Your mind went straight to "diet" as the solution. But consider:

> Diets do not lead to sustained weight loss or health benefits for the majority of people. (Wolpert, 2007)

It's a well-known fact in the diet industry that *diets don't work.* Pharmaceutical companies bank on it, plastic surgeons rely on it, your doctor is saddened by it, insurance companies deal with it, and the food industry loves it. The only people who don't seem to know this "inconvenient truth" are the *billions* of overweight people of the world who spend *trillions* to lose weight.

*Diet Industry Insider Secret: Most traditional diet programs now hide the fact they are promoting a diet and have rebranded themselves to remove the word "diet" from their names and logos.*

## Determinants of Weight

The same people who know that dieting doesn't work also know what *does* work, and it looks something like this:

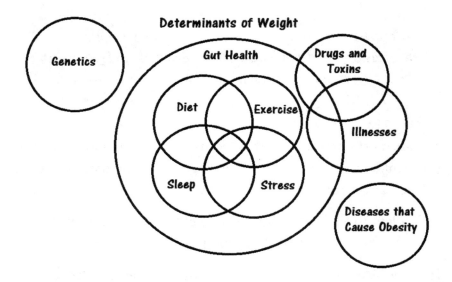

There are many factors that decide a person's weight. Genetics and certain diseases stand alone and have an impact on your weight completely outside of anything you do to try to lose weight. Your genes will mostly determine where you store fat and how much muscle you can ever hope to gain. Certain (somewhat rare) diseases will cause a person to become overweight or obese; these conditions are hard to diagnose and often lead to years of frustration as the person attempts in vain to lose weight. We'll address genetics and disease, but I want to focus mainly on the determinants of weight that are within our control.

You'll see from this diagram that "diet" is only a small piece of the puzzle and overlaps considerably with exercise, sleep, and stress. To focus singularly on any one of these items is a waste of everyone's time. Dieting for the purpose of weight loss is a very shortsighted venture as "everyone" knows. More than 95% of dieters will regain the weight lost, with many regaining *more* than they lost (Atkinson, 2003).

Underlying everything is the gut. To lose weight, we oftentimes destroy our own gut. The gut—meaning your stomach, small intestine, large intestine, colon, and supporting structures—is vital to our overall health and weight maintenance (Simon, 2019). Keeping the gut happy is paramount to enjoying a long, healthy life (Brandsma, 2019). Medications, antibiotics, and illnesses often impact the gut and will disrupt weight stability no matter how hard you try to lose weight (Tokuhara, 2019).

## What Is Dieting Good For?

Special diets are good for many things:

- Disease management (e.g., celiac disease, diabetes)
- Medical conditions (e.g., high blood pressure, high cholesterol)
- Weight gain (e.g., for cancer patients, malnourishment)
- Weight loss (e.g., for overweight or obese people)

We can easily devise a diet for therapeutic purposes when the root can be traced to a particular food source. It's as easy to design a diet for weight loss as it is to design a diet for celiacs.

## Wait. What? Weight Loss Diets Are Easy?

Yes! You can easily lose weight by following a weight loss protocol. Study after study shows that overweight people, with an otherwise healthy metabolism, can lose weight on any well-designed diet they can follow for 6–12 months (Yannakoulia, 2019). And this bears out in a real-world setting as well. The diet industry would not survive if most customers didn't lose weight as promised. Happy customers ensure the industry thrives. But no one highlights the dismally low long-term success rates.

The evidence is clear: weight loss is highly probable when you adhere to a special diet designed to decrease food intake.

> Recent reviews suggest that most diets are equally effective, a message very different from what the public hears in advertisements or expert pronouncements ... This supports the practice of recommending any diet that a patient will adhere to in order to lose weight. (Johnston, 2014)

## What's the Problem, Then?

The problem is that weight loss is not the endgame. Once the weight comes off, it goes right back on unless all the determinants of weight gain are kept stable. Excessive and inappropriate dieting can impact gut health, aggravate underlying medical conditions, or create other imbalances that make *keeping the weight off* impossible.

As I'll lay out in excruciating detail, *weight loss is not the problem* ... keeping it off is the problem. When researchers say that "95% of diets fail," they are talking about meaningful, lasting weight loss. Some put the number even higher, estimating that only 1–3% of dieters successfully keep their weight off (Atkinson, 2003).

*Weight Loss Industry Insider Secret:* "While hundreds, if not thousands, of weight-loss strategies, diets, potions, and devices have been offered to the overweight public, the multi-factorial etiology of overweight challenges practitioners, researchers, and the overweight themselves to identify permanent, effective strategies for weight loss and maintenance." (Atkinson, 2003)

Weight loss diets are very effective at causing weight loss, just like high-calorie diets cause malnourished children to gain weight. But as a gluten-free diet does not cure celiac disease, a weight loss diet will not cure obesity.

Just about everyone can summon the willpower to do what it takes to lose excess weight, but most of these attempts will be in vain because as soon as the dieting stops, the weight comes right back. Subsequent attempts to lose weight will be even harder.

## What's the Trick?

The trick is to lose weight safely and timely, then switch to a weight maintenance diet while simultaneously focusing on all the determinants of weight (in this order):

1. Diseases causing obesity/medical conditions/medications
2. Gut health
3. Diet
4. Exercise
5. Sleep
6. Stress
7. Genetics

First, focus on underlying medical conditions or diseases that might be hampering your efforts. Your doctor should be able to help come up with a plan of action that allows you to be healthy, even if you can never be at a normal weight.

Secondly, focus on gut health because without a healthy gut, everything you do may be futile.

> Emerging evidence suggests the human gut microbiota, a complex ecosystem residing in the gastrointestinal tract, may influence weight-gain through several inter-dependent pathways including energy harvesting, short-chain fatty-acids signaling, behavior modifications, controlling satiety and modulating inflammatory responses within the host. (Bliss, 2018)

Then start to dial in your diet, exercise, sleep, and stress levels all the while being mindful of your genes. If your mom, dad, grandpa, or grandma had big thighs or a big belly, chances are you will, too. Don't fight it; manage it. We can't all look like the people we see in weight loss ads, and quite frankly, we shouldn't.

## Conclusion

The rest of this book is devoted to hacking industry secrets to find a diet that works for *you*. And not just to lose a couple pounds for a week or two, but to lose substantial weight and keep it off forever. Weight loss diets work if you can find one that suits you *and* if you can stick to it long enough. Factors that will influence your success are oftentimes outside your control and need to be addressed first. We must also learn to differentiate between *looking good* and *being healthy*. Good looks are mostly a dream sold by advertisers. Good health comes from within.

# CHAPTER 2
## THE WESTERN DIET

**TL;DR:** *Most of us eat really bad food, called the Western diet. This diet lacks fiber and nutrients; it has too many chemicals and too much sugar, salt, and fat. Lobbyists fight to keep this diet legal so that big corporations can continue to rake in profits at our expense.*

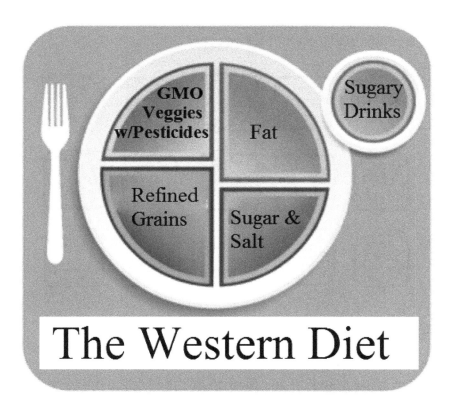

> A large body of research now supports the hypothesis that the Western Diet is causing changes in gut microbiota associated with obesity and metabolic disease. There also seems to be consensus that fixing the diet-induced dysbiosis is a possible approach in fighting the obesity epidemic. (Zinöcker, 2018)

There are hundreds of research papers that point to the Western diet as the *root cause* of most disease (Myles, 2014). The foods available are not only making us fat but are killing us. It's akin to getting trapped in a spider's web, eating like we do. We have easy access to cheap, tasty food that lasts forever. We hardly even have to *cook* anymore. If the food were *good*, this would be fine. But the food's *bad* (Hall, 2018). Sometimes I feel like the guy at Woodstock warning about brown acid.

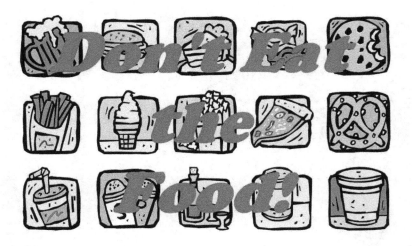

## Big Food

Food is an industry. From agriculture to stocking shelves, there's money in every step of the food chain. The food industry, or Big Food as they are lovingly called, is made of the corporations that develop and distribute the staples of the Western diet. Here's a list of the biggest of the big. Recognize any of these? I'll bet nearly all these companies have shelf space in your pantry right now. Go look. Am I right? With very few exceptions, if these names are on your packaged food, you'd be better off not eating it.

- Campbell Soup Company
- Conagra Foods
- General Mills
- Hain Celestial Group
- The Coca-Cola Company
- The Hershey Company
- Hormel
- Ingredion
- The J.M. Smucker Company
- Kellogg's
- Kraft Heinz
- Keurig Dr Pepper
- Mars, Incorporated
- T. Marzetti Company
- McCormick & Company
- Monarch Beverage Company
- Mondelez International
- PepsiCo
- Pinnacle Foods
- Post Holdings
- Rich Products
- Seaboard Corporation
- TreeHouse Foods
- Tootsie Roll Industries
- Tyson Foods
- WhiteWave Foods
- Zevia

These companies aren't evil; they fill a need. They spend billions on new techniques to make their products competitive in a market that relies on high volume and slim margins. My foray into the world of biotechnology helped me to understand exactly what lengths these companies go to in creating the perfect foods for Western tastes. We can use their tricks to our favor, but first let me show you just what's going on. Please keep in mind that these companies also bring us great food as well. They will happily provide us with organically grown papayas and hormone-free, free-range meat just as quickly as they will fill our larders with chemically flavored snacks that will sit in a pantry for a decade without spoiling. It's up to the consumer to identify what's healthy and what's not.

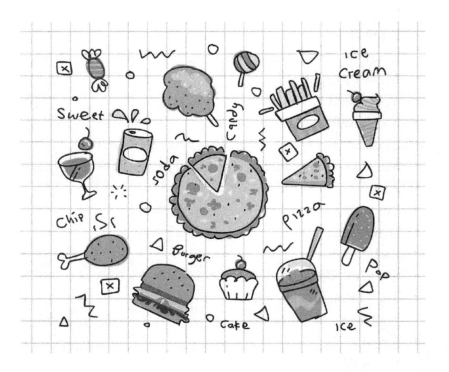

## Processed Food

In our desire for quick, cheap meals, we've created a huge demand for processed food. Most people have no idea the degree of processing that food undergoes. Over 75% of the modern diet (on a calorie-per-calorie basis) is made up of industrially formulated food. This food is low in nutrients and vitamins, and it drastically alters a healthy gut (Zinöcker, 2018). The fiber and natural nutrients that make humans healthy are replaced with man-made vitamins and minerals that minimally conform to government specifications. Chemically altered fat, man-made sugar, and heavy doses of salt are used along with chemical flavor enhancers, colors, and food additives to make processed food hyper-palatable and addictive (Morin, 2017).

## NOVA

A group of Brazilian nutritionists came up with a great idea. They've divided the food we eat into four categories based on processing. They call this classification system "NOVA." NOVA is a name, not an acronym. It means "a star burning bright" (da Costa et al., 2018).

| NOVA Food Category | Examples |
|---|---|
| Group 1—Unprocessed or Minimally Processed Foods | Fruits, vegetables, grains, legumes/beans, starchy roots and tubers, fungi, red meat, poultry, fish and seafood, eggs, milk, fresh fruit or vegetable juices (without added sugar, sweeteners or flavors), pasta, couscous, polenta, tree and ground nuts, seeds, spices, herbs, plain yogurt with no added sugar or artificial sweeteners, tea, coffee, drinking water |

| NOVA Food Category | Examples |
|---|---|
| Group 2—Processed Ingredients | Salt, sugar, molasses, honey, syrup (e.g., maple), vegetable oils crushed from olives or seeds, butter and lard obtained from milk and pork, starches extracted from corn and other plants |
| Group 3—Processed Foods | Canned or bottled vegetables, fruits and legumes/beans; salted, oiled, or sugared nuts and seeds; salted, cured, or smoked meats; canned fish/meat/poultry; fruits in syrup; cheeses; unpackaged freshly made breads |
| Group 4—Ultra-processed Foods | Carbonated drinks; packaged snacks, potato chips, pretzels, corn chips; ice cream, chocolate, candies (confectionery); mass-produced packaged breads and buns; margarines and spreads; cookies, pastries, cakes, and cake mixes; breakfast cereals, energy bars; energy drinks; milk drinks, "fruit" yogurts and "fruit" drinks; cocoa drinks; meat and chicken extracts and "instant" sauces; infant formulas, follow-on milks, other baby products; protein bars and drinks; meal-replacement bars and drinks; ready to heat products including pre-prepared pies and pasta and pizza; poultry and fish "nuggets" and "sticks," sausages, burgers, hot dogs, bacon, and other reconstituted/chemically preserved meat products, and powdered and packaged "instant" soups, noodles and desserts |

*Adapted from da Costa, 2018*

NOVA recommendations:

- Eat mostly from Group 1, flavored with Group 2.
- Eat sparingly from Group 3.
- Avoid Group 4.

Most of us have spent our lives eating mostly Groups 3 and 4. When you read through these food lists, it becomes clear where our problems lie. The problem is not too many potatoes, it's too much *other stuff.* It irks me to no end to see a popular diet that bans beans and rice but allows energy bars and bacon.

### Group 1—Unprocessed and Minimally Processed Food

Unprocessed food is found "around the edges" of the supermarket. Fresh fruit, vegetables, beans, rice, pasta, eggs, meat, fish, milk, and freshly made bakery goods. Most grocery stores have tons of unprocessed foods at our beck and call, but the siren song is from the many aisles of "healthy" cereals, snacks, and quick meals.

Organic food might be a step in the right direction, but conventional produce is fine if washed well. Sometimes it just gets to be too much to take in, but the crux of the argument is that we should be eating mostly unprocessed and minimally processed food. Just because a vegetable might have traces of pesticides does not mean it's entirely bad. It's not optimal, for sure, but it's better to buy veggies and wash them well than to buy a can of meal-replacement adult formula. Buy all organic if you can afford it; better yet, grow your own or befriend a farmer.

### Group 2—Processed Ingredients

A bit of sugar or salt makes some foods immensely more edible. This category is used to create dishes out of minimally processed food. Study the NOVA table ... you could make an entire Christmas dinner with items from the first two groups. All it takes is imagination and a bit of cooking prowess.

## Group 3—Processed Food

Group 3 of the NOVA table contains foods that are "mostly" okay, but you don't want to get all your calories from this category. It pays to read the labels of canned food. You can find many canned veggies that just have one ingredient, but others have oil, salt, and preservatives, making them lean awfully close to the next group. Plus, cans are not ideal for long-term storage of foods; glass is much better. Processed foods of Group 3 are often unreasonably salty or sugary. Preserving food in salt and sugar used to be an important part of food security, but now we just like the taste of salt and sugar a bit too much. Frozen foods are much closer to fresh than canned, especially when canning uses salt and other additives. Processed meats also have their own issues; nitrates, salt overload, and other preservatives, even if natural, are not ideal to eat to the exclusion of fresh meat. Use processed foods to augment the minimally processed foods in your meals or as small snacks and treats.

## Group 4—Ultra-Processed Food

Ultra-processed food has low nutritional quality and contains numerous additives, packaging contaminants such as BPA, and chemical alterations from production, processing, and storage (Steele, 2017). Ultra-processing is used to create food items that are easy to ship and last nearly forever. These foods are marketed as "ready-to-eat," "microwaveable," and "instant." More money is often spent on the packaging and advertising than the food itself. This requires the addition of firming, bulking, anti-bulking, defoaming, anticaking and glazing agents, emulsifiers, sequestrants, and humectants (Poti, 2017). These foods are designed to compete with unprocessed food for your attention and money. Who hasn't considered the merits of bananas compared to 100-calorie snack packs of potato chips for your lunchbox?

Ultra-processed food fills most of the aisles in your grocery store. Think Pop-Tarts, Cap'n Crunch, Wonder Bread, and Lean Cuisine. Many ultra-processed foods are made entirely of sugars, oils, and refined wheat—three of the world's cheapest foods (Steele, 2016). They contain many substances that exist merely to fool your taste buds: hydrogenated oils, modified starches, protein isolates, and other concoctions. Think Ho Hos, Diet Pepsi, Doritos, and Hawaiian Punch. Vegetables and meats are pressure extruded, molded, reshaped, deep-fried, and hydrogenated. Think Slim Jim, Pringles, Fish Sticks, and Hot Pockets. Ultra-processed foods are artificially flavored, artificially colored, and laced with chemicals that trick your brain into thinking it needs more. Think SweeTarts, Ben & Jerry's, Bologna that has a first name, and Cadbury Crème Eggs.

## Western Staples

"Staples" are food items purchased in bulk that make up most of your diet. Some staples commonly found in modern households are eggs, milk, bread, butter, sugar, flour, and rice. Yet most of our meals are not produced from the items we buy in bulk. Instead, our meals are hastily slapped-together concoctions of ready-to-heat or ready-to-eat meals, lunch meat, or meals purchased from restaurants (Pinho, 2018). Many households only incorporate "home-cooking" on rare occasions, and the depth of cooking that goes on in many homes is limited to bacon and eggs or pancakes on the weekend. *More than 70% of the food we eat is processed to some degree* (Steele E.M., 2017). The bulk foods we buy are used as additions to ultra-processed dry mixes (Rice-A-Roni, Hamburger Helper, cake mixes, etc.), and as replacements for fast-food (sandwiches, desserts, fried food).

## Make Ultra-Processed Food in Your Own Kitchen!

The Western diet is well-known for foods that are cooked by submerging them in superheated oil. French fries, donuts, egg rolls, and potato chips, for instance. This method of cooking is quite possibly the worst of the worst. I rail endlessly on Big Food for offering us a horrible array of altered food, but we deep-fry right in our own kitchens.

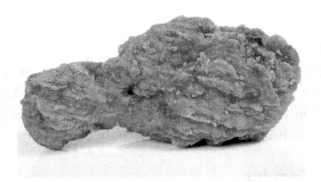

When oil, any oil, is heated over and over and used for frying meat, grain, and vegetables, it infuses highly inflammatory carcinogens into previously wonderful food. This is not big news. Researchers have known "forever" that fried foods are one of the worst features of the Western diet:

> Deep frying calls for high temperatures of approximately 350–370°F, usually using polyunsaturated seed/vegetable oils such as canola, corn and soybean oil, which are easily oxidized and generate potentially carcinogenic/mutagenic compounds such as aldehydes and acrolein. (Stott-Miller, 2013)

Our desire for tasty, hot food leads us to seek out fried foods. Electric deep-fryers are a common kitchen appliance across the civilized world. Would this still be the case if they carried a label that said,

"Eating deep-fried food is a leading cause of prostate cancer," or "Eating deep-fried food causes coronary heart disease, stroke, hypertension, diabetes mellitus, and obesity"? Shame on Big Food for selling Pringles to kids, but shame on *us* for feeding our family out of a FryDaddy (Gadiraju et al., 2015).

Oil itself isn't the problem. Oils can be part of a heart-healthy diet. But oil should never, ever be eaten after it's been heated to, or near, its smoking point and especially if repeatedly reused (Venkata et al., 2016). Big Food spends billions to suppress this type of information, much to the benefit of every fast-food restaurant and diner in the world.

## (Anything but) Natural Flavors

Staples in the average household also include an endless supply of cookies and candies. But Fall 2019 will be different. Who doesn't love pumpkin spiced coffee or banana bread? Seems it's everywhere. But in the United States, the FDA has banned six chemicals used as artificial flavors used to create the taste of cinnamon and spice, and also fruity, minty, and twangy vinegar (Choi, 2018). Wouldn't you think it would be easy to replicate the taste of cinnamon? Um, couldn't you use *cinnamon*? Apparently not.

The US Food and Drug Administration occasionally screens the items that Big Food uses. In October 2018, the FDA announced they are banning the use of six chemicals whose only labeling requirement is "artificial flavor." These six flavors are (FDA, 2018):

- Synthetically-derived benzophenone
- Ethyl acrylate
- Eugenyl methyl ether (methyl eugenol)
- Myrcene
- Pulegone
- Pyridine

And why are these ingredients being banned? They can cause cancer. Still, the FDA contends these additives are safe, "if used as intended." Otherwise, they've been known to cause cancer in humans and animals at higher doses (Choi, 2018).

The FDA regulates artificial flavors. The Code of Federal Regulations is the law of the land in governing everything that the government oversees. Title 21, Section 1, Subpart B, paragraph 101.22, states (FDA(2), 2018):

> (a)(1) The term artificial flavor or artificial flavoring means any substance, the function of which is to impart flavor, which is not derived from a spice, fruit or fruit juice, vegetable or vegetable juice, edible yeast, herb, bark, bud, root, leaf or similar plant material, meat, fish, poultry, eggs, dairy products, or fermentation products thereof. Artificial flavor includes the substances listed in §§172.515(b) of this chapter except where these are derived from natural sources.

§§172.515(b) lists these substances. Here's the list of artificial flavors that can legally be put in ultra-processed food and labeled simply as "artificial flavor":

Acetal; acetaldehyde diethyl acetal. Acetaldehyde phenethyl propyl acetal. Acetanisole; 4 ' -methoxyacetophenone. Acetophenone; methyl phenyl ketone. Allyl anthranilate. Allyl butyrate. Allyl cinnamate. Allyl cyclohexaneacetate. Allyl cyclohexanebutyrate. Allyl cyclohexanehexanoate. Allyl cyclohexaneproprionate. Allyl cyclohexanevalerate. Allyl disulfide. Allyl 2-ethylbutyrate. Allyl hexanoate; allyl caproate. Allyl a -ionone; 1-(2,6,6-trimethyl-2-cyclo-hex- ene-1-yl)-1,6-heptadiene-3-one. Allyl isothiocyanate; mustard oil. Allyl isovalerate. Allyl mercaptan; 2-propene-1-thiol. Allyl nonanoate. Allyl octanoate. Allyl phenoxyacetate. Allyl phenylacetate. Allyl propionate. Allyl sorbate; allyl 2,4-hexadienoate. Allyl sulfide. Allyl tiglate; allyl trans- 2-methyl-2- butenoate. Allyl 10-undecenoate. Ammonium isovalerate. Ammonium sulfide. Amyl alcohol; pentyl alcohol. Amyl butyrate. a -Amylcinnamaldehyde. a -Amylcinnamaldehyde dimethyl acetal. a -Amylcinnamyl acetate. a -Amylcinnamyl alcohol. a -Amylcinnamyl formate. a -Amylcinnamyl isovalerate. Amyl formate. Amyl heptanoate. Amyl hexanoate. Amyl octanoate. Anisole; methoxybenzene. Anisyl acetate. Anisyl alcohol; p- methoxybenzyl alcohol. Anisyl butyrate Anisyl formate. Anisyl phenylacetate. Anisyl propionate. Beechwood creosote. Benzaldehyde dimethyl acetal. Benzaldehyde glyceryl acetal; 2-phenyl -m- di- oxan-5-ol. Benzaldehyde propylene glycol acetal; 4- methyl-2-phenyl -m- dioxolane. Benzenethiol; thiophenol. Benzoin; 2-hydroxy-2-phenylacetophenone. Benzophenone; diphenylketone. Benzyl acetate. Benzyl acetoacetate. Benzyl alcohol. Benzyl benzoate. Benzyl butyl ether. Benzyl butyrate. Benzyl cinnamate. Benzyl 2,3–dimethylcrotonate; benzyl methyl tiglate. Benzyl disulfide; dibenzyl disulfide. Benzyl ethyl ether. Benzyl formate. 3-Benzyl-4-heptanone; benzyl dipropyl ke- tone. Benzyl isobutyrate. Benzyl isovalerate. Benzyl mercaptan; a -toluenethiol. Benzyl methoxyethyl acetal; acetaldehyde benzyl b -methoxyethyl acetal. Benzyl phenylacetate. Benzyl propionate. Benzyl salicylate. Birch tar oil. Borneol; d- camphanol. Bornyl acetate. Bornyl formate. Bornyl isovalerate. Bornyl valerate. b -Bourbonene; 1,2,3,3a,3b b ,4,5,6,6a b ,6b a -deca- hydro-1 a -isopropyl-3a a -methyl-6-meth- ylenecyclobuta [1,2:3,4] dicyclopentene. 2-Butanol. 2-Butanone; methyl ethyl ketone. Butter acids. Butter esters. Butyl acetate. Butyl acetoacetate. Butyl alcohol; 1-butanol. Butyl anthranilate. Butyl butyrate. Butyl butyryllactate; lactic acid, butyl ester, butyrate. a -Butylcinnamaldehyde. Butyl cinnamate. Butyl 2-decenoate. Butyl ethyl malonate. Butyl formate. Butyl heptanoate. Butyl hexanoate. Butyl p- hydroxybenzoate. Butyl isobutyrate. Butyl isovalerate. Butyl lactate. Butyl laurate. Butyl levulinate. Butyl phenylacetate. Butyl propionate. Butyl stearate. Butyl sulfide. Butyl 10-undecenoate. Butyl valerate. Butyraldehyde. Cadinene. Camphene; 2,2-dimethyl-3-methylene- norbornane. d- Camphor. Carvacrol; 2- p- cymenol. Carvacryl ethyl ether; 2-ethoxy -p- cymene. Carveol; p- mentha-6,8-dien-2-ol. 4-Carvomenthenol; 1 -p-menthen-4-ol;4-terpinenol. cis Carvone oxide; 1,6-epoxy -p- menth-8-en-2-one. Carvyl acetate. Carvyl propionate. b -Caryophyllene. Caryophyllene alcohol. Caryophyllene alcohol acetate. b -Caryophyllene oxide; 4-12,12-trimethyl-9-methylene-5-oxatricylo [8.2.0.0 4,6] dode- cane. Cedarwood oil alcohols. Cedarwood oil terpenes. 1,4-Cineole. Cinnamaldehyde ethylene glycol acetal. Cinnamic acid. Cinnamyl acetate. Cinnamyl alcohol; 3-phenyl-2-propen-1-ol. Cinnamyl benzoate. Cinnamyl butyrate. Cinnamyl cinnamate. Cinnamyl formate. Cinnamyl isobutyrate. Cinnamyl isovalerate. Cinnamyl phenylacetate. Cinnamyl propionate. Citral diethyl acetal; 3,7-dimethyl-2,6-octa- dienal diethyl acetal. Citral dimethyl acetal; 3,7-dimethyl-2,6-octa- dienal dimethyl acetal. Citral propylene glycol acetal. Citronellal; 3,7-dimethyl-6-octenal; rhodinal. Citronellol; 3,7-dimethyl-6-octen-1-ol; d- cit- ronellol. Citronelloxyacetaldehyde. Citronellyl acetate. Citronellyl butyrate. Citronellyl formate. Citronellyl isobutyrate. Citronellyl phenylacetate. Citronellyl propionate. Citronellyl valerate. p- Cresol. Cuminaldehyde; cuminal; p- isopropyl benz- aldehyde. Cyclohexaneacetic acid. Cyclohexaneethyl acetate. Cyclohexyl acetate. Cyclohexyl anthranilate. Cyclohexyl butyrate. Cyclohexyl cinnamate. Cyclohexyl formate. Cyclohexyl isovalerate. Cyclohexyl propionate. p- Cymene. g -Decalactone; 4-hydroxy-decanoic acid, g - lactone. g -Decalactone; 5-hydroxy-decanoic acid, d - lactone. Decanal dimethyl acetal. 1-Decanol; decylic alcohol. 2-Decenal. 3-Decen-2-one; heptylidene acetone. Decyl actate. Decyl butyrate. Decyl propionate. Dibenzyl ether. 4,4-Dibutyl- g -butyrolactone; 4,4-dibutyl-4-hy- droxy-butyric acid, g -lactone. Dibutyl sebacate. Diethyl malate. Diethyl malonate; ethyl malonate. Diethyl sebacate. Diethyl succinate. Diethyl tartrate. 2,5-Diethyltetrahydrofuran. Dihydrocarveol; 8 -p- menthen-2-ol; 6-methyl- 3-isopropenylcyclohexanol. Dihydrocarvone. Dihydrocarvyl acetate. m- Dimethoxybenzene. p- Dimethoxybenzene; dimethyl hydro- quinone. 2,4-Dimethylacetophenone. a , a -Dimethylbenzyl isobutyrate; phenyldi- methylcarbinyl isobutyrate. 2,6-Dimethyl-5-heptenal. 2,6-Dimethyl octanal; isodecylaldehyde. 3,7-Dimethyl-1-octanol; tetrahydrogeraniol. a , a -Dimethylphenethyl acetate; benzyl- propyl acetate; benzyldimethylcarbinyl ac- etate. a , a -Dimethylphenethyl alcohol; dimethyl- benzyl carbinol. a , a -Dimethylphenethyl butyrate; benzyl- dimethylcarbinyl butyrate. a , a -Dimethylphenethyl formate; benzyldi- methylcarbinyl formate. Dimethyl succinate. 1,3-Diphenyl-2-propanone; dibenzyl ketone. delta-Dodecalactone; 5-hydroxydodecanoic acid, deltalactone. g -Dodecalactone; 4-hydroxydodecanoic acid g - lactone. 2-Dodecenal. Estragole. r -Ethoxybenzaldehyde. Ethyl acetoacetate. Ethyl 2-acetyl-3-phenylpropionate; ethyl- benzyl acetoacetate. Ethyl aconitate, mixed esters. Ethyl acrylate. Ethyl r -anisate. Ethyl anthranilate. Ethyl benzoate. Ethyl benzoylacetate. a -Ethylbenzyl butyrate; a -phenylpropyl bu- tyrate. Ethyl brassylate; tridecanedioic acid cyclic ethylene glycol diester; cyclo 1,13-ethyl- enedioxytridecan-1,13-dione. 2-Ethylbutyl acetate. 2-Ethylbutyraldehyde. 2-Ethylbutyric acid. Ethyl cinnamate. Ethyl crotonate; trans- 2-butenoic acid ethyl- ester. Ethyl cyclohexanepropionate. Ethyl decanoate. 2-Ethylfuran. Ethyl 2-furanpropionate. 4-Ethylguaiacol; 4-ethyl-2-methoxyphenol. Ethyl heptanoate. 2-Ethyl-2-heptenal; 2-ethyl-3-butylacrolein. Ethyl hexanoate. Ethyl isobutyrate. Ethyl isovalerate. Ethyl lactate. Ethyl laurate. Ethyl levulinate. Ethyl maltol; 2-ethyl-3-hydroxy-4H-pyran-4- one. Ethyl 2-methylbutyrate. Ethyl myristate. Ethyl nitrite. Ethyl nonanoate. Ethyl 2-nonynoate; ethyl octyne carbonate. Ethyl octanoate. Ethyl oleate. Ethyl phenylacetate. Ethyl 4-phenylbutyrate. Ethyl 3-phenylglycidate. Ethyl 3-phenylpropionate; ethyl hydro- cinnamate. Ethyl propionate. Ethyl pyruvate. Ethyl salicylate. Ethyl sorbate; ethyl 2,4-hexadienoate. Ethyl tiglate; ethyl trans-2-methyl-2- butenoate. Ethyl undecanoate. Ethyl 10-undecenoate. Ethyl valerate. Eucalyptol; 1,8-epoxy -p- menthane; cineole. Eugenyl acetate. Eugenyl benzoate. Eugenyl formate. Eugenyl methyl ether; 4-allylveratrole; methyl eugenol. Farnesol; 3,7,11-trimethyl-2,6,10-dodecatrien- 1-ol. d- Fenchone; d- 1,3,3-trimethyl-2-nor- bornanone. Fenchyl alcohol; 1,3,3-trimethyl-2-nor- bornanol. Formic acid (2-Furyl)-2-propanone; furyl acetone. 1-Furyl-2-propanone; furyl acetone. Fusel oil, refined (mixed amyl alcohols). Geranyl acetoacetate; trans- 3,7-dimethyl-2, 6- octadien-1-yl acetoacetate. Geranyl acetone; 6,10-dimethyl-5,9- undecadien-2-one. Geranyl benzoate. Geranyl butyrate. Geranyl formate. Geranyl hexanoate Geranyl isobutyrate. Geranyl isovalerate. Geranyl phenylacetate. Geranyl propionate. Glucose pentaacetate. Guaiacol; μ -methoxyphenol. Guaiacyl acetate; μ -methoxyphenyl acetate. Guaiacyl phenylacetate. Guaiene; 1,4-dimethyl-7-isopropenyl- D 9,10- octahydroazulene. Guaiol acetate; 1,4-dimethyl-7-( a -hydroxy- isopropyl)- d 9,10-octahydroazulene acetate. g -Heptalactone; 4-hydroxyheptanoic acid, g - lactone. Heptanal; enanthaldehyde. Heptanal dimethyl acetal. Heptanal 1,2-glyceryl acetal. 2,3-Heptanedione; acetyl valeryl. 3-Heptanol. 2-Heptanone; methyl amyl ketone. 3-Heptanone; ethyl butyl ketone. 4-Heptanone; dipropyl ketone. cis- 4-Heptenal; cis- 4-hepten-1-al.

Heptyl acetate. Heptyl alcohol; enanthic alcohol. Heptyl butyrate. Heptyl cinnamate. Heptyl formate. Heptyl isobutyrate. Heptyl octanoate. 1-Hexadecanol; cetyl alcohol. w -6-Hexadecenlactone; 16-hydroxy-6- hexadecenoic acid, w -lactone; ambrettolide. g -Hexalactone; 4-hydroxyhexanoic acid, g -lac- tone; tonkalide. Hexanal; caproic aldehyde. 2,3-Hexanedione; acetyl butyryl. Hexanoic acid; caproic acid. 2-Hexenal. 2-Hexen-1-ol. 3-Hexen-1-ol; leaf alcohol. 2-Hexen-1-yl acetate. 3-Hexenyl isovalerate. 3-Hexenyl 2-methylbutyrate. 3-Hexenyl phenylacetate; cis- 3-hexenyl phen- ylacetate. Hexyl acetate. 2-Hexyl-4-acetoxytetrahydrofuran. Hexyl alcohol. Hexyl butyrate. a -Hexylcinnamaldehyde. Hexyl formate. Hexyl hexanoate. 2-Hexylidene cyclopentanone. Hexyl isovalerate. Hexyl 2-methylbutyrate. Hexyl octanoate. Hexyl phenylacetate; n- hexyl phenylacetate. Hexyl propionate. Hydroxycitronellal; 3,7-dimethyl-7-hydroxy- octanal. Hydroxycitronellal diethyl acetal. Hydroxycitronellal dimethyl acetal. Hydroxycitronellol; 3,7-dimethyl-1,7- octanediol. N- (4-Hydroxy-3-methoxybenzyl)-nonanamide; pelargonyl vanillylamide. 5-Hydroxy-4-octanone; butyroin. 4-( p- Hydroxyphenyl)-2-butanone; p- hydroxy- benzyl acetone. Indole. a -Ionone; 4-(2,6,6-trimethyl-2-cyclohexen-1- yl)-3-buten-2-one. b -Ionone; 4-(2,6,6-trimethyl-1-cyclohexen-1- yl)-3- buten-2-one. a -Irone; 4-(2,5,6,6-tetramethyl-2-cyclohexene- 1-yl)-3-buten-2-one; 6-methylionone. Isoamyl acetate. Isoamyl acetoacetate. Isoamyl alcohol; isopentyl alcohol; 3-methyl- 1-butanol. Isoamyl benzoate. Isoamyl butyrate. Isoamyl cinnamate. Isoamyl formate. Isoamyl 2-furanbutyrate; a -isoamyl furfuryl- propionate. Isoamyl 2-furanpropionate; a -isoamyl fur- furylacetate. Isoamyl hexanoate. Isoamyl isobutyrate. Isoamyl isovalerate. Isoamyl laurate. Isoamyl-2-methylbutyrate; isopentyl-2- methylbutyrate. Isoamyl nonanoate. Isoamyl octanoate. Isoamyl phenylacetate. Isoamyl propionate. Isoamyl pyruvate. Isoamyl salicylate. Isoborneol. Isobornyl acetate. Isobornyl formate. Isobornyl isovalerate. Isobornyl propionate. Isobutyl acetate. Isobutyl acetoacetate. Isobutyl alcohol. Isobutyl angelate; isobutyl cis- 2-methyl-2- butenoate. Isobutyl anthranilate. Isobutyl benzoate. Isobutyl butyrate. Isobutyl cinnamate. Isobutyl formate. Isobutyl 2-furanpropionate. Isobutyl heptanoate. Isobutyl hexanoate. Isobutyl isobutyrate. a -Isobutylphenethyl alcohol; isobutyl benzyl carbinol; 4-methyl-1-phenyl-2-pentanol. Isobutyl phenylacetate. Isobutyl propionate. Isobutyl salicylate. 2-Isobutylthiazole. Isobutyraldehyde. Isobutyric acid. Isoeugenol; 2-methoxy-4- propenylphenol. Isoeugenyl acetate. Isoeugenyl benzyl ether; benzyl isoeugenol. Isoeugenyl ethyl ether; 2-ethoxy-5- propenyl- anisole; ethyl isoeugenol. Isoeugenyl formate. Isoeugenyl methyl ether; 4-propenyl- veratrole; methyl isoeugenol. Isoeugenyl phenylacetate. Isojasmone; mixture of 2-hexylidenecyclo- pentanone and 2-hexyl-2-cyclopenten-1-one. a -Isomethylionone; 4-(2,6,6-trimethyl-2- cyclohexen-1-yl)-3-methyl-3-buten-2-one; methyl g -ionone. Isopropyl acetate. r -Isopropylacetophenone. Isopropyl alcohol; isopropanol. Isopropyl benzoate. r -Isopropylbenzyl alcohol; cuminic alcohol; r -cymen-7-ol. Isopropyl butyrate. Isopropyl cinnamate. Isopropyl formate. Isopropyl hexanoate. Isopropyl isobutyrate. Isopropyl isovalerate. r -Isopropylphenylacetaldehyde; r -cymen-7- carboxaldehyde. Isopropyl phenylacetate. 3-( r -Isopropylphenyl)-propionaldehyde; r -iso- propylhydrocinnamaldehyde; cuminyl ac- etaldehyde. Isopropyl propionate. Isopulegol; p- menth-8-en-3-ol. Isopulegone; p- menth-8-en-3-one. Isopulegyl acetate. Isoquinoline. Isovaleric acid. cis- Jasmone; 3-methyl-2-(2-pentenyl)-2-cyclo- penten-1-one. Lauric aldehyde; dodecanal. Lauryl acetate. Lauryl alcohol; 1-dodecanol. Lepidine; 4-methylquinoline. Levulinic acid. Linalool oxide; cis- and trans-2-vinyl-2-meth- yl-5-(1 ′ -hydroxy-1 ′ -methylethyl) tetra- hydrofuran. Linalyl anthranilate; 3,7-dimethyl-1,6- octadien-3-yl anthranilate. Linalyl benzoate. Linalyl butyrate. Linalyl cinnamate. Linalyl formate. Linalyl hexanoate. Linalyl isobutyrate. Linalyl isovalerate. Linalyl octanoate. Linalyl propionate. Maltol; 3-hydroxy-2-methyl-4H-pyran-4-one. Menthadienol; p- mentha-1,8(10)-dien-9-ol. p- Mentha-1,8-dien-7-ol; perillyl alcohol. Menthadienyl acetate; p- mentha-1,8(10)-dien- 9-yl acetate. p- Menth-3-en-1-ol. 1 -p- Menthen—9-yl acetate; p- menth-1-en-9-yl acetate. Menthol; 2-isopropyl-5-methylcyclohexanol. Menthone; p -menthan-3-one. Menthyl acetate; p- menth-3-yl acetate. Menthyl isovalerate; p- menth-3-yl iso- valerate. o- Methoxybenzaldehyde. p- Methoxybenzaldehyde; p- anisaldehyde. o- Methoxycinnamaldehyde. 2-Methoxy-4-methylphenol; 4-methyl- guaiacol; 2-methoxy -p- cresol. 4-( p- Methoxyphenyl)-2-butanone; anisyl ace- tone. 1-(4-Methoxyphenyl)-4-methyl-1-penten-3- one; methoxystyryl isopropyl ketone. 1-( p- Methoxyphenyl)-1-penten-3-one; a - methylanisylidene acetone; ethone. 1-( p- Methoxyphenyl)-2-propanone; anisylmethyl ketone; anisic ketone. 2-Methoxy-4-vinylphenol; p- vinylguaiacol. Methyl acetate. 4 ′ -Methylacetophenone; p- methylaceto- phenone; methyl p- tolyl ketone. 2-Methylallyl butyrate; 2-methyl-2-propenl- yl butyrate. Methyl anisate. o- Methylanisole; o- cresyl methyl ether. p- Methylanisole; p- cresyl methyl ether; p- methoxytoluene. Methyl benzoate. Methylbenzyl acetate, mixed o-,m-,p-. a -Methylbenzyl acetate; styralyl acetate. a -Methylbenzyl alcohol; styralyl alcohol. a -Methylbenzyl butyrate; styralyl butyrate. a -Methylbenzyl isobutyrate; styralyl iso- butyrate. a -Methylbenzyl formate; styralyl formate. a -Methylbenzyl propionate; styralyl propio- nate. 2-Methyl-3-buten-2-ol. 2-Methylbutyl isovalerate. Methyl p-tert- butylphenylacetate. 2-Methylbutyraldehyde; methyl ethyl acetal- dehyde. 3-Methylbutyraldehyde; isovaleraldehyde. Methyl butyrate. 2-Methylbutyric acid. a -Methylcinnamaldehyde. p- Methylcinnamaldehyde. Methyl cinnamate. 2-Methyl-1,3-cyclohexadiene. Methylcyclopentenolone; 3-methylcyclopen- tane-1,2-dione. Methyl disulfide; dimethyl disulfide. Methyl ester of rosin, partially hydrogenated (as defined in § 172.615); methyl dihydroabietate. Methyl heptanoate. 2-Methylheptanoic acid. 6-Methyl-3,5-heptadien-2-one. Methyl-5-hepten-2-ol. 6-Methyl-5-hepten-2-one. Methyl hexanoate. Methyl 2-hexanoate. Methyl p- hydroxybenzoate; methylparaben. Methyl a -ionone; 5-(2,6,6-trimethyl-2-cyclo- hexen-1-yl)-4-penten-3-one. Methyl b -ionone; 5-(2,6,6-trimethyl-1-cyclo- hexen-1-yl)-4-penten-3-one. Methyl D -ionone; 5-(2,6,6-trimethyl-3-cyclo- hexen-1-yl-)-4-penten-3-one. Methyl isobutyrate. 2-Methyl-3-( p- isopropylphenyl)-propionalde- hyde; a -methyl -p- isopropylhydro- cinnamal- dehyde; cyclamen aldehyde. Methyl isovalerate. Methyl laurate. Methyl mercaptan; methanethiol. Methyl o- methoxybenzoate. Methyl N- methylanthranilate; dimethyl an- thranilate. Methyl 2-methylbutyrate. Methyl-3-methylthiopropionate. Methyl 4-methylvalerate. Methyl myristate. Methyl b -naphthyl ketone; 2 ' -acetonaph- thone. Methyl nonanoate. Methyl 2-nonenoate. Methyl 2-nonynoate; methyloctyne car- bonate. 2-Methyloctanal; methyl hexyl acetaldehyde. Methyl octanoate. Methyl 2-octynoate; methyl heptine car- bonate. 4-Methyl-2,3-pentanedione; acetyl iso- butyryl. 4-Methyl-2-pentanone; methyl isobutyl ke- tone. b -Methylphenethyl alcohol; hydratropyl al- cohol. Methyl phenylacetate. 3-Methyl-4-phenyl-3-butene-2-one. 2-Methyl-4-phenyl-2-butyl acetate; dimethyl- phenylethyl carbinyl acetate. 2-Methyl-4-phenyl-2-butyl isobutyrate; dimethylphenyl ethylcarbinyl isobutyrate. 3-Methyl-2-phenylbutyraldehyde; a -isopropyl phenylacetaldehyde. Methyl 4-phenylbutyrate. 4-Methyl-1-phenyl-2-pentanone; benzyl iso- butyl ketone. Methyl 3-phenylpropionate; methyl hydro- cinnamate. Methyl propionate. 3-Methyl-5-propyl-2-cyclohexen-1-one. Methyl sulfide. 3-Methylthiopropionaldehyde; methional. 2-Methyl-3-tolylpropionaldehyde, mixed o-, m-, p-. 2-Methylundecanal; methyl nonyl acetal- dehyde. Methyl 9-undecenoate. Methyl 2-undecynoate; methyl decyne car- bonate. Methyl valerate. 2-Methylvaleric acid. Myrcene; 7-methyl-3- methylene-1,6-octa- diene. Myristaldehyde; tetradecanal. d- Neomenthol; 2-isopropyl-5-methylcyclo- hexanol. Nerol; cis- 3,7-dimethyl-2,6-octadien-1-ol. Nerolidol; 3,7,11-trimethyl-1,6,10-dodecatrien- 3-ol. Neryl acetate. Neryl butyrate. Neryl formate. Neryl isobutyrate. Neryl isovalerate. Neryl propionate. 2,6-Nonadien-1-ol. g -Nonalactone; 4-hydroxynonanoic acid, g - lactone; aldehyde C–18. Nonanal; pelargonic aldehyde. 1,3-Nonanediol acetate, mixed esters. Nonanoic acid; pelargonic acid. 2-Nonanone; methylheptyl ketone. 3-Nonanon-1-yl acetate; 1-hydroxy-3-nonanone acetate. Nonyl acetate. Nonyl alcohol; 1-nonanol. Nonyl octanoate. Nonyl isovalerate. Nootkatone; 5,6-dimethyl-8-isopropenyl- bicyclo[4,4,0]-dec-1-en-3-one. Ocimene; trans - b -ocimene; 3,7-dimethyl-1,3,6- octatriene. g -Octalactone; 4-hydroxyoctanoic acid, g -lac- tone. Octanal; caprylaldehyde. Octanal dimethyl acetal. 1-Octanol; octyl alcohol. 2-Octanol. 3-Octanol. 2-Octanone; methyl hexyl ketone. 3-Octanone; ethyl amyl ketone. 3-Octanon-1-ol. 1-Octen-3-ol; amyl vinyl carbinol. 1-Octen-3-yl acetate. Octyl acetate. 3-Octyl acetate. Octyl butyrate. Octyl formate. Octyl heptanoate. Octyl isobutyrate. Octyl isovalerate. Octyl octanoate. Octyl phenylacetate. Octyl propionate. w -Pentadecalactone; 15-hydroxypentadeca- noic acid, w -lactone; pentadecanolide; an- gelica lactone. 2,3-Pentanedione; acetyl propionyl. 2-Pentanone; methyl propyl ketone. 4-Pentenoic acid. 1-Penten-3-ol. Perillaldehyde; 4-isopropenyl-1-cyclohexene- 1-carboxaldehyde; p- mentha-1,8-dien-7-al. Perillyl acetate; p- mentha-1,8-dien-7-yl ace- tate. a -Phellandrene; r -mentha-1,5-diene. Phenethyl acetate. Phenethyl alcohol; b -phenylethyl alcohol. Phenethyl anthranilate. Phenethyl benzoate. Phenethyl butyrate. Phenethyl cinnamate. Phenethyl formate. Phenethyl isobutyrate. Phenethyl isovalerate. Phenethyl 2-methylbutyrate. Phenethyl phenylacetate. Phenethyl propionate. Phenethyl salicylate. Phenethyl senecioate; phenethyl 3,3-di- methylacrylate. Phenethyl tiglate. Phenoxyacetic acid. 2-Phenoxyethyl isobutyrate. Phenylacetaldehyde; a -toluic aldehyde. Phenylacetaldehyde 2,3-butylene glycol ace- tal. Phenylacetaldehyde dimethyl acetal. Phenylacetaldehyde glyceryl acetal. Phenylacetic acid; a -toluic acid. 4-Phenyl-2-butanol; phenylethyl methyl car- binol. 4-Phenyl-3-buten-2-ol; methyl styryl car- binol. 4-Phenyl-3-buten-2-one. 4-Phenyl-2-butyl acetate; phenylethyl meth- yl carbinyl acetate. 1-Phenyl-3-methyl-3-pentanol; phenylethyl methyl ethyl carbinol. 1-Phenyl-1-propanol; phenylethyl carbinol. 3-Phenyl-1-propanol; hydrocinnamyl alcohol. 2-Phenylpropionaldehyde; hydratropalde- hyde. 3-Phenylpropionaldehyde; hydrocinnamal- dehyde. 2-Phenylpropionalde-hyde dimethyl acetal; hydratropic aldehyde dimethyl acetal. 3-Phenylpropionic acid; hydrocinnamic acid. 3-Phenylpropyl acetate. 2-Phenylpropyl butyrate. 3-Phenylpropyl cinnamate. 3-Phenylpropyl formate. 3-Phenylpropyl hexanoate. 2-Phenylpropyl isobutyrate. 3-Phenylpropyl isobutyrate. 3-Phenylpropyl isovalerate. 3-Phenylpropyl propionate. 2-(3-Phenylpropyl)-tetrahydrofuran. a -Pinene; 2-pinene. b -Pinene; 2(10)-pinene. Pine tar oil. Pinocarveol; 2(10)-pinen-3-ol. Piperidine. Piperine. d- Piperitone; p- menth-1-en-3-one. Piperitenone; p- mentha-1,4(8)-dien-3-one. Piperitenone oxide; 1,2-epoxy -p- menth-4-(8)- en-3-one. Piperonyl acetate; heliotropyl acetate. Piperonyl isobutyrate. Polylimonene. Polysorbate 20; polyoxyethylene (20) sorbitan monolaurate. Polysorbate 60; polyoxyethylene (20) sorbitan monostereate. Polysorbate 80; polyoxyethylene (20) sorbitan monooleate. Potassium acetate. Propenylguaethol; 6-ethoxy -m- anol. Propionaldehyde. Propyl acetate. Propyl alcohol; 1-propanol. p- Propyl anisole; dihydroanethole. Propyl benzoate. Propyl butyrate. Propyl cinnamate. Propyl disulfide. Propyl formate. Propyl 2-furanacrylate. Propyl heptanoate. Propyl hexanoate. Propyl p- hydroxybenzoate; propylparaben. 3-Propylidenephthalide. Propyl isobutyrate. Propyl isovalerate. Propyl mercaptan. a -Propylphenethyl alcohol. Propyl phenylacetate. Propyl propionate. Pulegone; p- menth-4(8)-en-3-

one. Pyridine. Pyroligneous acid extract. Pyruvaldehyde. Pyruvic acid. Rhodinol; 3,7-dimethyl-7-octen-1-ol; l-citronellol. Rhodinyl acetate. Rhodinyl butyrate. Rhodinyl formate. Rhodinyl isobutyrate. Rhodinyl isovalerate. Rhodinyl phenylacetate. Rhodinyl propionate. Rum ether; ethyl oxyhydrate. Salicylaldehyde. Santalol, a and b . Santalyl acetate. Santalyl phenylacetate. Skatole. Sorbitan monostearate. Styrene. Sucrose octaacetate. a -Terpinene. g -Terpinene. a -Terpineol; p- menth-1-en-8-ol. b -Terpineol. Terpinolene; p- menth-1,4(8)-diene. Terpinyl acetate. Terpinyl anthranilate. Terpinyl butyrate. Terpinyl cinnamate. Terpinyl formate. Terpinyl isobutyrate. Terpinyl isovalerate. Terpinyl propionate. Tetrahydrofurfuryl acetate. Tetrahydrofurfuryl alcohol. Tetrahydrofurfuryl butyrate. Tetrahydrofurfuryl propionate. Tetrahydro-pseudo-ionone; 6,10-dimethyl-9- undecen-2-one. Tetrahydrolinalool; 3,7-dimethyloctan-3-ol. Tetramethyl ethylcyclohexenone; mixture of 5-ethyl-2,3,4,5-tetramethyl-2-cyclohexen-1- one and 5-ethyl-3,4,5,6-tetramethyl-2-cyclo- hexen-1-one. 2-Thienyl mercaptan; 2-thienylthiol. Thymol. Tolualdehyde glyceryl acetal, mixed o, m, p. Tolualdehydes, mixed o, m, p. p- Tolylacetaldehyde. o- Tolyl acetate; o- cresyl acetate. p- Tolyl acetate; p- cresyl acetate. 4-( p- Tolyl)-2-butanone; p- methylbenzylace- tone. p- Tolyl isobutyrate. p- Tolyl laurate. p- Tolyl phenylacetate. 2-( p- Tolyl)-propionaldehyde; p- methylhydra- tropic aldehyde. Tributyl acetylcitrate. 2-Tridecenal. 2,3-Undecadione; acetyl nonyryl. g -Undecalactone; 4-hydroxyundecanoic acid g -lactone; peach aldehyde; aldehyde C–14. Undecenal. 2-Undecanone; methyl nonyl ketone. 9-Undecenal; undecenoic aldehyde. 10-Undecenal. Undecen-1-ol; undecylenic alcohol. 10-Undecen-1-yl acetate. Undecyl alcohol. Valeraldehyde; pentanal. Valeric acid; pentanoic acid. Vanillin acetate; acetyl vanillin. Veratraldehyde. Verbenol; 2-pinen-4-ol. Zingerone; 4-(4-hydroxy-3-methoxyphenyl)-2-butanone.

Catching on yet? Six of these hundreds of allowable chemicals were recently found to cause cancer. I highlighted the six. How many others might be as dangerous or worse? Keep in mind there's a similar table of allowable artificial *colors* as well.

## White Power: Titanium Dioxide

Snacky staples are purchased on impulse because they look tasty. For some reason, consumers are in love with bright-white snacks (Schüz, 2015). The creamy center of a Twinkie or snow-white cake frosting is not at all what you'd expect.

I've been warning about the dangers of processed foods for many years now. Recently an article on the dangers of a common food additive titanium dioxide caught my attention. Titanium dioxide is used widely by the food industry as a coloring agent. Titanium dioxide, also known as Ti02, is extracted from certain rocks in mines around the world. When purified, Ti02 makes an excellent pigment for paint, paper, and plastic. Over 4.6 million tons of Ti02 are produced annually around the world. So, what does this have to do with food?

According to the FDA, Ti02 is generally recognized as safe (GRAS) when a food product contains less than 1% of Ti02. The FDA calls Ti02 a "mica-based pearlescent pigment," and allows it in all kinds of foods. The FDA allows Ti02 in ANY food if it does not exceed 1% of the total weight of the food and is labeled accordingly (FDA(3), 2015). Ingredient lists on packaged food generally disclose "other colors added" to indicate the use of Ti02.

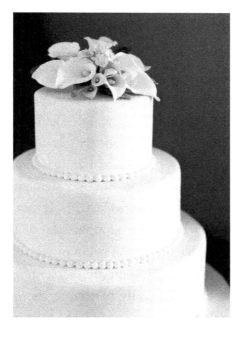

Ti02 is hidden in your candies, chewing gums, powdered donuts, frosting, coffee creamer, vanilla pudding, chocolate bars, mayo, cottage cheese, toothpaste, lotions, sunscreens, pills, and anything else that is a brilliant white color. Perhaps you think your product does not contain Ti02? Wrong! *There is no alternative.* If you are using a product that has been colored white, it contains Ti02. Very few of the foods we eat are naturally white. Whole milk is white, but when made into low-fat milk it turns gray—Ti02 solves *that* problem. Egg whites can be beaten to a bright-white consistency, but it doesn't preserve well. With very few exceptions, any food that's bright-white and found in a wrapper or carton has TiO2 in it whether listed on the ingredients or not. The manufacturers of processed snack foods know that people want to eat colorful foods, like found "in nature," (e.g., snow, rice, potatoes, cauliflower). We've come to expect a certain look for birthday cakes and chewing gum, and the only way to achieve this is with TiO2.

## The Problem with TiO2

Research indicates that TiO2 is not as safe as the FDA thinks (Gillois, 2018). Toxicology studies show that TiO2 can cause cell damage, genotoxicity, inflammation, and immune response due to its small (nanoparticle) size (Skocaj, 2011). Another study shows that TiO2 can be absorbed through the gut of mammals and will accumulate in body tissues much like mercury and lead. Further, yet another study showed that spleen and liver damage can occur when enough TiO2 accumulates (Jovanović, 2015). If that's not enough, it's also been proven that when these nanoparticles of TiO2 cross the gut barrier they can cause lesions in the colon or worsen existing lesions (INRA-France, 2018). Finally, even yet *another* research team found that TiO2 nanoparticles not only penetrate the gut wall, but also white blood cells where they are seen by the human body as foreign invaders. This prompts an immune response and creates inflammation throughout the body. Further, this team noted that when TiO2 is consumed by people with ulcerative colitis, a fairly common gut disease, they have an increased concentration of TiO2 in their blood (University of Zurich, 2018).

Why is this still allowed in our food? Mostly because the FDA has not gotten around to reviewing TiO2 as a safe food colorant. Dunkin' Donuts has stopped using TiO2 in their products (Maynard, 2015), and France is set to ban its use in their country soon (Chemycal, 2018).

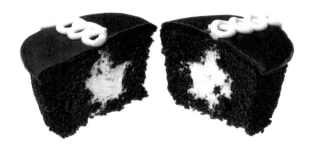

While Big Food still says Ti02 is quite safe "when used as directed," you can take some steps to avoid it. Most Americans eat a pound or more of Ti02 in any given year. Steer clear of processed foods for you and especially your kids! Break the habit of eating colorful snack foods, especially the bright-white ones. I have no doubt that Ti02 (and many other "safe" chemicals) will soon also be banned here and around the world as food coloring.

*__Food Industry Insider Secret:__ Polysorbate is an emulsifier added to many ultra-processed foods to make them feel better in your mouth. Polysorbate 80, for instance, makes ice cream smoother and melt slower. Polysorbate 60 is put in powdered cocoa to make it seem less "instant" and last longer on the shelf. These and other emulsifiers have a profound effect on your gut, resulting in low-grade inflammation of the gut lining and have been linked to obesity, colitis, metabolic syndrome, and more (Chassaing, 2017) (Viennois, 2018) (Lock, 2018) (Gillois, 2018).*

## Food Lobbyists

The reason I'm harping on Big Food, the Western diet, and ultra-processed food is because I want you to have a firm idea of what I mean when I say *bad food*. Ultra-processed food isn't poisonous, per se, but it cannot be consumed in excess without dire consequences. Ultra-processed food most certainly should not make up the bulk of our staple food items as it does. The food industry spends billions lobbying in Washington to keep certain research from tainting what they sell to the unsuspecting public.

The US Office of Disease Prevention and Health Promotion (ODPHP) releases a set of guidelines every five years outlining the state of eating in the United States and gives recommendations on things like school lunch programs, food labeling, and nutrition requirements. The last ODPHP Dietary Guidelines for Americans was released in 2015. Despite many years of scientific papers warning about the dangers of ultra-processed food, there is no mention of the dangers in this guideline. The key recommendations from the 2015–2020 guidelines are as follows (Department of Health and Human Services, 2015):

## Key Recommendations

**Consume a healthy eating pattern that accounts for all foods and beverages within an appropriate calorie level.**

**A healthy eating pattern includes:**[2]

- A variety of vegetables from all of the subgroups—dark green, red and orange, legumes (beans and peas), starchy, and other

- Fruits, especially whole fruits

- Grains, at least half of which are whole grains

- Fat-free or low-fat dairy, including milk, yogurt, cheese, and/or fortified soy beverages

- A variety of protein foods, including seafood, lean meats and poultry, eggs, legumes (beans and peas), and nuts, seeds, and soy products

- Oils

**A healthy eating pattern limits:**

- Saturated fats and *trans* fats, added sugars, and sodium

Key Recommendations that are quantitative are provided for several components of the diet that should be limited. These components are of particular public health concern in the United States, and the specified limits can help individuals achieve healthy eating patterns within calorie limits:

- Consume less than 10 percent of calories per day from added sugars[3]

- Consume less than 10 percent of calories per day from saturated fats[4]

- Consume less than 2,300 milligrams (mg) per day of sodium[5]

- If alcohol is consumed, it should be consumed in moderation—up to one drink per day for women and up to two drinks per day for men—and only by adults of legal drinking age.[6]

Why such weak language in the key recommendations for a policy that *shapes national health strategy*? Food industry lobby groups. There have been some famous battles on Capitol Hill; one infamous example is that frozen pizza was classified as a vegetable so that it could be featured on school menus around the nation. This was a billion-dollar win for the food industry (Jalonick, 2011).

> We are outraged that Congress is seriously considering language that would effectively categorize pizza as a vegetable in the school lunch program, it doesn't take an advanced degree in nutrition to call this a national disgrace.

Similar battles for school lunches include the classification of French fries, ketchup, and relish as "servings" of vegetables (Haskins, 2005). School lunch programs cost taxpayers $9.5 billion dollars a year, most of which goes to the food giants Tyson, Nestlé, and others. School lunches are the gateway drug for a lifetime of dependence on ultra-processed foods and nutritional confusion. French fries and ketchup are *not* two servings of vegetables.

## GMA

Grocery Manufacturers Association (GMA) is the most powerful lobbying group of the food industry. This group collects billions of dollars from Big Food to fight any new regulation or decision that might influence how America eats.

One of the GMA's current battles is to sway the labeling of genetically modified foods (GMO) as natural (Wikipedia, 2018). But any legislation that affects the bottom-line for the food industry is in their sights.

Michelle Obama famously addressed the GMA in 2010, urging them to "move faster and go farther" in making healthier food for kids.

> We need you not to just tweak around the edges but entirely rethink the products you are offering, the information that you provide about these products, and how you market those products to our children.

While her speech was well-received by the GMA and seen as a great move, it did not result in sweeping changes thanks to the powerful food lobby. In fact, the First Lady's initiative is now widely seen as a win for the food industry, as they have found new markets for ultra-processed snacks packaged in 100-calorie packets aimed at kids who eat them by the boxload. The fact is, the food industry already had healthy food options, but nobody wants them compared to the demand for Goldfish crackers, potato chips, and energy drinks (Warner, 2010).

## How about the Rest of the World?

Every economic region and country has its own special rules regarding food additives, food safety, and labeling requirements. The EU, for instance, is much tougher than the US on using food additives, GMOs, herbicides, and several other food safety concerns. Other countries have relatively few rules.

> At present, there are up to 2500 food additives being used worldwide. A large number of studies have confirmed that consuming excessive amounts of synthetic food additives may cause gastrointestinal, respiratory, dermatologic, and neurologic adverse reactions (Ghany, 2015).

Ghany also suggests that as processed foods make up to 75% of most people's diet, we each consume on average *8–10 pounds* of food additives per year!

## Lack of Fiber

This chapter wouldn't be complete without a brief talk about fiber. Fiber isn't food for you, it's food for the trillions of bacteria that live inside your intestines. This is a very important distinction.

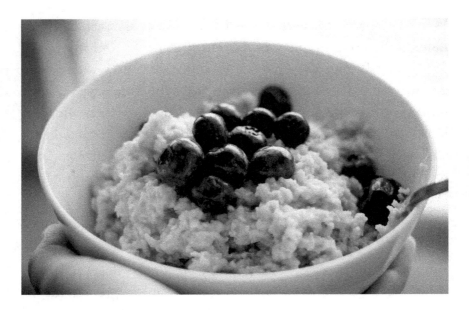

Fiber can be classified in several ways: soluble, insoluble, fermentable, or by other physical characteristics. Some types of fiber you might have heard of include:

- Beta-glucans
- Cellulose
- Dextrin
- FOS
- Inulin
- Lignin
- Pectin
- Psyllium
- Resistant Starch

Here's the catch ... don't worry about fiber if you eat multiple servings of fruit and vegetables every day. The official recommendation is to get about 30 grams of fiber per day. Most Americans on the Western diet get 15 grams or less. Believe me, it's a rabbit hole not worth going down. Just eat *lots of fruit and veggies*.

*Food Industry Insider Secret: Over 80% of the US popula-
tion fails to eat five servings of fruit and vegetables daily. Five
servings per day is the minimum recommended amount to
ensure good health (Kopf, 2018).*

Lack of fiber has been clearly associated with the onset of obesity
and conditions that cause obesity. Getting lots of fiber has many
benefits (Anderson, 2009):

- Benefits gastroesophageal reflux disease, duodenal ulcer, diver-
  ticulitis, constipation, and hemorrhoids
- Encourages better stools
- Enhances immune function
- Enhances weight loss
- Helps to prevent diabetes, obesity, and gastrointestinal diseases
- Improves insulin sensitivity
- Increases feeling of fullness after meals
- Lowers LDL cholesterol levels
- Lowers risk for developing coronary heart disease, stroke, and
  high blood pressure
- Lowers blood pressure

The distinct lack of fiber in the Western diet is perhaps its greatest
downfall. Big Food knows this, too, so they add refined fibers to
packaged food. But refined fibers are never enough; they need to be
eaten alongside the plant they came from for all these effects to be
realized (Singh, 2018).

Want fiber? Eat plants. It really is so simple even a caveman can do it.

## Scared Now?

Feeling guilty? Feeling bad for eating ultra-processed food and feeding it to your kids, your spouse, and your friends? Don't be. Be mad. Be pissed off. And make changes! You can still eat M&Ms, frozen burritos, and Honey Buns if you like, just be hyper-aware that these things are not to be your meals or pantry staples, just occasional snacks.

Ultra-processed food is bad, not only because of the many chemicals it contains, but mostly because it contains too much sugar, oil, refined wheat, and little fiber. Additionally, ultra-processing ruins most of the natural goodness found in whole foods. High heat, extrusion, and other industrial processes ruin the structure of starch molecules and vitamins, making them unusable in the body.

If you would stop eating ultra-processed food and start eating mostly minimally processed and whole food, you could stop reading right here and never need to diet again. You'll live a long and healthy life, and you won't know the pains of obesity-related disease. But you probably won't, so I'll keep on writing.

But, seriously, think hard the next time you choose Hamburger Helper or Burger King for dinner over salmon, spinach, and potatoes. Grab grapes, not grape-flavored taffy. Stop being a customer of Big Food, and start feeding yourself.

Enough of food for now. Dieting is not just about food, but I wanted to discuss food first. I hope I've sparked something in you. We are being duped by Big Food into thinking that packaged foods are healthy and should become your staples. Quick, easy, tasty? Yes. Healthy? Hardly.

## Conclusion

The Western diet wreaks havoc on all populations that eat it. The Western diet consists mainly of processed foods; these foods are filled with chemical additives that make cheap ingredients highly addictive and fattening. Even "natural" additives can be dangerous and are often banned after many decades of unrestricted use. "Big Food," the food industry, spends billions on lobbying efforts to ensure that staple food items in your house consist more of Hot Pockets and Reese's Pieces than beans and rice. Eating the Western diet is usually the beginning of a downward spiral in health; it ends in the smoking crater of metabolic syndrome, obesity, cancer, and many other diseases that affect affluent societies.

The good news is, each person has the capacity to reverse this trend. Instead of eating ultra-processed food, opt instead for minimally processed, whole foods. Western diets typically consist of 75% or more of processed food and 25% unprocessed food. The ratio needs to be closer to 90% or more of minimally processed food and 10% or less of ultra-processed food. Those who partake of the Western diet are ingesting close to *10 pounds of chemical adulterants annually*. Worst of all, the Western diet is nearly devoid of the fiber so desperately needed to have a healthy gut. This is totally unacceptable and incompatible with good health.

# CHAPTER 3

# HOW EXERCISE AFFECTS WEIGHT

**TL;DR:** *A good exercise program is vital to staying healthy. Exercising is not as hard as you might think.*

Your *diet* is the food you normally eat; but *going on a diet* is eating and behaving in a specific way to lose weight. Most people miss that to *lose weight*, many other factors besides food are involved. We need to start thinking of dieting not as a food makeover but a lifestyle intervention.

## Move It!

Exercise is an important piece to the healthy weight puzzle, yet the most often overlooked (Spring, 2018). When people exercise, every other aspect of health is much more forgiving. Your diet does not need to be so strict, you sleep better, and you have less stress in your life. Remove exercise from the equation, and you'll need to try extra, extra hard to watch what you eat, leading to more stress and poor sleep.

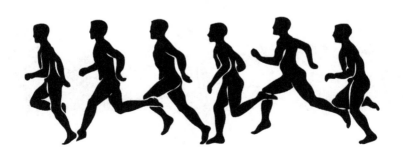

Okay… you might be thinking, *Gah! I hate exercise! Not gonna do it.* And if you're thinking you can cheat on this part, you do it at your peril. Please don't try to cheat by skipping the exercise part. This is the key to making your weight loss diet work.

## Jack LaLanne

As Jack LaLanne famously said:

> Exercise is king. Nutrition is queen. Put them together and you've got a kingdom.

Truer words were never spoken. Jack "The Godfather of Modern Fitness" LaLanne was ahead of his time, inventing weight lifting machines and home workout videos, and popularizing the entire "gym" lifestyle. Unfortunately, Jack came to us at a time when Big Food was just learning to make cinnamon flavor out of *Eugenyl methyl ether* and TV dinners were new and amazing. While Jack was a total beast in the gym (and on the stage, on the land, and in the water), you don't need to be Mr. Universe to get the same benefits of exercise.

## Why Exercise?

Before I tell you *what* you need to do, I'm going to tell you *why* you need to do it. According to researchers:

> Physical inactivity is a modifiable risk factor for cardiovascular disease and a widening variety of other chronic diseases, including diabetes mellitus, cancer (colon and breast), obesity, hypertension, bone and joint diseases (osteoporosis and osteoarthritis), and depression. (Warburton et al., 2006)

In other words, lack of exercise puts you at increased risk of developing diabetes, cancer, obesity, high blood pressure, arthritis, and depression. Let that sink in for a minute. Perhaps you have never exercised and have one or more of these disease states already. It's not too late. Even if you are in a wheelchair or hospital bed, you can exercise.

Humans seem to want to take the easy path. Maybe this was an evolutionary adaptation. Why burn unnecessary calories when food is hard to come by? The hard truth is that modern humans don't get enough physical activity in their daily lives. In one study, "people who went from unfit to fit over a five-year period had a reduction of 44% in the relative risk of death compared with people who remained unfit" (Blair et al., 1995). That's huge, in the grand scheme of things.

## Why Not to Exercise

Many people exercise to burn excess calories. One should not exercise for the purpose of subtracting calories from food. Any calories burned during exercise should be looked at as a dividend in the long-term plan, not a short-term deficit. Your exercise routine should be scheduled far in advance, not as an ad hoc punishment for overeating.

Other people start an exercise program to lose weight. Without addressing other factors, especially food, exercise is more likely to lead to weight gain (Foster, 2012). Do not exercise for the purpose of masking a poor diet.

## The Exercise Industry

Gym memberships, personal trainers, home exercise equipment, videos, books, and motivational products are a trillion-dollar industry. Like the Diet Industry, they don't really care that you get fit, just that you pay your dues.

By the numbers, there are roughly 250 million people in the United States over the age of 20. Fifty-four million people paid gym membership dues last year. Yet 70% of Americans over 20 are overweight with 35% being obese (Wells, 2015). This trend in gym memberships has remained stable for decades while the obesity rate skyrocketed. If joining a gym meant you *would* reduce your weight, the numbers would look different. But joining a gym just means you *can* lose weight, and that's the hook.

## Let's Exercise

Exercise has two components: muscles and heart. There are two types of exercises we need to do: *aerobic exercise* and *strength training*.

## Aerobic Exercise

Remember the aerobics craze of the '80s? Anyone over the age of 40 has images of Jane Fonda in her high-cut leotards emblazoned in their brain.

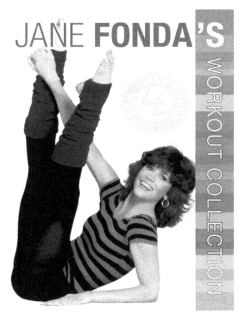

*Picture from Amazon.com*

Flash forward to 2018 and we've moved from carefully choreographed routines to flipping huge tires until you puke.

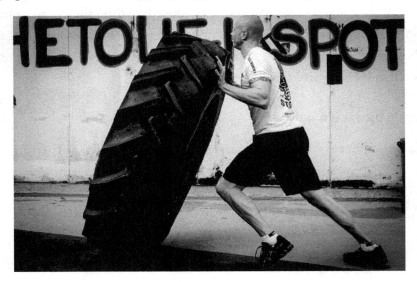

Quality, meaningful aerobic exercise does not have to be sexy or beastly; somewhere in the middle is best. The American Heart Association recommends we get at least 150 minutes per week of moderate-intensity aerobic activity or 75 minutes per week of vigorous aerobic activity, or a combination of both, preferably spread throughout the week.

Or:

- 30 minutes, 5 days a week of light-duty (moderate) exercises (walking, gardening, etc.), and/or
- 15 minutes, 5 days a week of (vigorous) exercises that will make you sweat and get out of breath a bit (jogging, bicycling, etc.).

Aerobic exercise needs to be intentional, timed, controlled, and meaningful. I'll show you some good aerobic routines later in the book. For now, just know that aerobic exercise is crucial to your health and needs to be part of your fitness routine.

## Aerobic versus Cardio versus Endurance Exercise

What's the difference between aerobic, cardio, and endurance exercise? Nothing! These words all mean the same thing, so please don't be confused if you find an article somewhere that says you need to do more cardio or endurance exercises. It's all the same. These words all refer to exercises that work your heart and lungs. I just happen to prefer the term "aerobic," possibly because of my age. Performing aerobic exercise can be done at different levels of exertion depending on how hard you exert yourself. As you work more vigorously, you'll begin to sweat and breathe harder. This is perfect training for the heart and leads to greater endurance.

## Why Aerobic Exercise?

Besides the obvious heart benefits, aerobic exercise also helps with:
- Blood volume and circulation
- Breathing/lung health
- Cardiovascular efficiency
- Decreased risk of coronary artery disease, cancer, and diabetes
- Decreased anxiety and stress
- Enhanced fat-burning metabolism
- Improved body composition
- Increased cardiac output
- Lowered resting heart rate
- Strengthened ligaments, tendons, and bones
- Stronger muscles

## Final Thoughts on Aerobic Workouts

According to the National Institutes of Health, less than 1% of Americans between the ages of 20 and 39 have coronary heart disease. But, among 40- to 59-year-olds, the number jumps to almost 6%. Aerobic exercise is the key to keeping your heart healthy (Benjamin, 2017).

After a while you'll really enjoy this and look forward to your aerobic sessions. People around you will see the results and want to exercise, too. You will be an inspiration for your friends, family, and even strangers. Being healthy isn't just about how much jiggly fat you carry on your body, it's about how well your heart pumps blood, how strong your bones are, and how good you feel.

## Strength Training

We'll start with advice from the United States government:

> Add muscle-strengthening activity (such as resistance or weights) on at least 2 days per week (Lichtenstein, 2006).

This recommendation is perfect. Even the Fitness Industry agrees on this, for the most part. Working our muscles is different than working our heart. Muscle strength training requires you to *overwork* a set of muscles, whereas aerobic workouts always *underwork* the heart. In aerobic exercise, the advice is always to keep your heart rate at 50–85% of the maximum, whereas strength training should include exercises that "train to failure."

A good strength-training program can include just simple bodyweight exercises or be a structured machine workout in a gym. As you get stronger and healthier, you might want to progress to using weights, resistance bands, and machines. Strength training needs to include all the major muscle groups:

- Arms
- Back
- Chest
- Core
- Legs
- Shoulders

Our core is of vital concern when developing a strength-training program. The muscles of your core area, or torso, help align the spine, ribs, and pelvis. Your core muscles control your posture as well.

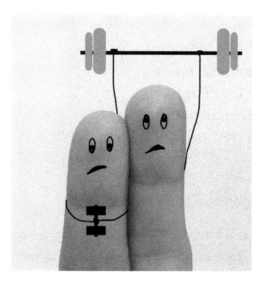

Getting *started* with a strength-training program is the hardest part. I suspect most people reading this have never lifted weights or done many bodyweight exercises, even when on a diet program that asked you to. Strength training can be incorporated through:

- Bodyweight exercises
- Resistance bands
- Weight machines
- Lifting weights

If you've never done *any* strength training before, you are going to have to buy a few things or join a gym. Many workplaces now have free exercise areas for employees, or you could start one where you work, if possible. Strength training is a bit more difficult than aerobics, but only in the beginning. We'll discuss how to get started with strength training later in the book.

## Why Strength Training?

Keeping your muscles strong is one of the basic tenets of overall health and fitness. Properly done, strength training provides improvements in your overall health. Some notable benefits of strength training include:

- Improved cardiac function
- Improved joint function
- Increased bone density
- Increased bone, muscle, tendon, and ligament strength and resilience
- Increased metabolism
- Reduced potential for injury

Strength training is known as "*an*aerobic" exercise because it does not significantly increase your heart rate or breathing requirements while performing the basic movements. Athletes understand the power of strength training. Even sports that do not require extreme strength, such as running or baseball, recognize the benefits of regular strength training. The benefits of a proper strength-training program build upon those gained in aerobic conditioning. To embark on a fitness program and exclude the strength training portion is folly at best.

## It's Not as Hard as You Might Think!

Most people will be delighted to learn that adding strength training to their weight loss program does not require excessive sweating or grunting. Different people undertake strength training for different reasons. If you want great big muscles, you'd need to lift very heavy weights many times a week. If you want to train for an endurance sport, like swimming, you'd be lifting light weights many times over and over. But for strength training—and that simply means keeping your muscles toned and your bones strong—you just need to exert a medium level of effort a couple times a week, hitting most of the major muscle groups as you exercise. You'll be mad you didn't know all this once you see how easy it is.

---

***Medical Industry Insider Secret:*** *Performing strength exercises once or twice a week for as little as five minutes can lower your risk of heart attack or stroke by 40–70% (Liu, 2018).*

---

## Conclusion

I hope you now understand what a good exercise program is and why you need one, unpleasant as it may seem. It's not about burning calories; exercise is about improving your physical condition. Once you've begun, you won't want to stop. This is your insurance policy for a long and healthy life. A good exercise program will include both aerobic and strength-training exercises. If the program I'm going to show you later is too difficult to understand or too hard to complete, you won't want to do it, you'll quit, and we'll both be failures. I promise to show you a fitness program that you'll look forward to and that you won't feel awkward about. Plus, it can be as cheap as you like!

But we're not done talking about co-factors to diet just yet. There are still three other important co-factors that make dieting successful: sleep, stress, and your gut. The next three chapters will discuss how to further improve your chances of making your weight loss diet successful.

# CHAPTER 4

# HOW SLEEP AFFECTS WEIGHT

**TL;DR:** *Getting a good night's sleep is just as important as what food you eat or how much you exercise. Maybe even more so.*

Ten years ago, sleep researchers saw little evidence that poor sleep habits had anything to do with obesity. They cited the fact that there were just as many underweight people who slept less than six hours per night as there were overweight people who slept eight hours per night. In 2008, one preeminent sleep researcher even noted:

> The greater danger to health from inadequate sleep is not obesity and its consequences, but having an accident as a result of inadvertently falling asleep. (Horne, 2008)

A decade later, researchers are singing a different tune. Perhaps the widespread use of technology in bed has led to more study subjects, but now researchers are writing conclusions such as this:

> Individuals who regularly slept less than 7 hours per night were more likely to have higher average body mass indexes and develop obesity than those who slept more. (Cooper et al., 2018)

Humans, like our wild-animal relatives, require adequate sleep and adherence to day/night cycles in order to have a healthy metabolism. Disruptions in sleep or light at night confuse our sensory systems that detect day and night. As the sunlight fades, chemicals and hormones are released throughout our bodies to help us sleep and shift us to a slower metabolism. When we stay up late, the chemicals float throughout the body and wreak havoc with many different systems that regulate weight.

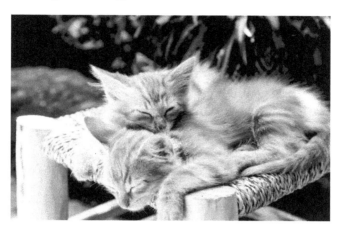

## What the Research Shows

Evidence-based medicine takes a three-pronged approach to treating patients using:

- The best available research
- Clinical expertise
- Patient preferences and values

There are hundreds of research papers published every year concerning sleep. Increasingly, many of these papers deal with the metabolic effects of sleep disturbances. Many other research papers from the last year show evidence-based connections between poor sleep and the obesity crisis. Here's a small sampling:

> "Sleep Duration and Excessive Daytime Sleepiness Are Associated with Obesity Independent of Diet and Physical Activity" (Maugeri, 2018): Short sleep duration (< 7 h) was associated with greater odds of being overweight (BMI > 25) and obesity (BMI > 30).

"Insomnia symptoms and sleep duration and their combined effects in relation to associations with obesity and central obesity" (Cai, 2018): Both short and long sleep duration, as well as insomnia symptoms, are associated with obesity and central obesity.

"Role of sleep duration and sleep-related problems in the metabolic syndrome among children and adolescents" (Pulido-Arjona, 2018): These findings suggested the clinical importance of improving sleep hygiene to reduce metabolic risk factors in children and adolescents.

## Causes of Poor Sleep

More than 40% of adults and 70% of college students surveyed said they don't feel well-rested most days (NIH, 2018). This is a leading cause of accidents, and not just fender-benders. Plane crashes, train accidents, and shipwrecks have been attributed to sleep—even the Chernobyl nuclear meltdown was attributed to sleepiness (Sleep Foundation, 2018)!

Some common causes of sleepiness and lack of sleep include:
- Caffeine
- Drugs
- Dyspepsia (GERD, IBS, etc.)
- Eating late
- Electronics (phones, readers in bed)
- Excess light (street lights, night lights, late summer sun)
- Exercising before bed
- Incontinence
- Lifestyle (up late partying, studying, gaming, etc.)
- Shiftwork
- Sleep apnea

## Sleep Apnea

Sleep apnea comes in two forms, central and obstructive. *Central sleep apnea* is caused when the brain fails to send breathing instructions while you're sleeping and is relatively uncommon. *Obstructive sleep apnea* occurs when the soft tissues at the back of the throat collapse during breathing, waking the sleeper and preventing deep sleep.

If you are a loud snorer or not feeling rested and waking up numerous times at night, ask your doctor about a sleep study to see if you have sleep apnea. Without treatment, sufferers of sleep apnea are at risk of:

- Accidents due to drowsiness
- Depression
- Diabetes
- Headaches
- Heart failure, irregular heartbeats, and heart attacks
- High blood pressure
- Stroke
- Worsening of ADHD

Take my word for it: it's not worth trying to suffer through sleep apnea. CPAP machines are covered by most insurance plans, and they'll help you get the sleep you so desperately need.

## Conclusion

You want your new diet to succeed, so please start by examining your sleep habits. If you're sleepy all the time, chances are you're also overweight. If this is the case, then making small changes to how you sleep might have a big impact on your goals. Lack of sleep has absolutely been identified as a major contributor to obesity. This is not insignificant. Mind your Zs if you want to lose some Lbs!

# CHAPTER 5

# HOW STRESS AFFECTS WEIGHT

**TL;DR:** *Stress as a cause of obesity is a new field of study. There are many proven connections. De-stress your life to regain control of your weight.*

US population surveyed: How did you try losing weight? Top answers on the board. Survey says:

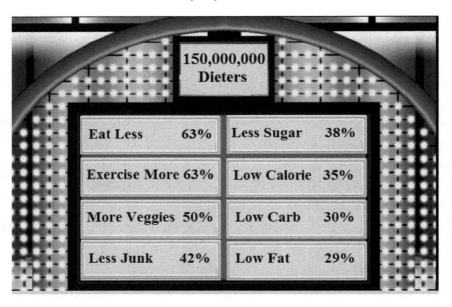

A recent survey showed that over 150 million people (49.3% of the US age 20 and older) tried to lose weight over the past 12 months (Centers for Disease Control, 2018). Less than 5% will succeed at losing weight.

This, my friend, is why I'm writing this book: Nearly 150 million people dieting, yet 140 million or more will fail at losing weight and keeping it off. I'm afraid that nearly all of them are doing it wrong. Many of these dieters are either following a popular diet plan or attempting to emulate a weight loss diet based on a headline or article they've recently read.

Researchers from the Centers for Disease Control (CDC) know what's wrong with our dieting habits: we are focusing on eating and not the more important "diet" factors of food quality, exercise, sleep, and stress-reduction.

> First off, we are more sedentary than ever before. Our enter-tainment is more likely to occur while we are sitting—in front of the TV, in front of a computer, in bed with our phones in our hands. Next, we're not cooking our own food as much, we're eating out more. And they add more fat, more sugar, more salt. Increasing stress levels can also play havoc with our metabo-lisms and that can prompt people to overeat. Sleeplessness is another known risk factor for poor eating. (CDC, 2018)

Not exercising, eating ultra-processed foods, getting poor sleep, and feeling stressed. Where have we heard that before? Stress-related obesity is a relatively new area of study, so I was pleased to see the CDC mention it in this interview. Studying the stress connection is even newer than studying sleep as a cause of obesity. But the connection is real. Control your stress, control your weight.

## Evidence-Based Connections

Lots of great research papers from the past couple years point to the mechanisms behind stress-related obesity. Until recently, everyone just thought that stress caused people to eat more; now we see it's much more complicated. The brain's reactions to stress are very similar to the biological processes involved in eating disorders and drug addiction. Chemical signals released from the brain during periods of stress affect how, when, and how much we eat as well as how our metabolism burns or stores these extra calories.

According to "Stress as a common risk factor for obesity and addiction" (Sinha, 2013):

> As stress promotes food craving and binge eating, stress reduction interventions may be useful in effective weight management programs, and some pilot behavioral stress reduction studies in obesity and type 2 diabetes mellitus are showing positive effects on improving stress, food craving and physiologic function.

A 2016 study, "Stress, cortisol, and obesity: a role for cortisol responsiveness in identifying individuals prone to obesity," (Hewagalamulage, 2016) explains:

> There is a strong inter-relationship between activation of the hypothalamo-pituitary-adrenal axis and energy homeostasis. Patients with abdominal obesity have elevated cortisol levels. Furthermore, stress and glucocorticoids act to control both food intake and energy expenditure. In particular, glucocorticoids are known to increase the consumption of foods enriched in fat and sugar.

And in "Stress and Eating Behaviors" (Yau, 2013), we read:

> Stress is an important factor in the development of addiction and in addiction relapse, and may contribute to an increased risk for obesity and other metabolic diseases.

## In Plain Words

There are a lot of big words in those papers. If you are not adept at reading medical literature, I'll explain in layman's terms. Stress causes overeating in the same way that stress causes addiction to drugs and alcohol (or other dangerous obsessions). During periods of stress, certain areas of the brain and adrenal glands activate and cause chemicals to be released that change our behavior. But not just our behavior, these chemicals also affect how we burn calories and store fat. The behavioral changes that occur lead us to choose high-fat, sugary, and refined foods that deliver instant satisfaction. "Emotional eating" is a real thing.

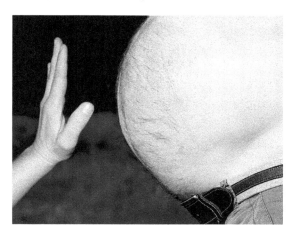

## Abdominal Obesity

Abdominal obesity is the accumulation of fat around our organs that give even lean people a big belly. When you scan the crowd at an airport, ball game, or any large public gathering, you see big bellies on just about everyone. You could call these "stress bellies" and not be far off. When you see skinny arms and legs with a protruding stomach, that's quite likely from stress, too.

## Cortisol

*Cortisol* is a chemical that comes from the adrenal glands in response to stress. High cortisol levels are nearly always present in people with excessive abdominal fat. Cushing's syndrome is a rare disease in which the adrenal glands produce too much cortisol, and those afflicted have symptoms that include big bellies, mood changes, diabetes, and high blood pressure. With Cushing's, cortisol is high all the time, causing the symptoms to appear rapidly. During periods of stress, cortisol is normally released in small, controlled doses to stimulate the immune system and metabolism, but during periods of *prolonged* stress, cortisol begins to act against our best interests, stymieing even the best diet plan.

## Causes of Stress

Stress is how our bodies react to threats. These threats can be physical or mental. Several common causes of stress in our modern lives include:

- Dieting
- Over-exercising
- Loss of job
- Relationships/breakups
- Money
- Noise
- Light
- Legal troubles
- Death of loved ones
- Moving
- Illness or injury
- Emotional issues
- Kids screaming
- Dogs barking
- Cats puking on the bed every day
- Boss being a jerk
- Computer crashing

Some stress in your life is okay; we all have it. But some of these stressors spin out of control and turn into chronic stress. Day after day, the cortisol accumulates, and we get Cushing-like symptoms; in turn we gain weight.

## Keep Calm and Read My Conclusion

It turns out that *dieting itself* is a stressful condition that causes us to store more fat, sleep less, and eat more. Is it any wonder that of the 150 some million people dieting, most will fail miserably? I think a smart marketer could create a new diet, *The Stress-Free Eating Diet: Sleep Your Way to a Flat Belly!* This diet would focus almost completely on getting better sleep and reducing stress. It would work. Until then, let's think of ways to reduce the stressors that *can* be reduced, manage the ones that *can't* as best we can, and not take on new stressors like eating too little or exercising too hard.

# CHAPTER 6

# MEDICAL CONDITIONS CAUSING OBESITY

**TL;DR:** *Medical conditions can cause you to become overweight no matter how hard you try.*

So far, we've discussed dieting hindrances that are somewhat controllable: Food intake, exercise, sleep, and stress are all external factors. However, there are numerous intrinsic factors (e.g., physical and psychological conditions) that cause weight gain as well. If you are obese or have gained weight very rapidly, please make an appointment with your doctor before you embark on a diet. There are some very real conditions that could explain your weight gain; it's best to tackle medical issues before you try toughing out a calorie-restrictive diet plan or starting an exercise program. Not addressing underlying issues will cause grave harm to your emotional state and hamper your attempts to lose weight.

## Medical Conditions

**Hypothyroidism:** An underactive thyroid will lower your metabolism. Hypothyroidism can be caused by an autoimmune condition called Hashimoto's (Hashi's) disease. With Hashi's, your own immune system attacks your thyroid gland, resulting in lowered levels of active thyroid hormones. This disease is common and easily treated. Left untreated, it will cause numerous metabolic symptoms, such as:

- Constipation
- Difficulty concentrating

- Drowsiness
- Dry skin, nails, and hair
- Fatigue
- Increased menstrual flow
- Increased sensitivity to cold
- Muscle soreness
- Weight gain

Hypothyroidism is treated with synthetic thyroid hormones (i.e., Synthroid) or natural thyroid hormones (i.e., Armour). Left untreated, hypothyroidism will lead to the formation of a goiter (enlarged thyroid gland).

The thyroid gland is a butterfly-shaped organ located in the base of your neck. It releases hormones that control metabolism, the way your body uses energy. The thyroid's hormones regulate vital body functions, including:

- Body temperature
- Body weight
- Breathing
- Central and peripheral nervous systems
- Cholesterol levels
- Heart rate
- Menstrual cycles
- Muscle strength

Yeah, that kind of stuff! If you are overweight, ask your doctor for a thyroid stimulating hormone (TSH) test. There is no cure for hypothyroidism other than thyroid replacement therapy. Some people do better on natural thyroid (Armour), while others do better on the synthetic drug (Synthroid). There is some debate about whether slightly elevated TSH requires treatment, but there is no debate about whether highly elevated (above 10) TSH or the presence of Hashi's antibodies require treatment (Mincer, 2018).

**Polycystic Ovary Syndrome (PCOS):** Sufferers of PCOS experience rapid weight gain and an inability to lose weight despite dedicated dieting attempts. PCOS is a disease found only in women, duh. Most likely, if you have PCOS, you already know it, but many experts believe that PCOS often goes undiagnosed or misdiagnosed for many years (Schulte, 2015). PCOS is an endocrine system disease that can cause, exacerbate, or facilitate metabolic problems (diabetes and cardiovascular diseases, mainly), reproductive issues, and anxiety and depression. Research suggests 40–70% of PCOS patients are obese (Schulte, 2015).

If you are wondering if you have PCOS and have not been to a doctor, initial symptoms include:

- Irregular periods or no periods
- Difficulty getting pregnant
- Excessive hair growth (hirsutism)—usually on the face, chest, back or buttocks
- Weight gain
- Thinning hair and hair loss from the head
- Oily skin or acne

If this sounds like you, get thee to a doctor, stat! PCOS is treated with drugs and lifestyle modifications. Treatment protocols sometimes address symptoms individually.

**Cushing's Syndrome:** This syndrome is caused by exposure to excess cortisol. Tumors on the pituitary gland (Cushing's disease) or taking steroid medications for too long are the top two causes (Chaudhry, 2017). Other tumors and inherited disorders can also cause Cushing's (Stratakis, 2007).

Common symptoms of Cushing's syndrome include (Chaudhry, 2017):

- Acne
- Bone loss, leading to fractures over time
- Cognitive difficulties
- Depression, anxiety, and irritability
- Headache
- Loss of emotional control
- Muscle weakness
- New or worsened high blood pressure
- Pink or purple stretch marks (striae) on the skin of the abdomen, thighs, breasts, and arms
- Severe fatigue
- Slow healing of cuts, insect bites, and infections
- Thinning, fragile skin that bruises easily
- Weight gain and fatty tissue deposits, particularly around the midsection and upper back, in the face (moon face), and between the shoulders (buffalo hump)

Symptoms specific to women include:

- Irregular or absent menstrual periods
- Thicker or more visible body and facial hair (hirsutism)

Symptoms specific to men include:

- Decreased fertility
- Decreased libido
- Erectile dysfunction

If you recognize any of these symptoms, please tell your doctor. Cushing's syndrome is very often underdiagnosed and requires many visits to the doctor. The symptoms of Cushing's syndrome often mimic obesity from overeating and a sedentary lifestyle. Cushing's syndrome is treated with medication, surgery, or radiation therapy. This is not a disease you want to leave untreated! Other medical conditions might cause weight gain and obesity, but it's always a "chicken or the egg" scenario. For instance, does type 2 diabetes cause obesity, or is it the other way around? If you find yourself overweight, it will pay to see a doctor to rule out underlying conditions first. Oftentimes the drugs your doctor prescribes have the side effect of causing weight gain.

## Drugs, Toxins, and Weight Gain

According to one study, the following drugs are associated with unwanted weight gain (Domecq, 2015) (Ness-Abramof, 2005). Please check your medications for the presence of any of these and discuss with your prescribing doctor or pharmacist:

- Amitriptyline
- Carbamazepine
- Clozapine
- Gabapentin
- Gliclazide
- Glimepiride
- Glyburide
- Hormone Replacement Therapy
- Lithium
- Mirtazapine
- Nateglinide
- Olanzapine
- Pioglitazone
- Quetiapine
- Risperidone
- Serotonin Reuptake Inhibitors (SSRIs)
- Sitagliptin

- Tolbutamide
- Valproate
- Valproic acid

In addition to drugs we may be prescribed to treat various medical conditions, there are "drugs" we take without even knowing. These environmental toxins are man-made and classified as "endocrine disruptors."

## Endocrine Disrupting Chemicals (EDCs)

EDCs have been implicated in obesity (McAllister, 2009). These chemicals are "obesogens" thought to interfere with natural weight-stabilizing hormones found in humans, such as estrogen and androgen as well as sperm production (Cook, 2019). Two of the most common EDCs in the environment are the flame retardant poly-brominated diphenyl ether (PBDE) and the plasticizer bisphenol A (BPA).

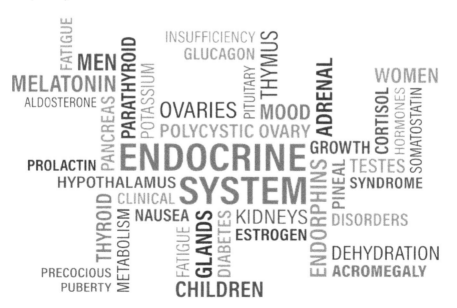

Polybrominated diphenyl ether (PBDE) was widely used during the 1980s, 1990s, and 2000s. It has now been banned in the United States and most parts of Europe (Vuong, 2018). PBDE was used to "fireproof" consumer goods such as electronics, furniture, carpets, carpet padding, gym mats, car seats, and hundreds of other products found in households across the United States. Studies show the presence of PBDE in the blood and bodily tissues of nearly every resident of the United States (Vuong, 2018). PBDE has been shown to damage thyroid function, reproductive capability, fetal development, and brain development in children (Vuong, 2018). PBDE is a known carcinogen and found on nearly every surface in homes and workplaces across the country. It's released from fireproofed products and floats like dust throughout homes and offices (Allen, 2016).

Plasticizer bisphenol A (BPA) is used to make plastic and is found *everywhere* (Stahlhut, 2018). BPA is also used to line cans, milk cartons, and other metal and paperboard containers used to package food and beverages. BPA leaches out of plastic containers and contaminates foods, beverages, and drinking water. Some other commonly found EDCs are contained in pesticides, herbicides, solvents, and even on cash register receipts. BPA is found in the blood of 95% of people (Cook, 2019). BPA has a solid connection with metabolic syndrome and other metabolic disease states (Stahlhut, 2018). The FDA contends that BPA is safe when used as intended, but this will most likely change as the dangers of BPA are exposed.

Sometimes it feels like we should just throw our hands up and surrender if we're overweight. How can we get ahead of the obesity monster if "obesogens" are found in our food, water, and air? While this may seem the stuff of conspiracy theory websites and bad movies, endocrine disruptors are real, and they're everywhere. The National Institutes of Health, a governmental agency, recognizes the presence of EDCs in our environment and confirms the problems they cause (Tox Town, 2018):

The following comes from a National Institutes of Health flyer for public information:

## How can I be exposed to Endocrine Disruptors?

Endocrine Disruptors commonly enter(s) the body through:

**Ingestion (swallowing)**

- Swallowing food, beverages, or medicines that contain endocrine disruptors

**Inhalation (breathing)**

- Breathing air contaminated by endocrine disruptors

**Skin contact**

- Touching products made with endocrine disruptors

## What happens when I am exposed to Endocrine Disruptors?

Exposure to endocrine disruptors even at low levels can affect human health.

Exposure to endocrine disruptors can cause:

- Cancer or an increased risk of cancer
- Changes in the development and behavior of infants and children
- Changes in a developing fetus
- Interference with the body's natural hormones
- Changes in reproductive organs and function
- Infertility and endometriosis
- Disturbances in the immune and nervous system functions
- Heart disease and stroke
- Asthma

Unfortunately, there is no sure way to clear the body of EDCs, though some studies suggest that EDCs are eliminated from the body through sweat (De Coster, 2012). This is the price we pay to be modern humans, sad as that may sound. However, avoiding ultra-processed food, food packaged in plastic, and plastic utensils, and staying away from areas where heavy chemical use is prevalent (agriculture, factories, etc.) are steps we can take to avoid EDC overload (Cook, 2019).

Having a healthy gut is essential to combating the presence of EDCs. My advice: Don't be a victim. Don't blame EDCs for your health woes. Be as healthy as you can by eating good food, exercising, sleeping well, and de-stressing your life. Avoid ultra-processed food as much as you can. Work up a good sweat now and then.

## Conclusion

There are valid medical reasons for weight gain. The most common disease for both men and women is hypothyroidism, in fact Synthroid for hypothyroidism is the most widely prescribed drug in the United States, with over 120 million people currently taking the drug. Hypothyroidism is easily checked by your doctor. If your thyroid is okay, have the doc rule out other medical conditions. Medication itself can also cause weight gain. Lastly, be aware of the presence and effects of environmental toxins called endocrine disruptors; these are found everywhere and can affect people differently. If you are concerned, please bring this up to your doctor as well.

Most people can become weight-stable by adhering to the principals of eating less, exercising more, sleeping better, and de-stressing their lives. Unfortunately, many people have medical issues that prevent easy weight loss. Some medical conditions might prevent exercise, such as arthritis, but there are ways around this. And some medical conditions might be stressful in and of themselves; the treatment of cancer or chronic back pain often leads to overeating and a sedentary existence. Seek assistance, overcome, and adapt!

# CHAPTER 7

# DISEASES CAUSED BY OBESITY

**TL;DR:** *You don't have to be skinny to be healthy. But being overweight is a risk factor in many diseases.*

A doctor friend of mine once motioned toward the patients in his waiting room and remarked, "None of these people would be here if they ate right." What *I* saw was a group of middle-aged to elderly folks, mostly obese, carrying various canes and walkers, a bottle or two of oxygen, and plastic bags filled with prescription bottles. One elderly couple was sharing lunch from a McDonald's bag, and others were drinking sodas and eating candy bars. It dawned on me that none of these people were connecting their *ill health* with the *food* they were eating. Sometimes I think the doctors are to blame; they treat the symptoms of obesity—not the cause. But I also understand how frustrating it must be to be a doctor. Who would really take their advice? And that's all it would be, friendly advice. A doctor cannot prescribe a healthy diet, exercise, a good night's sleep, or a stress-free lifestyle. And so, we go, 'round and 'round.

> Although many diseases associated with obesity include those directly related to excess adiposity, including sleep apnea, osteoarthritis, and stress incontinence, other diseases like insulin resistance/diabetes, fatty liver disease, dyslipidemia, and hypertension appear to be secondary diseases that develop in the chronic inflammatory milieu associated with obesity. (Albaugh, 2018)

Earlier we discussed medical conditions that cause obesity; now we're going to look at some of the diseases and other medical conditions that obesity itself can cause. Becoming and staying overweight leads to many preventable problems, which are often called "modern diseases." This is why we should be dieting. As with everything, prevention is key. If you are overweight and on the fence about dieting, perhaps reading this will spark something within you and you'll be convinced that it's time to change your ways. If you've dieted continually and are still overweight or obese, much of this will look familiar.

When the human body accumulates too much fat, especially around the organs, it starts to fail. Carrying excess weight has been associated with numerous medical problems, including (Hruby, 2016) (Kreuter, 2018) (Sarica, 2019) :

- Cancer
- Depression
- Fatty liver disease
- Gout
- Heart disease
- High blood pressure
- High cholesterol
- High triglycerides
- Inflammatory bowel diseases
- Kidney disease
- Kidney stones
- Osteoarthritis
- Pregnancy problems
- Sleep apnea
- Strokes
- Type 2 diabetes

Dieting (*and that's more than just eating right!*) needs to be about living life without this list of medical problems. It's not about looking good or losing a few pounds for summer. This list is what Big Pharma loves about the obesity epidemic; each condition creates billions of dollars' worth of revenue for everyone in the medical industry. I personally was on meds to treat six of these conditions in the not-so-distant past. Surely someone lost out on a new Mercedes-Benz because I got healthier. So sad.

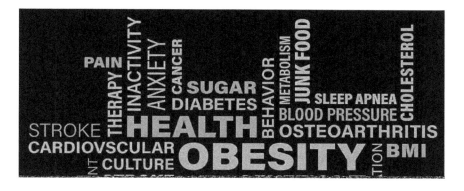

Some of these conditions have sort of a "chicken or the egg" dilemma. Which came first? And, truthfully, sometimes it's hard to tell. Sleep apnea, for instance, can be both caused by and a cause of obesity. Sometimes the medicines prescribed to treat a disease of obesity only serve to make things worse. It can be a long road, treating symptoms. Drug interactions when you're taking multiple drugs can be a real bear, too. But no matter how you slice it, losing weight will help with all of these.

## Overweight and Healthy

It's completely possible to be overweight, even obese, and healthy—"fit-but-fat," as it's called in some circles (Loprinzi, 2014). Approximately 10% of the overweight and obese populations of the United States are fit-but-fat (Duncan, 2010). This condition is characterized by BMI and weight in the overweight/obese categories combined with a low resting heart rate, healthy lungs, great muscles, and absence of the diseases associated with being overweight.

Most fit-but-fat people have some things in common: exercise, adequate sleep, low stress levels, and a healthy gut. This should give great hope to those who start a diet program but can't lose weight no matter how hard they try. Blame your genes but keep exercising! The statistics are grim: Tens of millions of obese people in the United States will never escape the obesity label. The vast majority who diet might expect to lose 10% of their bodyweight only to regain it within five years. The pressure to lose weight is more often psychological than medical. This adds stress to an already stressed person (MacLean, 2011).

One goal of a good diet program should be to get off the medicines you take to counter the effects of being overweight. This requires a long talk with your doctor and a good assessment of your true health. Losing just 10–15% of your bodyweight is a good starting point, and health benefits are seen at that level of weight loss (MacLean, 2011). But don't worry if you are not losing weight at the rate you desire. Continue the course of exercising daily, eating good food, sleeping well, and de-stressing your life. You'll see benefits beyond needing to buy new clothes. Your heart will thank you.

## Metabolic Syndrome

Metabolic syndrome is the start of a death spiral. Metabolic syndrome is a cluster of conditions that occur together:

- Excess body fat around the waist
- Fatty Liver
- High blood pressure
- High blood sugar
- High cholesterol
- High triglycerides

These conditions greatly increase your risk of heart disease, stroke, cancer, and diabetes. As with other diseases of Western society, Western medicine simply treats each symptom as if it were an independent variable. Normally, metabolic syndrome begins with weight gain in your thirties as your metabolism begins to slow down from its heyday in your twenties. You continue to eat like a teenager, but your activity level slumps. You're working 40–50 hours a week, maybe on a night shift. Your kids may be growing and creating more problems. Your marriage might be rocky. There's never enough money to go around. Suddenly your 34" jeans no longer fit, and you're buying them in "Husky" sizes. A visit to the doc reveals you have a serious "statin deficiency" causing your high cholesterol, so you get a couple new prescriptions. You have heartburn every night, keeping you awake. Sex becomes a chore.

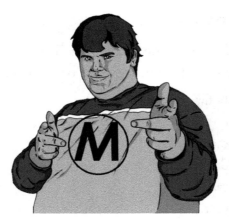

*Met-Syn Man*

And so it goes: one thing leads to another, and trips to the pharmacy become even more frequent. This is metabolic syndrome. In most cases it's completely reversible with diet, exercise, sleep, and stress-reduction. Sometimes just cleaning up the diet helps, and it should be your starting point for sure.

Left untreated, metabolic syndrome will plague you with discomfort for years, culminating in a trip to the hospital where you may (or may *not*) leave with a nice zipper-scar to remind you of the quadruple bypass you just received. Stents, catheters, pills, and injections are your new lifeblood.

*Healthcare Industry Insider Secret: Doctors treat the symptoms of Metabolic Syndrome not the cause.*

*In fact, it is easier to prescribe a drug to lower blood pressure, blood glucose, or triglycerides rather than initiating a long-term strategy to change people's lifestyle (exercise more and eat better) in the hope that they will ultimately lose weight and tend to have a lower blood pressure, blood glucose, and triglycerides. (Kaur, 2014)*

## Conclusion

Being overweight carries considerable consequences. Obesity is associated with numerous diseases and medical conditions. Metabolic syndrome is a cluster of disease states found in overweight patients. Not everyone will be able to lose all the weight they desire, but this can be mitigated by a good diet program that encompasses the things I've been mentioning: food, exercise, sleep, and stress. Medically speaking, yo-yo dieting is not a good practice. Better to learn to manage your weight through exercise and other means, even if you are not as thin as you'd hoped. Know your health markers, and look at ways you've become healthier that might not show on the scale. Even modest weight loss will lower your blood pressure, heart rate, and cholesterol levels. Doctors know the secret to making you healthy, but they also know that most people won't be receptive to the idea. Instead, they prescribe drugs to treat each new symptom.

# CHAPTER 8

# GENETICS AND WEIGHT

**TL;DR:** *How and where you store fat is genetic. Most people have unreal expectations of what they can achieve by dieting. DNA testing for weight loss is a rip-off.*

*Diet Industry Insider Secret:* *Your body shape and propensity to gain weight are largely determined by your genetics, not how much you eat and exercise (Rask-Andersen, 2019).*

The shape of your body and where you store fat are determined by your genes more than any other factor (Rask-Andersen, 2019). This doesn't mean that we should throw our hands up and surrender; it means we need to have realistic expectations about how far dieting will get us in the pursuit of a "perfect" body. It also means that we need to find our *own* way when it comes to losing weight and staying healthy.

Food, exercise, sleep, and stress are controlling factors in determining how our bodies will adjust to our genetic blueprint. Some people will naturally respond better to dieting or exercise than others. Some people will be more stressed than others. Some people will sleep better than others. No diet plan works equally well for everyone who tries it. Therefore, I'm taking a much different approach to dieting in this book. Most people will be able to find a diet program that works for them, especially if they are mindful of all the aspects that determine weight and health.

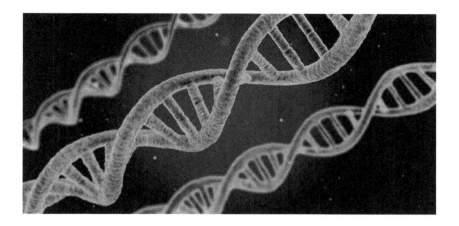

## Genetics 101

Our understanding of genetics has exploded in the last decade, and you might have even seen ads for genetic test kits that not only determine your ancestry but also give insights to your health and longevity. It's a heady subject, for sure. I think it will benefit everyone if I don't gloss over this topic like I'd love to do. Instead, I'm going to cram a college degree's worth of information into a couple of paragraphs here so that we are on the same page.

## DNA

Your DNA determines nearly everything about you, such as eye color, hair color, and the shape of your nose. You inherit DNA from your parents. The genetic information stored within you is encoded on strands of DNA found in nearly every cell in your body. These DNA strands contain about three billion combinations of just four chemicals: adenine (A), guanine (G), cytosine (C), and thymine (T). These four chemicals combine in unique ways to make us human (or make birds birds). We inherit certain combinations of DNA from generation to generation, making it more likely that some of us will have blue eyes and others brown, depending on the eyes of our ancestors.

### Genes

Genes are made up of DNA. Genes have different purposes. Some genes create things you need to live, such as insulin, sweat, and gastric juices, while other genes act as regulators of these bodily functions. We each have about 30,000 genes that *create* things (coding DNA) and billions of genes that *regulate* (non-coding DNA). About 99% of our genes are similar to those of other humans; it's the 1% that makes us each unique. The differences in genes are called "alleles."

### Chromosomes

Deep inside nearly every cell in your body is a packet of DNA called a chromosome. Humans have 46 chromosomes packaged as pairs, or 23 pairs of chromosomes. Each one of these chromosomes, when examined, contains numerous genes. Scientists have figured out what most of these genes do by observing them. They've given the 23 pairs of chromosomes names (well, numbers, actually) and have named most of the 30,000 or so genes they've discovered as well. For example, a unique gene allele on chromosome 7 is found in people with cystic fibrosis. This gene is called the "cystic fibrosis transmembrane conductance regulator," and its symbol is CFTR.

### There's an App for That!

With modern computers, scientists can now unravel your DNA with just a few cells found in skin, saliva, or blood. They run the cells through a powerful computing program, and the DNA can be mapped out to show which gene alleles you have on your chromosomes. The alleles can be cross-referenced in a database to show the likelihood of being blue-eyed or having a propensity for high blood pressure, for instance.

## Is It Useful?

DNA testing is still used mainly to establish identity and paternity, but this new science of unraveling and decoding your DNA is still too new to be of much use to the average dieter. While we might have a couple of coding genes that show we have a propensity for diabetes, there might be thousands of noncoding genes that protect us. The leader in home DNA testing is 23andMe. They offer a full line of genetic testing to determine your ancestry and give insights into your health. Their website contains the following disclaimer: "When it comes to your health and traits, DNA is only part of the story. Other variables come into play, including non-genetic factors, such as your environment and lifestyle."

Medical professionals can use DNA reports to confirm or rule out hereditary diseases like Huntington's disease or Down syndrome, and insurance companies would love to get their hands on everyone's DNA report to predict individual liability. But beyond that, DNA testing services are just for fun.

The Diet Industry is already selling DNA testing kits to help you in your pursuit of a perfect physique. For instance, the Jenny Craig™ website proclaims: "The new DNA test will not only further personalize your weight loss plan but focus on your overall health and well-being. Based on your genetic markers our highly trained personal consultants will design a multi-faceted plan unique to you in a one on one setting."[4]

And from the website of GenoVive™: "GenoVive takes customization much further by using DNA testing to design the best diet for your patient's unique metabolism … Knowing our genetic

---

4    "Our Latest Innovation: A personalized weight loss approach powered by your DNA," Jenny Craig, accessed February 23, 2019, https://www.jennycraig.com/dna-innovation.

predispositions is the key to an effective customized weight loss program. That's why understanding our individual genetic variations is essential to choosing the best foods and types of physical activity that our body needs."[5]

## DON'T FALL FOR IT!

This is a scam. I get it, though. Investors want to sell more products, so they jump to the newest thing, in this case DNA testing, and try to look like a leader in the industry. For now, DNA testing is simply a numbers game. They'll get some right, most wrong. There is simply too much going on with our DNA and genes to use the results of a test to tailor a specific diet beyond the advice to eat a balanced diet and restrict calories to lose weight.

If you'd like to get a DNA test anyway, just to see what the fuss is all about, I highly recommend using the services of 23andMe. For under $200, you'll get a full report that explores your genome and gives insights to your ancestry, possible hereditary diseases you may be susceptible to, and genes you have that predispose you to certain health concerns. DNA testing is still in its infancy, so don't expect miracles.

### Genetics and Weight Gain

We're all different. This includes how we gain and store fat. I know a family with two sets of twin boys. One set of twins is tall and skinny like the mother. The other set is short and chubby like the father. It's a hilarious sight to see, these very different sets of twins. They were fed from the same table and raised under the same conditions, with completely different outcomes. What could be going on in their genetic code that made them that way?

---

5  "Why DNA Test?" GenoVive, accessed February 23, 2019, https://www.genoviveusa.com/dna-test/.

In 1952, a prominent geneticist developed the "Thrifty Gene Hypothesis" to explain why some groups of people were more prone to type 2 diabetes than others. This hypothesis was later expanded to explain why obesity was also prevalent in certain cultures and not others. The theory was that some groups throughout history had better survival rates if they stored more fat when food was plentiful and that other groups never experienced food shortages, and thus did not need to store fat.

Then in October 2018, scientists identified gene SGLT1. This gene controls how carbohydrates are absorbed in the small intestine and explains why some people can eat loads of carbs and not have diabetes while others must restrict and still have problems. Today's melting pot of societies has resulted in children of the same family inheriting these different genes from the Wayback Machine that is our DNA.

## The Obesity Paradox

It's easy to explain weight gain. When a person eats more calories than they burn, they'll store the excess as fat. With enough overeating and under-exercising, a person will become overweight and obese. What's hard to explain is why some people can eat all they want, not exercise, and stay lean. Genetics is the key to understanding weight gain. The holy grail of obesity research is to identify a gene that causes us to gain weight and then invent a drug or gene-editing method that changes this gene.

Researchers have identified over 50 genes associated with weight gain since 2006 (Butler, 2015). Most of the genes have very small effects when looked at individually and are thought to act together and with environmental conditions (e.g., sleep, stress) to cause obesity. Other researchers have uncovered evidence that this genetic fat-storage code is related to our gender as well (Rask-Andersen, 2019).

## CRISPR

Ever heard of it? CRISPR has been in the news a lot this year. Clustered Regularly Interspaced Short Palindromic Repeats (CRISPR) can be used by genetic researchers to edit a gene (Pawluk, 2018). Scientists are now using CRISPR to create better plants for agriculture, but the science has also been extended to animals and even humans.

Oddly enough, the day after I wrote this, every news organization was reporting that a Chinese company had successfully edited the genes of a human baby using CRISPR. While highly controversial, CRISPR could one day be used to create humans that are immune to weight gain or epilepsy, or could design babies that have perfect blond hair and blue eyes. Let's all just hope CRISPR is used for good and that there are no hidden consequences of such a powerful tool. When you see CRISPR in the news, pay attention. This is bound to be one of the biggest topics in science very soon, you can expect much lively debate and many new laws in response to tinkering with genes.

## Body Somatotypes

Science aside, there are some very real implications to genetics and dieting. Mostly, this has to do with "body types" and expectations.

*Diet and Fitness Industry Insider Secret: You cannot change your body type to any significant degree. Humans have three basic shapes called "somatotypes" (Koleva, 2002).*

### Mesomorphic Build

Mesomorphs have athletic builds, muscular bodies, good skin, and great posture.

### Ectomorphic Build

Ectomorphs are thin, lightly muscled, and flat chested with thin skin and very few fat deposits under the skin.

### Endomorphic Build

Endomorphs are rounder, shorter, and softer than the other body types. They store fat easily and have great appetites.

These body types are sometimes even further categorized when a person doesn't conform completely. There are four subtypes: mesomorph-ectomorphs, mesomorph-endomorphs, mesomorphic ectomorphs, and ectomorphic mesomorph types.

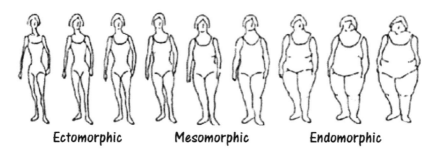

Ectomorphic    Mesomorphic    Endomorphic

*Adapted from Li (2010)*

Sounds crazy, no? But look around. Do you think any of the people in the fitness ads started out as short and fat? I remember pondering over body types when I was a young boy. Why did I need the Husky jeans, whereas my brother was skinny? And as a young man, why didn't I have six-pack abs like some of my Air Force flight-mates?

And even now, at 53, why must I diet so hard to keep from being overweight?

Doctors never mention this. You rarely read about the basic body types in diet programs. But there *is* a group that's highly interested in somatotypes: the athletic community. There are hundreds of research papers written on the somatotypes of various sports athletes. For instance, the research paper, "Somatotypes of Weight Lifters" discusses the body types of the different classes of weight lifters. The authors noted, "Weight lifters in the lighter weight classes are found to be ectomorphic or balanced mesomorphs, while those in the heavier weight classes tend to be endomorphic mesomorphs" (Oranová, 1990). There are similar papers discussing the body types of golfers, swimmers, and every other Olympic athlete. I'm sure this interest in body type is so talent scouts and coaches can single out potential athletes and weed out people who are never going to be an elite athlete, based on a trained glance at a young person's build.

There are a few papers that discuss health problems of the different body types. In one study, 524 men and 250 women were categorized into five somatotypes and studied for chronic diseases (Koleva, 2002). The authors concluded that body type was a good predictor of certain diseases, but simply using the BMI (body mass index) chart was a better predictor than body type. Every body type can become overweight and obese. Even the most physically fit athletes lose their musculature if they stop training. And the skinnier and rounder body types can become elite athletes in sports suited to their physical nature; for instance, runners are generally tall and skinny while weight lifters are shorter and stockier.

## **Should We Care about Our Somatotype?**

The short answer is no.

The longer answer is not so easy. If you ever come across a diet plan that promises to change you from an endomorph into a mesomorph, run. Can't be done. But a pudgy person who's never exercised or eaten right can certainly transform themselves into a leaner, healthier, more confident person. We all know that (within limits) we cannot change our height or where we store fat. People are sometimes classified as "pear shaped" or "apple shaped" to describe where they store fat. The apples are always going to store fat around their midsection and pears on their thighs. Hormonal changes can play funny tricks on menopausal women who often note drastic fat storage changes, but younger women and most men of all ages are stuck with what they were born with.

Body image is a huge topic. The media usually depicts the perfect female body as being very lean with large breasts, and the perfect male body as athletic with defined abs and big biceps. Only a small percentage of the human population can achieve these attributes. This mismatch is often blamed for eating disorders and behavioral problems in adolescents (Morris, 2003). It doesn't stop there.

The Diet and Fitness Industry is continually messing with your mind. Any fitness guru worth his salt sports washboard abs, has a thick head of hair, and boasts veiny arms that look like they could bend steel. Most likely that person looked that way their whole life. The industry is not going to show you a room full of listless overweight folks—there'd be no motivation. People want most what they *can't* have; it's just basic human psychology. What I think most people need to understand is how far they can get with the cards they were dealt.

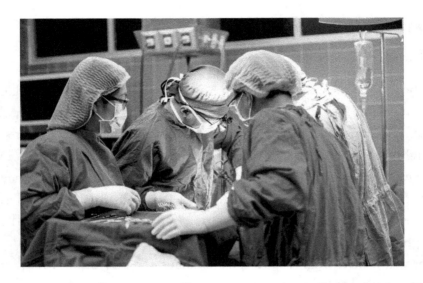

There's another industry that knows this only too well: the Cosmetic Surgery Industry. If it were easy to lose weight or change a body type, there'd be no plastic surgeons. Americans spent over $15 billion in 2016 on "beauty procedures" including breast augmentation, liposuction, and nose jobs (MedicalXpress, 2018).

## Conclusion

*The Diet Hack* is not about getting *pretty*—it's about getting *healthy*. Being obese is not healthy. It's hard on the joints and heart, and it can lead to serious medical conditions. The real hack is getting *ahead* of obesity by starting a diet program that addresses exercise, sleep, and stress as well as medical conditions *and* food. The Diet and Fitness Industry would like you to believe that you can look like a Baywatch Babe or Magic Mike, but Mother Nature has other plans. The best bet is to be the best *you* you can be.

# CHAPTER 9

# HOW GUT HEALTH AFFECTS *EVERYTHING*

**TL;DR:** *Having a healthy gut is vital to health and weight stability. We know very little about how to create a healthy gut beyond eating lots of high-fiber fruits and veggies. Gut testing is a rip-off.*

Everything I've written so far has been against the backdrop of gut health. Anyone who's been around me any length of time quickly learns that I'm fascinated with the human gut. I've been blogging and writing about gut-related illnesses and quick fixes for years. But as the years wear on, I realize that nobody knows much about the gut, and all the quick fixes we came up with only helped a small portion of the people who tried them. I've come to the conclusion that there are no quick fixes, but there are things you can do to improve your gut health. The most important are eating good quality food, exercising, getting plenty of sleep every night, and living a stress-free life. Do all that and your gut will be the best it can be.

I couldn't have said this better myself:

> The human gut microbiota consists of up to 100 trillion microbes and possesses at least 100 times more genes than are present in the entire human genome. These microbes serve a number of important functions including: producing additional energy otherwise inaccessible to the host by breaking down soluble fiber; producing vitamins such as biotin, folate and vitamin K; metabolizing xenobiotics such as the inactivation of heterocyclic amines formed in meat during cooking; preventing colonization by pathogens; and assisting in the development of a mature immune system. (Davis, 2016)

## Gut Health, Antibiotics, and Weight Gain

Many experts feel that damage to the gut from widespread use of antibiotics in children is a major contributor to the obesity epidemic (Ville, 2017). Luckily for us, the use of antibiotics has seen a dramatic decline over the last 20 years; still, most children are prescribed one or two courses of antibiotics per year for the first decade of their lives (Vaz, 2014) (Hicks, 2015). We should consider ourselves lucky to have access to antibiotics. Most antibiotics for children are prescribed for conditions that simply cannot be treated any other way. Ear infections, respiratory tract infections, and skin or other bacterial infections can easily maim or kill children if left untreated. The Centers for Disease Control indicates that approximately 30–50% of all antibiotic prescriptions are not needed (CDC, 2016), but most doctors feel the rewards outweigh the risks and caution on the safe side. There are many dangers to overprescribing antibiotics, weight gain being just a minor one. Whereas thousands of experiments have been conducted on using antibiotics for fattening farm animals, hardly any research has been done to study the effects of antibiotics as a "fattening agent" for humans (Ville, 2017).

*Healthcare Industry Insider Secret: Livestock farmers fatten their animals for market by feeding them antibiotics. The antibiotics alter the bacteria in the guts of animals, which causes massive changes to how the animals absorb nutrients and store body fat. Thousands of experiments have been conducted on the use of antibiotics for livestock fattening programs, and they've gotten it down to a science. Medical researchers have known for many centuries that the gut is an important organ not just for digestion but also as the mediator of weight stability (Li, 2017).*

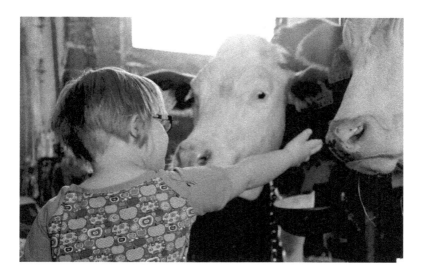

The solution isn't to ban antibiotics; it's to feed kids better. After most children are weaned and transitioned to processed foods, their gut health starts going downhill. Gerber's baby food isn't much better than Carl's Jr. in terms of quality, and once kids start eating real food, it gets even worse. Hot dogs, Hot Pockets, and Hamburger Helper are not appropriate foods for growing children.

## Gut Problems Got You Down?

By "gut," I am talking about your intestines, mostly, and the bacteria that reside within (called "gut flora"). Most people never consider their *gut* as a cause for weight gain, but it's quite possibly the most important piece of the puzzle. By the time you've become quite overweight you've also most likely developed gut problems. A bad gut is not doing you any favors, but instead is treating you like a sheep being led to slaughter. It causes you to stay hungry and store fat where it doesn't belong (Davis, 2016). Gut problems usually start out slowly.

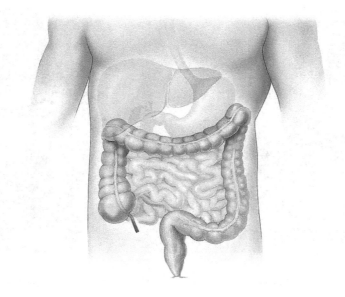

We've become the Pepto Bismol generation: "Heartburn, nausea, indigestion, upset stomach, diarrhea … Hey! Pepto Bismol!" It's a funny jingle, but once your gut is trashed, it's very hard to recover. This is the modern dyspeptic gut. This list of common gut problems is saddening:

- C. diff infections
- Celiac disease
- Crohn's disease
- Diverticulitis
- Gastroesophageal reflux disease (GERD)
- Inflammatory bowel disease (IBD)
- Irritable bowel syndrome (IBS)
- Ulcerative colitis

Having any of these gut issues can make life miserable, and the treatments are often harsh, requiring surgery or multiple rounds of antibiotics and a special diet. It's better to try to get ahead of gut disease. For the overweight and obese, the gut is a ticking time bomb.

If you've avoided these common problems thus far in your life, consider yourself lucky because 60–70 million people in the United States are affected by these diseases (Clearinghouse, 2013). Learn from the risk factors to prevent becoming a statistic. Common causes of gut disease are: (Cabré, 2012):

- Lack of sleep
- Medication
- Obesity
- Smoking
- Stress
- Western diet

Does this list look familiar? It should, we've been discussing these exact things for the past 40 pages! The causes of gut disease are the same things that cause obesity. Coincidence?

## Gut Guardians

Your gut is home to your immune system, and it converses regularly with your brain (Tokuhara, 2019). I could fill volumes telling you how amazing your gut is, but the words are long and the concepts are quickly lost on everyone but the most well-studied microbiologists. Researchers have learned a lot about our gut microbiome; they know the common inhabitants, the good and the bad. Most bacterial genes have been cataloged, and we even know how bacteria and yeast interact to cause disease. But what we *can't* do is define exactly what a *good* gut flora looks like. All we can do is tell you that you need to eat more high-fiber plants and fewer Western foods (Diether, 2019).

*Healthcare Industry Secret: Even the scientists and experts don't really know how this all works. The gut holds lots of mysteries.*

*The hormonal control of appetite and metabolism is complex and involves a mix of both brain and gut hormones, including insulin, leptin and ghrelin. Release and control of these hormones can be considered akin to an orchestra, with levels of each hormone changing rhythmically in response to each other. However, whether the brain or the gut has more influence, like the conductor of an orchestra has not been established. (El Aidy, 2015)*

## A Bit of Advice

In my experience, people should look first at all of the other issues in their life before tackling gut problems *unless* they have a serious gut disease. If the gut is compromised, that takes priority. Many times, however, people are convinced by slick marketers and internet "doctors" that the root of all their problems lies within the gut. This leads to years of gut-tinkering: unneeded gut tests, consultations, specialized diets, pills, herbs, or more invasive techniques requiring colonics, enemas, and oftentimes harmful detoxing protocols.

The overweight and unhealthy should instead focus on the external factors they control directly (eating, exercise, sleep, stress) before tackling "leaky gut" or "SIBO." Most often these undiagnosable conditions are eliminated by switching to a better diet and other controllable variables (Quigley, 2016).

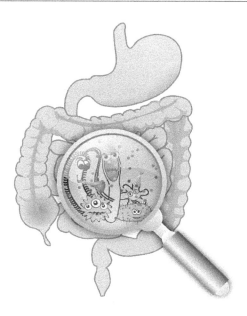

## Probiotics

The probiotics industry generated $35 billion in 2015 (Jarde, 2018). Marketers will tell you that you need probiotics in order to have a healthy gut. Probiotics are living bacteria that, when eaten, colonize your gut and make you and your gut healthier … hopefully. There are thousands of probiotic pills and foods for sale. Many of the probiotics on the market are a complete waste of money, but others are quite effective. It's nearly impossible for the average consumer to make wise purchases by reading product labels. The FDA regulates the sale of probiotics very loosely, and sellers take advantage (Quigley, 2019). Many wild claims are made about probiotics with zero supporting evidence. Buyer beware.

The Healthcare Industry (aka "Big Medicine") is not an ardent fan of probiotics. Nor is Big Pharma. Probiotics are sold as dietary supplements; there are no prescription-only probiotics. Big Pharma has been trying for many years to construct a probiotic that only *they* control, but to no avail. Probiotics are a natural entity, and therefore regulated as food. The FDA has not approved a single probiotic for preventing or treating *any* health conditions, and insurances will not cover them; for this reason, doctors are not particularly fond of prescribing probiotics [Liu (2), 2018]. Some pharmacies carry probiotics, and many doctors will prescribe or recommend probiotics for health concerns such as (Ciorba, 2012):

- Acute onset infectious diarrhea
- Antibiotic associated diarrhea
- Irritable bowel syndrome
- Inflammatory bowel diseases

There is much research to support the use of probiotics in medical care and for general well-being and weight loss. I suspect that probiotic therapy will become more widespread in the future, especially if they are one day covered by insurance providers.

## Prebiotics

The bacteria in your gut eat special kinds of fiber, this fiber is called "prebiotic" fiber, meaning it feeds bacteria. Prebiotics have been studied for anti-obesity effects for many years, and there is no doubt that a well-fed gut flora is a key regulator of human health and weight (Markowiak, 2017). The Western diet is almost completely devoid of the proper types of fiber for feeding the gut.

Supplement manufacturers have jumped on the bandwagon and now offer countless concoctions containing numerous blends of prebiotic fibers that bacteria are known to eat. But you know what your gut bacteria really like to eat? Plants. Your gut flora doesn't want to be fed powders and pills any more than you do. Your gut residents want real food—plants. Beans, potatoes, rice, bananas, cauliflower, chocolate, nuts, corn, apples, and every other edible plant. Did I mention chocolate? Gut bacteria especially loves chocolate (Hayek, 2013).

*Supplement Industry Insider Secret: A cheap cooking ingredient, potato starch, is quite possibly the best prebiotic supplement available. Adding 1–2 tablespoons of uncooked potato starch per day will supply vital fermentable fiber required for optimal gut health (Baxter, 2019).*

If you think doctors are reluctant to prescribe *pro*biotics, just wait until you ask them about *pre*biotics. The term itself, *prebiotic*, is like a foreign word in the world of Big Medicine even though researchers have been studying the health effects of prebiotics for over 30 years.

Prebiotic supplements have only just recently started showing up on store shelves. The world is largely clueless to the concept. Fiber has been successfully marketed for decades, but most of the fiber sold is not prebiotic fiber, rather just "bulking" fiber that helps make old people poop better.

## Conclusion

Gut health is quite possibly more important to weight maintenance and human health than all the other factors we've discussed so far put together. Gut health is more important than food, exercise, sleep, stress, medications, smoking, and any other thing that affects our health. But here's the kicker: the health of your gut is a product of everything you do—how you eat, exercise, sleep, etc. You cannot expect to have good gut health eating the Western diet, neglecting exercise, feeling stressed all the time, or continually depriving yourself of sleep. Get everything else right and good gut health will follow. Pills and powders cannot replace fruit and veggies.

# CONCLUSION TO PART 1

Part 1, The Obesity Epidemic, was intended to show you that being overweight is not entirely your fault. Unless you have the genes to keep you lean, there's a high chance you're going to get fat. This is especially true if you eat the Western diet, don't exercise, sleep poorly, or live under stressful conditions. You might have an illness and take drugs that further exacerbate weight gain. And let's say you are doing *everything* right but are still overweight—you might have an undiagnosed disease that results in weight gain.

Let's not forget the gut! The gut is the most important piece of this whole puzzle, but we need not worry about it if we take care of all the other things. If we take care of our gut, our gut will take care of us. The first step in regaining our health is to lose weight. For this, we need a special weight loss diet. Diets have a poor track record of success. In Part 2, I'll tell you all about weight loss diets and how to create a diet plan that will work for you.

# PART 2
# LOSING WEIGHT

# INTRODUCTION TO PART 2

Diet books, ads, and websites are filled with stories of people who lose lots of weight—we commonly see stories of people losing 100 pounds or more. Stories of these big losses sell. *The Biggest Loser* is all about massive weight loss, and each episode attracts a viewing audience of over 7 million people. What would a diet book be without pages of before-and-after photos showing how the fat just melted off to reveal a svelte, younger-looking person inside?

If you think you know everything there is to know about dieting, I urge you to keep reading. I thought I knew it all, too. Then I started studying; turns out I didn't know much at all. Perhaps you'll learn something new if you read on.

Here in Part 2, I want to help you lose weight by showing you the key elements of some very successful weight loss programs. I'll show you how you can develop your own program using tried-and-true tactics of the diet and medical industries. I'll even give you a brand-new diet that rivals anything you've ever seen.

# CHAPTER 10

# MEET THE MODERN-DAY WEIGHT LOSS DIET

**TL;DR:** *Weight loss diets can be commercial programs, self-directed, or medically supervised. All diets follow one of three styles: Low-carb, low-fat, or balanced meals. Any diet can work for weight loss if it can be adhered to long enough. To ensure success, weight loss diets must follow a set pattern that involves healthy eating, support, goals, exercise, and personalized advice.*

The term *diet* has negative connotations, especially if you've been overweight most of your life. Dieting is seen as a punishment for overeating, so we go on a diet with the mindset that we brought this all upon ourselves and don't deserve the right to feel good about what we are doing. There is nothing shameful about getting healthy! In fact, the word "diet" is so dreaded that most *diet* companies have changed their names and are loath to even utter the word. *Dieting* should be viewed as a *positive* step in the right direction, and "diet" should not be treated like a four-letter word. Regaining health is a highly rewarding endeavor. Who doesn't want to get off medication and be healthy? My goal is to take the mystery out of dieting and empower you to take control of your health. And it's quite possible you don't need to diet at all!

*Weight Loss Industry Insider Secret:* Want some proof that diets aren't to be trusted? Medicare and other insurance giants would benefit greatly if people could self-prevent obesity. Medicare pays nothing for diet programs. They know that most people will fail. Therefore, most insurance providers only pay for three obesity treatments (Zomosky, 2015): weight loss counseling, bariatric surgery, and FDA-approved weight loss drugs.

## Why We Diet

Many people don't consider dieting until they are well overweight, and often the first dieting attempts fail. Most people find a tipping point that causes them to start (or restart) a diet:

- Can't fit into clothes
- Changes in life-status (divorced, married, retired, etc.)
- Doctor's orders
- Harsh words from others
- As a requirement for surgery
- Low energy levels
- Unhappy with appearance
- Worried about health

These are all good reasons to lose weight, but weight loss diets are not right for every circumstance. Weight loss diets are a big deal; they're not to be taken lightly. I only recommend weight loss diets for people who are *quite* overweight (more on this in a bit).

## Three Kinds of Diets

- **Weight Loss Diets:** Weight loss diets are used by overweight people in an attempt to drop excess weight for health or vanity. Weight loss diets require a great deal of attention and effort to ensure success. Weight loss diets work by restricting food intake, but exercise is generally encouraged too. Weight loss diets are low in calories (hypocaloric) and should only be used for short periods of time, approximately 4–12 months. These diets are typically designed to create a loss of 1–3 pounds of weight per week. Weight loss diets also reduce inflammation, which can account for a portion of the weight that is lost. Heavy caloric restriction can lead to loss in lean body (muscle) mass when done to the extreme.

- **Maintenance Diets:** Maintenance diets are not "diets" in the traditional sense. They are used for weight stability, nourishment, and to fuel activity. Also known as "eating right" or "way of eating." There are many different maintenance diets. Many overweight people achieve meaningful weight loss by switching from the Western diet to a maintenance diet, forgoing a weight loss diet altogether. See Part 3 for detailed information on weight maintenance diets.

- **Special Diets:** Certain health conditions call for special diets. Often, these special diets result in weight loss and are adopted by weight loss or maintenance dieters in the (often wrongful) belief that the special diet would benefit them. Special diets are tailored to individual health needs and should only be used under direct supervision of a doctor. Examples of special diets are those used by people with celiac disease (gluten-free diets), allergies (e.g., dairy, egg, nut, soy, seafood), epilepsy (ketogenic diets), diabetes (sugar-free), or gut diseases (fiber-free, low residue, "FODMAP" diets).

Which is best? If you are not experiencing a rapid decline in health due to your weight, it's best to first try a maintenance diet that suits your eating habits and lifestyle. If your weight is affecting your health or you've become greatly overweight, it will be beneficial to use a weight loss diet. Special diets should only be used for verified health conditions.

## Three Methods of Weight Loss Dieting

- **Commercial Diet Programs:** Commercial diet programs are trademarked and rely on mass-marketing to attract clients. These programs either require upfront payment to learn the techniques of weight loss or entice you to buy products associated with the program. Many commercial programs supply prepared meals or meal-replacements (shakes, bars, etc.). Most commercial programs offer a range of support options. Completion rates for commercial diets are generally low (high dropout). Success rates can be quite high when the diet is followed (Lemstra, 2016). Some examples of commercial diet plans are WW™ (formerly Weight Watchers™), Atkins™, Jenny Craig™, and Nutrisystem™.

- **Self-Directed Diets:** The majority of dieters attempt to lose weight by devising their own plans. The strategies used are most often based on diets described in books, articles, ads, or by word-of-mouth. Numerous books, apps, and computer-based tools exist to aid in self-directed weight loss. Self-directed dieting is just as effective as using commercial programs if the same pattern is followed (Tang, 2014). For self-directed dieting, people commonly turn to paleo, low-carb, keto, or Mediterranean diets, among others.

- **Medically Supervised (Clinical) Diets:** Medical treatment of obesity is most typically done via weight loss surgery or drugs. Medically supervised weight loss diets generally rely on the use of low-calorie meal replacement formulas, behavior modification, and exercise counseling. These diets have a much better long-term success rate than commercial or self-directed diets (Krishnaswami, 2018).

Which is best? All three have their place. Medically supervised diets and treatments are generally seen as a last resort after other diets have failed. Commercial programs need to be carefully evaluated to see if they are compatible with the dieter's needs. Self-directed diets can be successful if crafted mindfully. No method guarantees success or easy adherence.

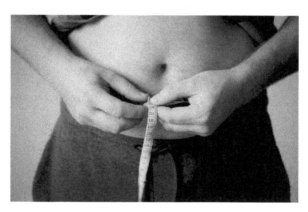

## Dieting for Vanity

There's absolutely nothing wrong with losing a couple pounds to look your best for times when you'll be on display. Family or class reunions, speaking engagements, job interviews, or first dates are times when your looks can be very important to you. If you normally eat well and exercise but your weight has crept up, it's easy to change your eating habits to drop 10–15 pounds. Nearly every women's magazine shows you how to do this with their "Lose 10 Pounds in

10 Days" cover stories. Unfortunately, these "crash diets" don't result in lasting weight loss, so you might be disappointed when the weight comes right back on.

## Bariatric Surgery

Weight loss surgery is the only treatment for obesity that results in substantial long-term weight loss (Albaugh, 2018). Most people who undergo this procedure maintain a 25% weight loss even after 20 years. It also improves or cures type 2 diabetes, cardiovascular risk factors, fatty liver disease, and muscle/bone pain (Willmer, 2018). However, bariatric surgery has risks and is only used for certain patients after attempts at dieting have failed (Willmer, 2018) (Albaugh, 2018). If your attempts at dieting have failed and your health suffers, talk to your doctor to see if bariatric surgery is right for you.

## Three Styles of Weight Loss Diets

Weight loss programs operate from one of three basic principles:

- **Low-Carbohydrate:** By restricting "carbs," people tend to eat less. Carb restriction is generally accomplished by limiting the weight (in grams) of carbs eaten. For example, 70g/day, or maintaining carbs below a percentage of total food intake (e.g., 20% of total calories). Low-carb diets are becoming increasingly popular for diabetics and for those with Metabolic Syndrome (Wylie-Rosett, 2013). Low-carb diets are sometimes referred to as "keto" or "high-protein" diets for advertising purposes.

- **Low-Fat:** By restricting fat, people tend to eat less. Fat restriction is accomplished similarly to low-carb diets, either by grams per day or as a percentage of total calories eaten. Low-fat diets have been preferred by doctors and nutritionists for many decades mainly due to the belief that dietary fat is stored as body fat and that low-fat diets protect against heart disease (Jéquier, 2002).

- **Balanced Eating:** Many weight loss methods do not track fat or carbs but instead focus on eating healthy food and restricting overall calories. Balanced plans will offer a selection of foods with higher fat or higher carb content but limited in portion size. Meal replacement drinks and shakes are typically designed to have a balance of fats and carbs. Balanced plans are based on the belief that there are both healthy carbs (e.g., whole grains, tubers) and healthy fats (e.g., olive oil, omega-3) (Koliaki, 2018). Balanced plans are generally easier to adhere to since no major food groups are eliminated.

Which is best? All three styles have shown good results (Hamdy, 2018). Focusing intently on limiting either carbs or fat can be self-defeating for many dieters, as the preoccupation with examining every bite is both cumbersome and difficult. Overweight people with metabolic syndrome or insulin problems may benefit from low-carb diets. People who do not have blood sugar issues typically respond better to low-fat diets or balanced eating (Hu, 2012). Balanced meals are easier to prepare, and focus is placed on food quality rather than microscopic details of food chemistry.

## Cheat Days

Many diet plans and programs incorporate "cheat days." There is evidence that suggests the lowering of metabolism during weight loss may be reversed a bit by periodically overeating during the diet (Trexler, 2014). This is most often accomplished by including one day per week where you can eat excess calories, most often in the form of simple carbs (e.g., sugar, bread, cereal) (Jenkins, 1997) (Dirlewanger, 2000). A well-planned cheat day would be one where you go slightly above your normal diet-level of calories by eating some whole grain bread, rice, or potatoes. For instance, if you've been keeping calories at 1,800/day, once a week eat an additional 500–750 calories of carb-rich cheat food. The cheat food needs to be as high-quality as possible. Cheat days in diets date back to at least the '70s and are affectionately known as "piggy days," "refuel days," or "free days." Many people like to use these cheat days as an excuse to eat junk foods like greasy pizza, sugary ice cream, or other addictive treats. If that's what works for you, go for it. But those are the foods that got you here in the first place. Maybe it's time to wean off the Big Food teat?

## Components of a Good Weight Loss Diet

Not all diets are created equal. A diet that works perfectly for one might feel like torture to another. The National Weight Control Registry tracks thousands of people who've lost weight. Some common themes emerge when you ask these people how they lost their initial weight. Good weight loss diet plans provide (Bond, 2009):

- Food variety
- Social support
- Personalized advice
- Realistic goals

If you ask researchers who study weight loss, they will add some other important factors of a good diet (Vakil, 2017):

- Must be hypocaloric (low in calories); 1,300–1,800 calories per day for most females and 1,500–2,000 calories for most men
- Must include high-quality food; must be adequate protein, low in added sugars, and low in ultra-processed foods, with a high intake of fiber from fruit, vegetables, and whole-grain products

- Weight loss rate should be 1–3 pounds per week, 6–10 pounds per month
- Hypocaloric diets should last no more than 6–12 months
- Must also include aerobic exercise and strength training

And a couple requirements of my own:

- Must be affordable
- Must not use meal replacement shakes or bars; only real food allowed
- Must not rely on supplements or other special products

> In general, scientific evidence about what constitutes a healthy [weight loss] diet is both consistent and straightforward: a healthy diet is a varied diet rich in fruits, vegetables, whole-grain products and high-quality proteins and poor in added sugar, refined grains, and highly-processed foods. Most importantly, the best [weight loss] diet is a diet that people can comply with for a long period of time without significant weight regain, so whatever facilitates this effort is greatly appreciable (Koliaki, 2018).

Diet marketers will try hard to set their diet apart from the others by making fantastical claims, but there are simply no tricks to weight loss other than the aforementioned basic diets, which all rely on cutting calories to elicit fat loss. What makes diets successful is how well followers can adhere to the diet.

## The Downside of Dieting

### Loss of Muscle/Lean Body Mass

Weight loss diets are a drastic measure, hard on the body and mind, and must be done with great care. Restricting calories is the only way to mobilize and remove fat tissue without using surgery, liposuction, or freezing techniques (Ingargiola, 2015). Unfortunately, restricting calories not only removes fat, but also breaks down muscle, heart, liver, and kidney tissues as well as causing hormonal disturbances (Weiss, 2017) (Heymsfield, 2014). Calorie restriction also causes bone loss and a reduction in heart size (Weiss, 2017). These effects may be lessened to a large degree by ensuring adequate protein intake and implementing a cardio and strength-training program along with the calorie restriction (Calbet, 2017) (Weiss, 2017) (Heymsfield, 2014).

## Slowed Metabolism

During calorie restriction, your body wants to conserve energy. To do so, it will try to maximize the food you eat by slowing your metabolism. The more you restrict and the longer you diet, the more your metabolism will slow (Johannsen, 2012). This slowing is not well understood, even by the most brilliant scientists (Smith, 2018). Diet gurus will promise *their* diet keeps the metabolism "boosted," but this is mostly hype. If it were that easy, Big Pharma would already have a drug for it. The truth is, there are so many intertwined metabolic systems at play that no one has figured out how to solve this problem, from hormones to cells, there are problems along every step of the way when humans ingest fewer calories than required. Lowered metabolic rate is a problem with any type of weight loss that restricts calories and reduces bodyweight (e.g., bariatric surgery, fasting, dieting) (Smith, 2018).

To maintain a faster metabolism and prevent the loss of lean body mass, diets should emphasize these factors (Sutherland, 2005):

- Not cutting calories too far
- Eating a balanced, whole-food diet with adequate protein
- Exercise
- Sleep

- Stress reduction
- Incorporating "cheat" days

## The Dreaded Plateau

A weight loss plateau is a stall in weight loss. This usually occurs after about 3–6 months of steady weight loss and can be quite frustrating to dieters. Weight loss forums are inundated with requests for help in "breaking a stall." There are two schools of thought on what causes this plateau effect (Thomas, 2014):

1. Metabolic changes prevent further weight loss at the present calorie level
2. Not accurately tracking calories/poor diet adherence

Both ideas hold weight. In strictly controlled clinical diets there are often plateaus that must be dealt with by reducing calories. In the real world, dieters often start to get lax in their eating after several months and "slip up" in tracking calories. This makes breaking a stall much more difficult because now there are two problems (Thomas, 2014). The appetite is a formidable foe and hard to ignore for long (Hall, 2018). The estimated calorie counts for weight loss are always based on bodyweight. After several months of losing weight, the calories needed for continued weight loss must be reduced (Hall, 2018).

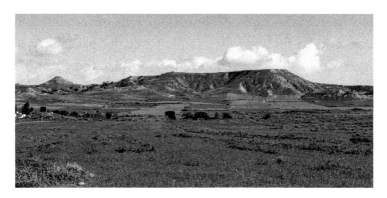

Most likely, plateaus are caused by a combination of both lowered metabolism and not adhering well to the diet plan. To effectively break a stall, one must carefully assess their calorie needs based on bodyweight and activity levels AND accurately track calories for the remainder of the diet, reducing calories as weight drops (Hall, 2018) (Thomas, 2014).

Plateaus are a fact of life for dieters. The savvy dieter will see the plateau as a way marker for change. Unfortunately, many dieters are mentally unprepared, and the stall leads to the end of dieting and weight regain ensues (Chaput, 2007). Weight loss diets need to be continually reassessed to ensure the downward trajectory of weight loss. Eventually, all diets should end in a plateau that signifies the desired weight has been reached.

## When to Give Up on Dieting

For some people, it's just not meant to be. There are thousands upon thousands of overweight and obese people who've tried everything and cannot lose weight no matter what. Beyond eating "right," exercising, sleeping well, de-stressing, and treating medical conditions that may cause weight gain, there's not a whole lot left to try. But before you give up completely, read through the rest of my book and give it some thought. Then have a long talk with your doctor and see what needs to be done. If you are obese and gaining, and your health is in rapid decline, then your physical and mental health depend on finding relief. Do not rule out psychiatry, weight loss surgery, or FDA-approved weight loss drugs. There is more than one way to skin a cat.

## Conclusion

Weight loss diets should only be used when necessary. Otherwise, just start eating right. Many people find that they can lose weight when they move from the Western diet to a diet that contains ample nutrition from fruit, vegetables, fiber, and whole grains. Research shows that just about any diet will work for weight loss if it can be followed for 6–12 months. Dieters find equal success with both commercial programs and self-directed weight loss diets. Medically supervised weight loss is usually a last resort to prepare a patient for surgery or to prevent serious medical conditions requiring weight loss. Successful weight loss programs should follow a pattern that includes a variety of nutritious, hypocaloric menus; support systems; obtainable time and weight goals; exercise; and a plan for transitioning from weight loss to weight maintenance. Calorie restriction is very hard on the human body. Lean body mass (muscle and other tissue) will be reduced, and metabolism will be altered. Exercising and ensuring adequate protein intake are two of several proven ways to combat these effects. Read on to learn more about dieting and how to find a plan that will work for you.

# CHAPTER 11

# DIET RIGHT

**TL;DR:** *Don't take dieting lightly!*
*Don't diet unless you absolutely must.*

The medical community has devised weight loss diets for hundreds of years. In a clinical setting, weight loss is easy. Just restrict calories until an overweight person depletes their body fat stores (See Appendix: The Minnesota Starvation Experiment). Most clinicians have given up on this treatment for obesity because it's too hard to do. It's easier to perform bariatric surgery than to cloister a person in a treatment facility for months on end monitoring every morsel they eat. Forced caloric restriction is one of the cruelest medical treatments ever devised. Doctors of the past have reported having to *whip* patients into compliance!

*Weight Loss Industry Insider Secret: Statisticians examined the medical records of over 175,000 dieting obese and morbidly obese people. They worked out the probability of attaining a normal weight over a nine-year dieting history (Fildes, 2015):*

- *Chances of an obese person (BMI 30–35) dieting to a normal weight: 1 in 215*
- *Chances of a morbidly obese person (BMI 40–45) dieting to a normal weight: 1 in 1,000*
- *Chances of an obese person losing 5% of their bodyweight over nine years: 1 in 7*

Weight loss is an important step in regaining health. Experts agree that ridding the body of inflammatory fat is the first step in a long process for returning to a normal weight (Botchlett, 2017). But it's nearly impossible to go from obese to a healthy weight on your own.

## The Intensive Weight Loss Intervention Model

Through many decades of trial and error, weight loss researchers devised a commonly accepted medical approach to weight loss known as *the intensive weight loss intervention* (Hollis, 2008). It works like this:

- Provide a tailored approach based on each person's goals, starting point, and current health.
- Provide education in nutrition, physical activity, problem solving, and goal setting.
- Develop a menu based on the patient's preferred eating style.
- Reduce portion sizes to limit calorie intake to an appropriate number for age, sex, and activity levels.
- Eliminate ultra-processed foods.
- Increase consumption of minimally processed food, especially fruit, vegetables, and whole grains.
- Limit alcohol consumption.
- Keep accurate logs of food intake, bodyweight, and physical activity.
- Provide group interaction with like-minded dieters.
- Provide social support.

This style of dieting is used when patients need to lose considerable weight prior to surgery or for other health reasons where rapid initial weight loss is required. It works extremely well (Espeland, 2013). Weight loss interventions like this are designed to cause a loss of 5–10 pounds per month and to be used for periods of 6–12 months. Intensive weight loss interventions are stopped when the patient has lost the desired number of pounds or when it's demonstrated that the patient is not responding as expected.

This is also how *successful* commercial programs work. It's not a "cookie cutter" approach but is centered completely around the person in need of losing weight. If any of these elements are missing, the likelihood of failing increases dramatically (Brantley, 2008).

## Clinical versus Commercial versus Self-Directed Approaches to Dieting

The difference between a medically supervised *clinical* approach to weight loss and a *commercial* approach is that the trademarked diet programs want to keep you around long after the weight is gone, and they don't want you to leave, even if you are not losing weight. Clinical weight loss has an end point; once the weight has been reduced sufficiently, you are moved to another treatment center for further evaluation.

Commercial diet programs don't want to lose you. Their business model relies on having customers that are "addicted" to the diet and continue buying branded meals, supplements, and merchandise as well as paying membership fees. A savvy dieter needs to know when to stop a commercial plan (and whether to even start in the first place).

The goal of self-directed diets is the same as the clinical approach: to lose weight and move on to a maintenance diet. When self-directed dieters use the methods of a commercial plan, they find they cannot easily get away. Self-directed dieters need to take a clinical approach rather than a commercial approach. This means only dieting when medically necessary and establishing a firm end point.

## Unnecessary Dieting

Many normal-weight people start diet programs (mainly for vanity reasons), but they don't need to. Many overweight people think they can use "one weird trick" or tweak their eating just a bit to lose weight. If you are healthy and just a few pounds overweight, simply changing your eating style to avoid ultra-processed food and improving gut health is enough. Combine that with exercise, better sleep, and all the rest we've talked about and you won't ever need to go on a diet. But if your weight is causing health problems, you should go *all in* on a *real* diet. Simple tricks are not enough.

*Medical Industry Insider Secret:* There are two types of fat; subcutaneous and visceral. Subcutaneous fat is found under the skin and does not present much of a problem. Visceral fat forms around organs such as the kidneys, intestines, liver, and pancreas. Subcutaneous fat is relatively harmless. Visceral fat is highly active and secretes chemicals that make one prone to diabetes, fatty liver disease, high blood pressure, high cholesterol, and more (Wajchenberg, 2000).

Dieting is a drastic step that should only be undertaken by people who truly need to lose weight for health reasons. How do you know if dieting is for you? The big diet companies want *everyone* to be on a diet. But dieting is hard on a body and can lead to some long-term health issues if done incorrectly (Lowe, 2004). Only diet if absolutely necessary. An easy way to determine if you *need* to diet is to use the BMI chart, waist measurement, and some key health markers.

## BMI

The Body Mass Index (BMI) is used by doctors, researchers, insurance providers, and pharmaceutical companies to quickly determine if a person is in a healthy weight range. BMI is also used to differentiate between underweight, normal, overweight, and obese classifications.

There is just one BMI chart, used by men and women alike. At first glance, it seems ludicrous to have just one standard when there are so many variables to consider. For instance, the BMI chart will indicate that some elite athletes are obese even though they have very little body fat. The BMI chart was made with the entire global population in mind, so it misses outliers. However, when researchers tracked over 60,000 people for 15 years, they found that BMI was a better predictor for heart disease and weight-related health concerns than directly measuring body fat (Ortega, 2016).

The ranges within the BMI scale are fairly accurate for determining a healthy weight for most people. Simply line up your height with your weight and voilà, there's your BMI.

| BMI | Healthy Weight | | | | | | Overweight | | | | | Obese | | | | | |
|---|---|---|---|---|---|---|---|---|---|---|---|---|---|---|---|---|---|
| | 19 | 20 | 21 | 22 | 23 | 24 | 25 | 26 | 27 | 28 | 29 | 30 | 31 | 32 | 33 | 34 | 35 |
| Height | Weight (in pounds) | | | | | | | | | | | | | | | | |
| 4'10" | 91 | 96 | 100 | 105 | 110 | 115 | 119 | 124 | 129 | 134 | 138 | 143 | 148 | 153 | 158 | 162 | 167 |
| 4'11" | 94 | 99 | 104 | 109 | 114 | 119 | 124 | 128 | 133 | 138 | 143 | 148 | 153 | 158 | 163 | 168 | 173 |
| 5'0" | 97 | 102 | 107 | 112 | 118 | 123 | 128 | 133 | 138 | 143 | 148 | 153 | 158 | 163 | 168 | 174 | 179 |
| 5'1" | 100 | 106 | 111 | 116 | 122 | 127 | 132 | 137 | 143 | 148 | 153 | 158 | 164 | 169 | 174 | 180 | 185 |
| 5'2" | 104 | 109 | 115 | 120 | 126 | 131 | 136 | 142 | 147 | 153 | 158 | 164 | 169 | 175 | 180 | 186 | 191 |
| 5'3" | 107 | 113 | 118 | 124 | 130 | 135 | 141 | 146 | 152 | 158 | 163 | 169 | 175 | 180 | 186 | 191 | 197 |
| 5'4" | 110 | 116 | 122 | 128 | 134 | 140 | 145 | 151 | 157 | 163 | 169 | 174 | 180 | 186 | 192 | 197 | 204 |
| 5'5" | 114 | 120 | 126 | 132 | 138 | 144 | 150 | 156 | 162 | 168 | 174 | 180 | 186 | 192 | 198 | 204 | 210 |
| 5'6" | 118 | 124 | 130 | 136 | 142 | 148 | 155 | 161 | 167 | 173 | 179 | 186 | 192 | 198 | 204 | 210 | 216 |
| 5'7" | 121 | 127 | 134 | 140 | 146 | 153 | 159 | 166 | 172 | 178 | 185 | 191 | 198 | 204 | 211 | 217 | 223 |
| 5'8" | 125 | 131 | 138 | 144 | 151 | 158 | 164 | 171 | 177 | 184 | 190 | 197 | 203 | 210 | 216 | 223 | 230 |
| 5'9" | 128 | 135 | 142 | 149 | 155 | 162 | 169 | 176 | 182 | 189 | 196 | 203 | 209 | 216 | 223 | 230 | 236 |
| 5'10" | 132 | 139 | 146 | 153 | 160 | 167 | 174 | 181 | 188 | 195 | 202 | 209 | 216 | 222 | 229 | 236 | 243 |
| 5'11" | 136 | 143 | 150 | 157 | 165 | 172 | 179 | 186 | 193 | 200 | 208 | 215 | 222 | 229 | 236 | 243 | 250 |
| 6'0" | 140 | 147 | 154 | 162 | 169 | 177 | 184 | 191 | 199 | 206 | 213 | 221 | 228 | 235 | 242 | 250 | 256 |
| 6'1" | 144 | 151 | 159 | 166 | 174 | 182 | 189 | 197 | 294 | 212 | 219 | 227 | 235 | 242 | 250 | 257 | 265 |
| 6'2" | 148 | 155 | 163 | 171 | 179 | 186 | 194 | 202 | 210 | 218 | 225 | 233 | 241 | 249 | 256 | 264 | 272 |
| 6'3" | 152 | 160 | 168 | 176 | 184 | 192 | 200 | 208 | 216 | 224 | 232 | 240 | 248 | 256 | 264 | 272 | 279 |
| 6'4" | 156 | 164 | 172 | 180 | 189 | 197 | 205 | 213 | 221 | 230 | 238 | 246 | 254 | 263 | 271 | 279 | 287 |

*National Institutes of Health, 2018*

## Waist Measurement

Waist circumference is also a good predictor of overall health, especially when combined with BMI (Højgaard, 2008). The National Institutes of Health recommend people should first assess their BMI and then waist measurement. If your BMI shows you are overweight, and your waist is greater than 35" (for women) or 40" (for men), you should "take action." I think this is very good advice. As you get into the "overweight" zone, it's time to start working on the quality of your diet, eat right, and examine your lifestyle and exercise habits (Upadhyay, 2017). If you're in or nearing the "obese zone," with a too-large waist, you most likely will need to use a weight loss diet.

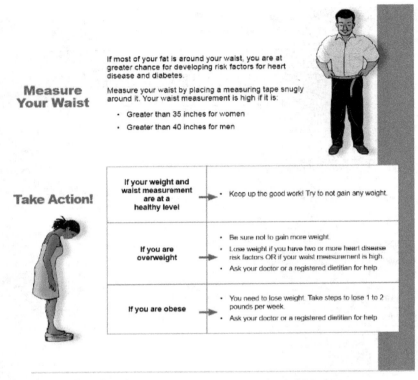

**Measure Your Waist**

If most of your fat is around your waist, you are at greater chance for developing risk factors for heart disease and diabetes.

Measure your waist by placing a measuring tape snugly around it. Your waist measurement is high if it is:

- Greater than 35 inches for women
- Greater than 40 inches for men

**Take Action!**

| | |
|---|---|
| If your weight and waist measurement are at a healthy level | • Keep up the good work! Try to not gain any weight. |
| If you are overweight | • Be sure not to gain more weight.<br>• Lose weight if you have two or more heart disease risk factors OR if your waist measurement is high.<br>• Ask your doctor or a registered dietitian for help. |
| If you are obese | • You need to lose weight. Take steps to lose 1 to 2 pounds per week.<br>• Ask your doctor or a registered dietitian for help. |

*Adapted from National Institutes of Health, 2018*

The waist measurements criteria ignore your height, build, and age. The prevailing theory is that when any man or woman gets a waist bigger than recommended (i.e., 40" or 35", respectively), it indicates the person is accumulating fat around their organs. This so-called abdominal (or visceral) fat is the deadliest type of fat, as it interferes with how your organs function. Back in the old days, we were simply told that you should only be able to "pinch an inch" of fat around your waistline. This advice was wrong because it only considered fat that was under the skin and not the fat on your liver, kidneys, and intestines.

## Blood Tests

While you can get a good idea of your general health and weight by looking up your BMI number and measuring your waist, your doctor has some other tools to really dial this all in. The regular set of blood tests drawn during routine checkups can tell you a lot about the effectiveness of your diet and exercise program and your overall health.

Your doctor should be tracking your cholesterol levels, triglycerides, blood pressure, and fasting glucose, among others. If some or all of these are out of range, and you are overweight with a waist circumference that's over the limit, you qualify as a person who needs to be on a weight loss diet (Chadid et al., 2018). If you are at a normal weight, but you have bad blood test results, you should look first at your diet and exercise routine. Your doctor should attempt to rule out any medical or genetic condition that might be the root problem.

## A Sane Approach to Dieting

Weight loss diets should only be used as a last resort. First, try to switch to a healthy maintenance diet and consider other lifestyle modification (exercise, sleep, stress, etc.). Valid medical concerns aside, don't even consider a weight loss diet unless you have a BMI over 27 or your waist circumference is over 35" (women) or 40" (men). If you have a BMI of 26 or less, and a waist measurement under 35"/40", then skip weight loss dieting and go straight to a maintenance diet. Weight loss diets are drastic and time consuming. Maintenance diets are mostly just about eating right and exercising.

Once you've determined you need to go on a diet, these steps will help you to successfully lose weight:

- Set reasonable goals: pounds to lose, time frame, etc. Know that 5–10 pounds per month is reasonable; 20–30 pounds in a month is not. Dieting for longer than 12 months is not rec-ommended; 4–12 months is best.

- Decide on a diet plan/type/method to use. Have a backup plan in mind.
- Fully immerse yourself in the diet plan you decide on. Join the online forums, and introduce yourself. Read all you can about the diet strategies used.
- Develop an exercise program appropriate for your physical fitness level.

If you do this right, you'll be able to get to a healthy weight in well under a year. It will be a wild emotional rollercoaster ride, and your entire life may change. People will look at you differently. People will talk about you. Your doctor will be *so* proud.

## Effectiveness versus Efficacy

*Diet Industry Insider Secret: Commercial diet programs are not subject to any type of regulatory oversight. For perspective, Big Pharma must put new drugs and medical therapies to rigorous testing before the Food and Drug Administration will approve them for humans. Two such tests are known as efficacy and effectiveness.*

*Efficacy* refers to how well a drug or therapy works in a clinical setting. For instance, if a new cancer drug cures 98% of the patients who take the drug, it gets high efficacy scores. If the drug only cures 10% of patients, it would score low in efficacy.

*Effectiveness* refers to how well a drug works in a real-world setting. For instance, if the cancer drug that cured 98% of cancer patients costs over $1 million per day, no one could afford it, and it would not be an effective therapy. But if the drug was cheap and had very few side effects, it would be very effective.

If diet plans had to undergo this same scrutiny, most diets would pass the efficacy standards but fail on effectiveness. Humans can lose 1–2 pounds *a day* by fasting for extended periods (high efficacy), but fasting is not enjoyable and leads to bingeing, preoccupation with food, and nutrient deficiencies, so most people will not do extended fasts for weight loss (low effectiveness). Ketogenic diets change the way our bodies metabolize fat and have been shown to lead to weight loss (high efficacy), but ketogenic diets also ban major groups of food people love to eat, and cause bad breath, so hardly anyone will stick to this diet for long (low effectiveness).

## 3,500 calories equal 1 pound of fat

A doctor once told me in all seriousness that if I could just cut out 10 calories per day, I'd lose a pound a year. With an excited grin, he then said that if I cut out 100 calories a day, I'd lose 10 pounds a year. He used M&Ms as an example. "Just one M&M," he said, "could be the difference between gaining and losing weight!"

I said, "No way it can be that easy, Doc!" And it's not. Don't fall for this old wives' tale. This line of reasoning comes from the fact that one pound of lard, butter, oil, or human body fat contains exactly 3,500 calories. Further reduced, if you eat 3,500 calories extra, it will all turn to fat, causing exactly 1 pound of weight gain.

Mammalian metabolism doesn't work this neatly. When we change our eating habits, there are numerous metabolic feedback circuits that will influence how we burn, store, or replace the nutrients in question. Hormones deliver powerful messages to increase appetite and decrease satiety. *Increasing* food intake might actually cause weight *loss* if it affects basal metabolism. *Reducing* food intake might cause paradoxical weight *gain* through similar actions (Hall, 2018).

The only way to use calories as a weight loss tool is to determine how many calories you are currently eating and then reduce that amount by several hundred until your weight starts to drop. This requires careful monitoring and meticulous tracking of everything you eat. It's physically impossible to accurately guess how many calories you eat in a day. Luckily there are apps for that.

## Counting Calories

I know I'm going to be chastised for using calories as a weight loss tool, but I am firmly convinced this is the best way to lose weight. One could try eating in a way that leads to weight loss without counting calories as some popular diets promote, but from my experience, I've not seen much success come from diets that allow unlimited eating without some type of caloric control.

Let's look at this from another angle. You should be able to go to bed and wake up on your own about 7–8 hours later. Your body naturally regulates your sleep, much as it should regulate your weight. But how successful would you be in life if you refused to look at a clock or set an alarm? Not very. Modern-day humans cannot be trusted to eat freely. They will almost always overeat. The only way to accurately limit how much you eat is to track your calories (read more on calorie counting in Chapter 10). This is an extremely effective weight loss tool. But for the long-run, after you've lost weight it's best to just learn to eat in moderation and not worry so much about the calorie content of every meal.

## Conclusion

Weight loss diets are not to be taken lightly. If you don't need to diet, don't. If you are unsure, talk to your doctor. Perhaps you just need to work on your normal eating and exercise or focus on some lifestyle factors like sleep, stress, or drinking. Maybe your medications are making you gain weight. Once you've decided to go on a weight loss diet, you need to *fully commit* yourself to success. You should immerse yourself in the new diet and do everything it takes to stick to it. Take full advantage of any support or personalized plans offered. If you pay for a membership, pay for the best plan you can afford. Look at this as a short-term, high-return investment. The goal of a weight loss diet needs to be *losing weight*. If you don't see results that meet your expectations, find a different diet. Don't let anyone talk you into sticking with a plan that's not working.

# CHAPTER 12

# COMMERCIAL WEIGHT LOSS PROGRAMS

**TL;DR:** *There are many commercial diet plans. For best results do some research; then pick a plan that suits your lifestyle and eating habits. Don't get stuck on a program that doesn't produce results. Stay away from diets that insist you eat ready-made food. Three good commercial plans are Atkins, Weight Watchers, and Slimming World.*

## Hallmarks of the Modern Commercial Weight Loss Diet

Diet marketers have created a strange reality: they want everyone to be on a diet, even though they know their diet will only work for a fraction of the people who try it. They also know that many of the people who start a diet don't need to be on a diet at all. Most people know very little about how dieting or the diet industry works. If more people knew how ineffective dieting really was, the diet industry would disappear. There are thousands of diet books and dozens of branded, trademarked diets. These diets aren't approved by regulatory agencies, and only in very rare cases are diet marketers held to any standards or liability.

*Weight Loss Industry Insider Secret: The Kimkin Diet promoted a very low-carb, low-calorie plan. The Kimkin's website was filled with fraudulent claims and made-up testimonials. A class action lawsuit for fraud and unjust enrichment was filed. The courts ruled in favor of the plaintiffs, and the owner* *was ordered to pay over $2 million in restitution. Had this class action lawsuit not been filed, Kimkin would still be operating today.*

## Marketing

Commercial diets are heavily marketed affairs. Diet ads feature thin, happy-looking people who have presumably lost weight using the plan. Celebrity spokespeople are used by the bigger diet companies: Oprah Winfrey, Kirstie Alley, Marie Osmond, Valerie Bertinelli, Queen Latifah, and others have graced the airwaves, extolling the virtues of one diet or another, oftentimes with a spectacular failure or two. Weight Watchers, Jenny Craig, and Nutrisystem are the top three spenders for TV weight loss commercials; together they spend over $50 million dollars a year.

Most commercial plans have started to move away from the word "diet," instead focusing on the wellness or healthfulness that their weight loss plan brings. But let's not fool ourselves. They are *diets*. Period.

## Branding

Most commercial diet programs have their own lines of diet products such as ready-to-eat meals, bars, shakes, snacks, clothing, and merchandise. According to MarketResearch.com, the weight loss industry is valued at over $60 billion. Weight Watchers is the leader, raking in profits of over $300 million a year. The names of these diets are household words. Who hasn't heard of Weight Watchers (now WW™), Jenny Craig, or Atkins? It's a numbers game for the diet industry—the more people they can lure to their websites, the more money they make. The modern diet is filled with ever-changing buzzwords. "Low-fat" was replaced by "low-carb," which has been replaced by "keto."

## Books

Most commercial weight loss programs have a large library of cookbooks, updated methods, challenges, or "reset" programs. There are also thousands of standalone diet books that are not associated with a commercial weight loss plan. Be careful when reading diet books; many are based on faulty research or fringe methods of weight loss. Buyer beware when embarking on a diet written by an unknown author. Many diet books are written to describe the latest fad in dieting.

## Fad Diets

Fad diets are those that are widely shared and enjoy intense, though often short-lived, enthusiasm. Fad diets aren't necessarily unhealthy; paleo, low-carb, and other widely accepted diets started as fads.

A consistent hallmark of modern dieting is the use of viral marketing to promote the latest trends. The latest fad diet is the keto diet. "Keto" is short for ketosis or ketogenic, a diet that's been used to treat epilepsy since the 1920s (Paoli, 2013). Modern keto diets are just a rebranding of the low-carb diet fad popularized in the 1980s. Fad diets often promise effortless weight loss based on pseudoscience. People who embrace fad diets are called "faddists," and they will defend their diet tooth and nail, so be careful when approaching them on forums or in real life.

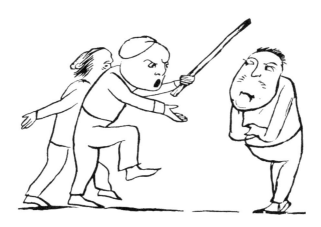

## Commercial Diets Get Results

I know what you're thinking: "You've been saying 95% fail! Why bother?" Yes, most diets do fail, but only at *long-term* weight maintenance. In the short-term, weight loss diets can do exactly as they are designed to do.

While trying to determine the best commercial diets for weight loss, clinicians conduct experiments to see which diets work best. Guess what they find time after time? Most weight loss diets work (Bray, 2012). The only thing that sets one diet apart from the others is how well people can *adhere* to the diet. Diet marketers have been debating the merits of low-carb versus low-fat or other aspects peculiar to one diet over another since the first diet book was written. This is all for show. The diet that will work best is the diet that you can stick to for 4–12 months.

The hardest part about dieting is wading through countless diet websites and picking a good one. Most diet plans boast a near 100% success rate in losing significant amounts of weight over a 4–12-month period, but only if you count the people who *do* the diet as intended. For every successful dieter, there are 80–90 people who started a diet but couldn't complete it.

Commercial diet programs are good for people who need structure in their lives. Also, people who've tried dieting on their own often turn to a commercial program after failing to lose weight.

## The Plans

There were approximately 15 trademarked/branded diet programs in operation at the time of writing this book. Some non-trademarked diets appear to be commercial programs, but upon closer examination they are just diet books or websites disguised as commercial programs. There are also meal-delivery services that look like weight loss programs but are not.

*Note: I have not received any compensation from any of these diet companies!*

| Brand Name | Where Found; Costs | Style |
|---|---|---|
| **Low-Carb** | | |
| Atkins | Website; free | Low-carb |
| Dukan | Website; $29.95/mo | Low-carb |
| Ideal Protein | Website; $450/week | Low-carb/Meal replacements |
| South Beach | Website; $300–400/mo | Low-carb |
| **Low-calorie, balanced and/or low-fat meals** | | |
| Beachbody | Website; $99+/mo | Low-calorie + supplements |
| Mayo Clinic Diet | Website; $25/mo | Low-calorie |
| Nutritarian | Website; $49.95/mo | Low-calorie /Vegan |
| Slimming World | Website; $10/mo | Low-calorie |
| Weight Watchers | Website; $20–$50/mo | Low-calorie |

| Brand Name | Where Found; Costs | Style |
|---|---|---|
| **Prepared/Delivered Meals** | | |
| Jenny Craig | Website; $19.95/mo, $99 Enrollment | Low-fat |
| Fast Mimicking Diet | Website; $225/week | Low-calorie |
| HMR Program | Website; ~$100/week | Low-fat |
| Medifast | Website; $400+ monthly | Low-calorie |
| Nutrisystem | Website; $300–$400/mo | Low-calorie |
| Slim Fast | Website; Various costs | Meal replacement shakes |

## My Top Three

If you are looking for a commercial weight loss program, you should narrow your search to these three:

| Plan | Style | Cost | Free Trial | Free Stuff | Easy Access | Active Forums | Personal Plans | Staff Available |
|---|---|---|---|---|---|---|---|---|
| Atkins | Low-carb | Free | n/a | Yes | Yes | Yes | No | Yes |
| Weight Watchers | Balanced | $20–$50/mo | Yes | Yes | Yes | Yes | Yes | Yes |
| Slimming World, US | Balanced | $10/mo | Yes | Yes | Yes | Yes | Yes | Yes |

## Runners Up

There were several programs that might be worthy but didn't make my cut:

- Mayo Clinic Diet
- Nutritarian
- Dukan

Try these if you like, but I cannot vouch for how they will work. The Mayo Clinic Diet requires up-front payment to see what the plan entails. Nutritarian's website was extremely hard to navigate. The Dukan diet seemed too good to be true, and their claims rely on pseudoscience. It's very possible one of these might work for you. And there may be more; the diet industry is a morass of poorly designed websites, clickbait, and Error 404s. Stick with my top three picks if you want to remove weeks of stress from your life spent searching for a plan.

### Definitely Out

While weight loss might be possible, I recommend against the following plans due to their extensive use of ultra-processed food, supplements, and meal replacement shakes/bars:

- Beachbody
- Fast Mimicking Diet
- HMR
- Ideal Protein
- Jenny Craig
- Medifast
- Nutrisystem
- Slim Fast
- South Beach

Diet plans that feature prepared/delivered meals or push supplements should raise a red flag for health-conscious people. If you are dead set on trying one of these, feel free, but don't say I didn't warn you.

Look at reviews and nutritional data of the plans first. To me, these look worse than just eating at McDonald's. The Western diet is what gets most of us into trouble in the first place, eating the same diet with reduced serving sizes is not going to end well for long term weight stability, even if you manage to lose a few pounds quickly. There are much better ways to lose weight than with these ultra-processed, ultra-hyped plans.

## Getting Started

If you'd like to use one of my recommended programs (or any diet program, for that matter), it's easy to get started:

1. Visit the website and peruse the free information available to see if the plan looks like a match for your personality and lifestyle.
2. Decide on a program.
3. Sign up and get a free trial plan or pay for one month.
4. Get serious about doing the program as designed. Join the forums, download the apps, start tracking everything you can.

If you like structure, you'll love the three programs I recommended.

## Forum Survival Guide

During my weight loss journey, I used diet forums extensively. The weight loss forums that I once used (e.g., Low Carb Friends, Mark's Daily Apple, and The Cave) have all disappeared over the past four or five years. Facebook groups are now the standard setting to discuss diets and dieting, but most commercial weight loss programs still offer forums on their website.

Online forums are a great way to get the most out of a diet. You'll interact with others following a similar path as you. Be forewarned, though, forum "regulars" will eat you alive if you break protocol. To make navigating forums easier, here are some tips from a forum pro:

- Use your real name when registering. First name/last initial is fine. Silly aliases will not be taken seriously. If you can assign a picture, choose one where you look happy. Don't be creepy. Cats or flowers are also acceptable. Celebrity faces or muscular body pics are weird.
- Before you make your first post, spend several sessions looking through the posts to get a feel for acceptable behavior.
- Read the forum rules.
- Learn to use the search function. Look for answers to your question before asking, chances are people have already asked the same question many times. Forum regulars get testy when the same question is asked over and over by new members.
- Your first post should be an introduction; there will always be a forum section dedicated to new member introductions.
- Be polite, and don't engage with impolite people.
- DON'T TYPE IN ALL CAPS. This is considered yelling.
- If you make a long post, use paragraphs and proper punctuation; otherwise, no one will read.
- Learn the difference between "lose" and "loose." Never, ever ask "Why aren't I *loosing* weight?" You'll be branded a noob forever if you use *loose* in place of *lose*.
- Learn the acronyms. Ask if you don't know what is being said. Some common acronyms:
  - DH is "dear husband," DW is "dear wife," SO is "significant other"
  - AFAIK means "as far as I know"
  - TL;DR means "too long; didn't read"
  - IMHO means "in my humble opinion"
  - SMH means "shaking my head"
- Don't make unhelpful replies unless you're directly involved in a conversation. It's not helpful to add a reply such as, "I'd like to know, too." Or, "Try Google." Lots of people get email

notifications of new comments, and this type of comment is VERY ANNOYING.

- If you start a thread, check for replies. It's rude to leave people hanging.
- Have fun with it.

## Conclusion

Dieting is a seller's market. With nearly three-fourths of the world overweight or obese, it's child's play to attract new customers. Smart marketers are always looking for new buzzwords that will generate more clicks and hits, and in turn, more money. The latest fad diet is "keto," a rebranding of the low-carb diets of the 1980s. The diet industry relies on attracting new customers and keeping old customers by using all the tricks of mass marketing. Don't join a program on impulse or because you like the spokesman; research and talk to others before paying. Commercial programs like Atkins, WW, or Slimming World are well-structured yet provide flexibility. If you use a commercial diet program, get your money's worth by taking advantage of all the perks, free apps, forums, and personalized support provided. If the program is not working, don't stick with it for long—find a different diet.

# CHAPTER 13

# ATKINS

> **TL;DR:** Atkins is a time-tested low-carb program. The original keto diet.

## Portal

You can access information about the Atkins diet at www.atkins.com.

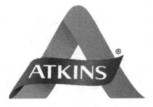

## The Promise

*"This is Today's Atkins™ It's not just a diet ... it's life well lived."*

## Background

In 1963, Dr. Robert C. Atkins, MD, was concerned that his fellow medical doctors were doing more harm than good by prescribing appetite suppressants and amphetamines for weight loss. Atkins came to believe that instead of restricting calories by treating hunger, overweight people could simply restrict the carbs they were eating to achieve desired weight loss.

In 1972, Dr. Atkins released his first book, *Dr. Atkins' Diet Revolution*. While not the very first diet to restrict carbohydrates for weight loss, Atkins became the first mainstream low-carb diet. Starting around

1990, Atkins began producing nutrition bars, drinks, frozen meals, shakes, and low-carb snacks. Today Atkins sells over $20 million dollars' worth of products in retail and online markets. Atkins is a public company in the portfolio of Simply Good Foods company (symbol: SMPL).

The Atkins Diet spawned numerous other low-carb diets throughout the years, and just about every low-carb or keto diet in existence is a reinvention of Atkins' works. The Atkins Diet was the first to use blood ketones as a marker for progress and adherence to a weight loss diet. Dr. Atkins used the term "ketosis" in his 1972 *Dr. Atkins' Diet Revolution*, and practitioners of the Atkins Diet are urged to measure ketones with Ketostix, a urine-activated test strip, to determine if they are eating the proper level of carbs for the diet.

## How It Works

The term "Atkins" has become synonymous with "low-carb," but upon closer examination, you'll find that the Atkins Diet is a multifaceted program that starts with low-carb eating and ends with a long-term maintenance plan where plentiful carbs are allowed.

### Atkins 20® and Atkins 40®

The Atkins Diet currently has two programs: one for people with more than 40 pounds to lose (Atkins 20), and one for people with less than 40 pounds to lose (Atkins 40). The 20 and 40 refer to the number of carb grams one can consume in the early phases of the program. By eating from the detailed allowable food lists and tracking the number of carbs you eat, you should see meaningful weight loss.

Both the 20 and 40 programs proceed through four phases, when a weight goal is achieved, you may progress to the next phase, where additional healthy foods are added to your allowable foods list. To begin, one simply accesses the Atkins website and signs up for the program they desire. The website is easy to navigate and allows users to register free of charge.

Once registered you are given numerous free downloads including food lists, meal planners, and apps. You'll also be given access to a very active forum where you can talk with others in real-time or spend hours and hours digging through old conversations on topics that interest you. If you've never participated in a diet forum, you'll be very surprised how helpful the other users are. Warning: Forums are addictive!

## Atkins Phases

Atkins plans proceed through four phases:

- **Phase 1:** Induction. Carbs are kept to a bare minimum, you'll eat several servings of protein daily including meat, fish, poultry, as well as plant-based protein sources. In addition, 4 ounces of cheese, and an ounce of nuts add to the protein sources. Healthy fats like butter, olive oil, and avocado oil are allowed during induction. Of vital importance is that you eat several servings of foundation vegetables (e.g., non-starchy veggies like broccoli, greens, mushrooms, etc.). You'll learn to count carbs and eat no more than 20–40g per day. Stay with Phase 1 for 2–3 weeks.

- **Phase 2:** Eat up to 50g of carbs per day. Include beans, whole milk, tomato juice, and berries. Stay on phase 2 until you are at your goal weight.

- **Phase 3:** Eat up to 80g of carbs per day. You are free to eat whatever you want, just limit the carb intake. Stay on phase 3 for at least a month as you learn to maintain your weight.

- **Phase 4:** This is considered the long-term maintenance phase. Eat up to 100g of carbs daily.

During all four phases, you must ensure you are eating lots of veggies. The biggest critique of low-carb diets by scientists, nutritionists, and doctors is that they do not provide enough plant matter, especially fiber. It's very easy to get into a rut with Atkins where you are eating fatty meats, cheese, nuts, and snack bars. This is *not* in keeping with the tenets of the Atkins Diet.

Atkins bills itself as a "whole foods" program, and the prepackaged foods they sell are NOT required to do the Atkins plan, but these might help in a pinch. These products are Atkins' foray into the world of diet food products and have been shown to help augment their diet plans. If you navigate through the website, you'll find a section called "meal plans." You'll find sample menus of nutritious low-carb meals. For each plan, there is a "foodie" menu, this is where you will find mostly whole-food ideas. Other plans recommend Atkins meals and bars for nearly every meal. Don't be tempted to take the easy way out! Cook your own food.

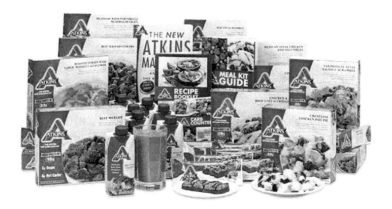

## Best For

The Atkins Diet is best for people who need structure and support and have time to use the online tools available. If you have a PC, laptop, or smartphone (and time to get online) you'll find Atkins quite enjoyable. Atkins is great for first-time dieters of all ages, shapes, and sizes. Atkins works equally well for men and women. You can also do Atkins on your own just by reading the books and sticking to the diet guidelines.

Low-carb diets are best for people with metabolic syndrome and blood sugar issues, such as pre-diabetes. Low-carb diets might not be recommended for some Type 1 diabetics. If you're unsure if it's right for you, it's best to check with your doctor first (Syed-Abdul, 2018).

## Costs

The Atkins 20® and Atkins 40® programs are free. You'll get free planners and calculators as well. Atkins makes money when you buy their books and food. Eating a low-carb diet may end up costing most consumers more than their previous diet because it requires that participants eat much more wholesome foods than most are accustomed to.

## Tech

Atkins has done a great job keeping up with our fast-paced, tech-heavy lifestyles. If you really want to "do" Atkins, you'll need to spend lots of time online using the free apps. After you've reached your goal weight, maintaining your weight becomes more intuitive, and the apps are not as crucial.

The Atkins online community is accessed through the "Community Forum." Here you can meet and chat with other Atkins dieters, get help with meal prep and recipes, or ask *anything* you like, really.

Nothing is off-limits, and the forum is very active. There are seven different forums:

- Getting Started
- Atkins for Life
- Ask a Nutritionist
- Talk to the Moderators
- Recipe Exchange
- Fitness and Health
- Community Lounge

All these forums have had active discussions every time I looked while researching Atkins. This is a good sign that support will be there when you need it. The tone of the group was very upbeat and helpful, and there was an even mix of men and women.

Once you've joined the Atkins community, you'll have access to numerous carb counters, apps, and a dashboard to help you track your goals. You don't have to use any of these, but you'll find they are addictive (in a good way) if you do. If you want to make the most of your Atkins experience, you'll find that becoming an active member of the community will help immensely.

## Pros

The Atkins Diet has been around for a long time. It's easy to succeed if you're willing to do what it takes and follow the phases as instructed. The Atkins Diet is very structured, a huge plus for many people who have had trouble with other diets. Unlike other low-carb diets, Atkins uses the lowest carb intake only for a short period as you become accustomed to giving up junk food.

There is a massive online support network for people who need inspiration from others, and the Atkins website is full of very useful tools and reading materials. The Atkins Diet does not require a membership, subscription, or up-front cash. One could easily follow the Atkins trademarked plans by simply signing up for the programs and taking advantage of all the free content on their website.

## Cons

Low-carb diets are very limited in food choices. Falling off the wagon often results in rapid, hard-to-reverse weight gain. It's very easy to do Atkins wrong. Many people mistakenly think that Atkins is a diet where butter and bacon are king. While many low-carb diets push these fat-bombs, Atkins is not a long-term high-fat diet. Atkins requires that you give the utmost attention to what you consume—you have to strictly adhere to lowering carbs, even on the maintenance phases of the diet. If you don't follow the plan closely, you can quickly become deprived of beneficial fiber, resulting in intestinal disturbances.

## Famous Practitioners

Atkins' current spokesman is Rob Lowe, who has purportedly followed the Atkins eating style for many years.

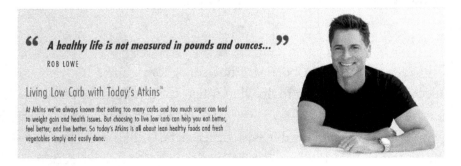

66 *A healthy life is not measured in pounds and ounces...* 99
ROB LOWE

Living Low Carb with Today's Atkins®

At Atkins we've always known that eating too many carbs and too much sugar can lead to weight gain and health issues. But choosing to live low carb can help you eat better, feel better, and live better. So today's Atkins is all about lean healthy foods and fresh vegetables simply and easily done.

Past spokespeople include Courtney Thorne Smith, Sharon Osborne, Alyssa Milano, Kim Kardashian, and singer Lauren Alaina.

## Recommended Reading

You only need one book: *Atkins: Eat Right, Not Less: Your Guidebook for Living a Low-Carb and Low-Sugar Lifestyle* (2017). The book is available through the Atkins website, Amazon, and most booksellers in hard cover and ebook formats. This newest book, published December 2017, was written by Colette Heimowitz, M.Sc. Vice President, Nutrition and Education, Atkins Nutritionals, Inc. This book builds on lessons learned from the previous books dating back to the original 1972 *Dr. Atkins' Diet Revolution* book.

## Bottom Line

Atkins has been around for 30 years. They have a solid reputation for achieving successful weight loss using a low-carb approach to dieting. Except for all the processed food they will tempt you with, I have no qualms in recommending Atkins as a primary weight loss program for people who want to try a low-carb/keto diet.

# CHAPTER 14

## SLIMMING WORLD

**TL;DR:** *Slimming World focuses on healthy eating for weight loss. Similar to Weight Watchers in structure, but without the multimillion-dollar advertising budget or endless lines of products. A good old-fashioned weight loss plan with 21st century technology.*

### Portal

Learn about Slimming World at www.slimmingworld.com.

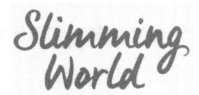

### The Promise

> *"Discover a world of weight loss without dieting."*

### Background

Slimming World™ was started in the United Kingdom in 1969 by Margaret Miles-Bramwell. This popular weight loss program was only available in the UK until recently. Slimming World has attracted a large following of Americans since its US debut in 2017. I'm not sure why it took nearly 50 years to make it "across the pond," but I'm glad it did. Slimming World's unique weight loss plan is exactly what America needs right now.

Slimming World is barely even a diet. This program emphasizes whole, nutritious, filling foods and yet allows for the treats we have all become addicted to. It's a complete weight loss program that incorporates education, social support, personalization, and exercise. Their website and ads don't feature the waif-like models we've become accustomed to seeing, and their online store is completely free of supplements, fake foods, and endless merchandise.

## How It Works

Access to Slimming World's weight loss program requires a $15 monthly membership fee. If you pay for three months, you'll only pay $10 a month. For the price of membership, you'll have access to hundreds of well-written weight loss articles, "Free Food" selection downloads, apps, planners, and a community message board. You'll also be invited (for no extra charge!) to a weekly online group chat where you'll meet a Slimming World representative and other members of the community.

Slimming World's program has three key elements: food, support, and activity.

## Food

The Food Optimizing plan, which is based on the science of energy density and satiety, helps you pick only the best food to eat. You'll learn to place food into three categories:

- Free Food
- Healthy Extras
- Syns

The "Free Food" list seems almost too good to be true, but it's based on very solid logic. These foods (e.g., meat, potatoes, eggs, fruit, and vegetables) are whole, unprocessed, energy-dense foods that are nearly impossible to overeat.

"Healthy Extras" are things like bread, dairy, canned foods, and nuts. This type of food is healthy but fattening if eaten in excess, so you are limited to about two servings per day. It's these healthy extras that create a balanced diet so sadly missing from other weight loss plans.

"Syns" are treats or cheats. Candy, ice cream, and junk food is eaten in moderation on the Slimming World program. You'll get several "Syns" a day to help you keep these foods *mostly* out of your diet without having to give them up completely.

You'll find three pdf files under a "Food Lists" tab; the first thing you should do is print these files for handy reference. These three files contain "Free Foods," "Healthy Extras," and "Syns."

## Support

You'll get all the support you need when you become a paid member. They've developed an online community where you can ask questions 24/7 and get quick answers from Slimming World staff and other members of the community. The first 12 weeks of the program are designed to help you settle into the Slimming World lifestyle as you slowly learn to eat according to the plan. At sign-up, you'll be asked to pick a time slot for your weekly meeting. This weekly meeting is an hour-long chat with staff and other members to educate and share ideas. In the UK, this meeting is done in person in a community setting.

## Activity

Slimming World doesn't push exercise very hard, but they have great recommendations. "Activity Awards" are given for how much exercise you do in a month.

- Bronze: 45 minutes per week
- Silver: 90 minutes per week
- Gold: 150 minutes per week

Other than these self-paced awards, there is no mandatory exercise plan, so you'll be on your own. People who have become accustomed to a sedentary lifestyle for many years could use these awards as motivation when starting their diet. The gold medal is given for 30 minutes of exercise, 5 days a week. If you really want to succeed with this plan, I suggest getting to the gold level very quickly and staying there. (See my exercise recommendations in Part 4.)

## Best For

Slimming World works best for people who cook most of their meals at home. Also, you'll need to be able to log into your account several times a day to track your food and activity. The apps make it easy to keep track on a smartphone or home computer. Slimming World is perfect for anyone who wants the freedom to select what they eat. Participants must be over 18 and shouldn't be pregnant or have an eating disorder. I get the feeling that Slimming World is geared to target women more than men, but I think men will benefit just the same.

## Costs

The cost to join Slimming World is $10/month.

## Tech

The Slimming World website is easy to navigate, and you can quickly become immersed in the well-presented data. The community section is not set up like a typical forum where you can see the threads and sub-threads, but more like a chat room where recent conversations are at the top of the page. You will be prompted to search for the answer to your question before making a new post. I think they could do a bit better on this, especially considering there's not a Facebook group dedicated to Slimming World.

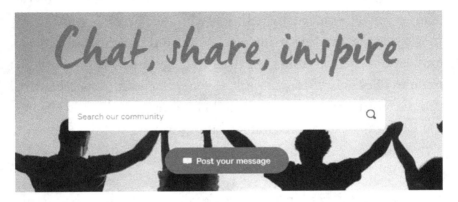

Slimming World does a good job keeping up with social media. You'll find them on Twitter, Facebook, Instagram, Pinterest, and LinkedIn.

Spend an hour playing around on the site and you'll be a pro. If you get stuck, ask an expert in the community. Too easy!

## Pros

The diet is nutritionally sound and doesn't require counting calories. It's very easy to follow if you stick to the Food Optimizing principals. The diet points out foods high in fiber and other important nutrients so you can easily pick the best food choices.

Slimming World has been around for 50 years! They've learned a trick or two in that time—no gimmicks, no supplements, no salesmen knocking down your door. A glitch-free browsing experience that gets you right down to the business of dieting.

## Cons

Slimming world is new to the US, if you visit the UK website (http://www.slimmingworld.co.uk/) you'll see a few features that don't appear on the US site. Perhaps when more Americans discover Slimming World there will be more perks to joining, or maybe there are just issues in the transition. However, I was pleased to see that recipes and weights were all expressed using terms Americans are familiar with (e.g., Fahrenheit versus Celsius, pounds versus grams).

Someone once said, "England and America are two countries separated by one language." I found some of the terms used a bit off-putting. For example, "syns" would come across better if they were called "cheats" or "treats." It would be very hard to discuss this diet with coworkers unfamiliar with Slimming World. And even the name, Slimming World, sounds like something out of the '50s, harkening to the days when Diet Rite soda and corsets ruled women's lives. But then again, it makes it kind of cool. Retro. A breath of fresh air in the world of dieting.

## Recommended Reading

There are no books to buy—something unheard of in the world of weight loss programs. For your membership fee, you'll get several books that explain the diet and recipes, and a food log and diary.

## Bottom Line

If you want to try a good old-fashioned diet plan that's stood the test of time, try Slimming World. If I were to design a commercial weight loss program, it would look much like Slimming World. The price of entry is dirt cheap for what you get in return. You won't find ads or hard-sell techniques to get you to buy things you hadn't considered. Slimming World is all about the diet. Use Slimming

World as a structured program to drop some pounds and learn good eating habits as you develop a lifelong plan that includes eating better and exercising. I don't think you'll be disappointed. I think it's great that this program has been around for so long and has finally made it to America. I have a feeling it will be here for a long time.

# CHAPTER 15

# WEIGHT WATCHERS

> **TL;DR:** *If you think you know Weight Watchers, chances are you don't. Weight Watchers still controls food intake by assigning point values to what you eat, but they've branched heavily into the entire realm of wellness and health. This diet giant has kept up with the times and has over four million users, their technology is second to none.*

## Portal

You can learn more about Weight Watchers at www.weightwatchers.com.

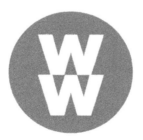

## The Promise

*"Wellness that Works™"*

## Background

Weight Watchers was founded in 1963 by Jean Nidetch, a New York City homemaker who was under-impressed with weight loss programs of the day. Nidetch developed her own unique program, trained others, and franchised the company in 1964. Since then, the company has undergone many changes to keep up with the times.

By the early 2000s, Weight Watchers began losing members and slipped in popularity until Oprah Winfrey became the company's spokesperson and partner in 2015. The company underwent a tech explosion and launched a new initiative called "Beyond the Scale," a lifestyle and fitness program that's proven immensely popular with a new generation of dieters. In 2017, Weight Watchers introduced "Freestyle," giving its members extreme flexibility beyond the long-running in-person meetings and weigh-ins.

Weight Watchers was rebranded as WW in 2018 and is now the highest-earning diet company in the world. WW earned over $300 million in 2018 with over four million members worldwide. In addition to its well-known diet program, WW also publishes a monthly magazine and sells numerous WW-branded foods, apps, services, and products.

## How It Works

WW enjoys immense name-brand recognition and attracts dieters to their website with innumerable offerings of products and free diet-related material. For a subscription fee, customers can receive many levels of support through one of three WW programs.

- **Digital:** An app-based experience that allows users to track food intake, activity levels, and weight changes. The Digital program offers 24/7 access to a WW coach and chat room.

- **Studio:** All the Digital benefits plus in-person weekly meetings in a WW studio. These meetings are led by a certified WW wellness coach.

- **Coaching:** Digital benefits, but instead of weekly meetings you'll be paired with a WW coach. You're given 24/7 access to your coach via unlimited phone calls and messages. Your coach will help you devise a personalized diet and exercise program and assist you with meeting your goals.

WW considers itself a health and wellness service rather than a weight loss program. The WW website is the center of all WW activity for its community of members. The WW weight loss strategy emphasizes fruits, vegetables, lean meat, and whole grains. While WW focuses on balanced eating, personalized plans can be developed for consumers who need vegan, low-carb, or other nutritional requirements.

WW uses a point-based system instead of counting calories for controlling food intake. They've continually updated their methodology through the years. Today's WW uses SmartPoints® and has over 200 ZeroPoint™ foods (e.g., eggs, skinless chicken breast, fish and seafood, corn, beans, peas) you may eat of freely throughout the day.

**Best For**

WW has something for everyone. Though 90% of WW members are female, they actively target men by using male actors and advertising during sporting events. Both men and women would benefit from WW's programs. Being tech-savvy is a requirement for taking full advantage of all WW has to offer, but if you have a smartphone or regular access to the internet, you'll be good to go.

**Costs**

- Digital: $4.22/week
- Studio: $9.61/week
- Coaching: $12.69/week

## Tech

## <u>WW App</u>

If you're into tech, you'll love WW. Even if you don't care anything about joining a WW group or chatting with others, the apps they've developed are nothing short of incredible. WW has smartphone apps that let you calculate SmartPoints by scanning food barcodes at the grocery store as well as tracking the food you eat by taking a picture of it for analysis. They've also created an app that lets you pre-track your meals so you can accurately plan what you'll be eating on a weekly basis. Better yet, the apps aren't just for food, they can also help you track your activity and wellness goals. It even syncs with Fitbits and other fitness devices! And get this—the WW app even integrates with online devices like Alexa and Google Assistant. Word has it they've partnered with Headspace, a meditation app, to help you control your stress levels as well. For the true techies out there, the WW app was developed by Ray Wu. Originally called Weilos, Wu sold the app to WW in 2015. The WW app is considered the gold standard in weight loss apps (Pai, 2015).

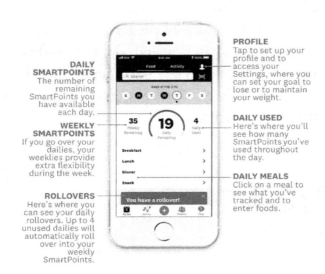

## Connect

WW's online community, called Connect, is the best social media platform ever developed for dieters. Connect is considered "the heart and soul" of WW. Expect more and more from Connect. WW has over 1.5 million US members, and Connect users post an average of 9,000 new posts with over 42,000 comments *per day*. The weight loss forums I used to frequent were lucky to get 25–50 new posts a day. Connect lets you join micro-communities based on age, interests, hobbies, or special diets among other things. When you consider they're competing against the social media giant Facebook for users, it's nothing short of miraculous what they've accomplished with Connect.

## Website

The weightwatchers.com website *is* WW. You won't find a single glitch anywhere. It's very obvious they have a top-notch web team. Even if you don't want to join WW, you'll find hundreds of free wellness articles at the "Daily Feed" tab on the top of the home page. WW puts their money where their mouth is, or in this case, where their website and apps are.

## Pros

The best thing about WW is that you are getting almost 60 years' worth of weight loss knowledge on a state-of-the-art website with apps that have no match. I'm a big fan of WW's focus on wellness versus weight and the fact that they don't push supplements or put skinny models all over their splash page. WW has a massive line of snack bars and ready-made meals, but I don't get the impression they hard-sell these foods to WW dieters.

## Cons

WW *is* Big Diet. It's impossible to even say who owns WW. Weight Watchers was owned by Heinz until 1999, then they went big league. At that time, Weight Watchers was worth $735 million. Now WW trades on NASDAQ as WTW, and the company was valued at over $8 billion in mid-2018. Oprah Winfrey is a 10% owner who has made many millions buying and selling her shares since she joined on in 2015.

WW will do anything to stay on top of the industry. Their new name, WW, is an attempt to erase 60 years of fat-shaming overweight housewives. But such is modern business. Weight Watchers sells. Oprah and the board of directors are banking on future generations buying WW.

## Famous Practitioners

From sports all-stars to movie stars, Playboy Bunnies, and royalty, celebrities of all stripes have signed on to WW over the years. WW is the king of celebrity spokespeople. Remember these?

- Lynn Redgrave, 1984
- Sarah Ferguson, 1997–2008
- Greg Grunberg (from *Heroes*), 2007
- Jenny McCarthy, 2009
- Jennifer Hudson, 2010
- Charles Barkley, 2011
- Jessica Simpson, 2012
- Oprah Winfrey, 2015
- DJ Khaled, 2018

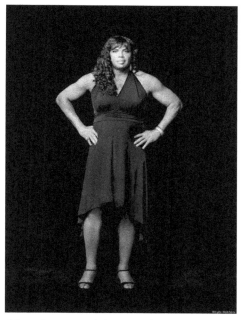

*Charles Barkley shows Weight Watchers is not just for women.*

## Recommended Reading

If you decide to go the WW route, there are literally hundreds of books that have been published by Weight Watchers over the years. These are available on the WW website, Amazon, or wherever books are sold. Due to the WW website's comprehensive nature and use of electronics, books are not required to learn about the diet, but you might like to browse their library if you want a cookbook or other specialty reading material.

## Bottom Line

Even though WW represents all that I hate about the Diet and Fitness Industry, this is a really good weight loss program. WW spent billions to create a sustainable weight loss platform and provide the tech needed to stay relevant in a tech-heavy market. If you long for the old Weight Watchers meetings, they still exist, too. My advice: If you want to try WW, jump in with both feet and give it a good two or three months. If you hate it, you're only out a hundred bucks. If you love it, stick with it as long as you like.

# CHAPTER 16

# SELF-DIRECTED DIETS

> **TL;DR:** *"Watching what you eat" is not a valid weight loss plan. Dieters need structure and support. Careful eating will work for weight maintenance but not weight loss.*

## DIY Dieting

More than 150 million Americans are on a diet. Yet WW, the largest commercial diet program in the United States, has just 1.5 million US customers. Only about 10 million people use any of the available commercial diet programs. The other 140 million people are just winging it. When asked about their dieting habits, most people say they are "watching what they eat," or "eating healthy." This approach doesn't bode well for weight loss (McLaughlin, 2018).

Self-directed diets fail to achieve *any* weight loss over 90% of the time. The reason for this dismal success rate is due mainly to lack of structure and support (Cook, 2017). For people with weight problems, it's nearly impossible to limit calories without carefully logging food intake. When people are asked to report what they've eaten from memory, their recall is likely to be 25% less than what they've actually eaten (van den Boer, 2017).

## Designing a Self-Directed Weight Loss Plan

To effectively lose weight, you must take it seriously. Doctors, dieticians, and the weight loss industry know that overweight people rarely lose weight without structure. Most people don't like structured diet programs, so they attempt to lose weight on their own. Self-directed diet plans can work quite well if steps are taken to mimic the programs developed by the medical and diet industries.

You read in chapter 2 about the intensive weight loss intervention approach researchers use (Espeland, 2013) (Hollis, 2008), but it's worth repeating here:

- Provide a tailored approach based on each person's goals, starting point, and current health.
- Provide education in nutrition, physical activity, problem solving, and goal setting.
- Develop a menu based on the patient's preferred eating style.
- Reduce portion sizes to limit calorie intake to an appropriate number for age, sex, and activity levels.
- Eliminate ultra-processed foods.
- Increase consumption of minimally processed food, especially fruit, vegetables, and whole grains.
- Limit alcohol consumption.
- Keep accurate logs of food intake, bodyweight, and physical activity.
- Provide group interaction with like-minded dieters.
- Provide social support.

This approach can easily be tailored to a self-directed diet when weight loss is crucial. Recall our earlier discussions of appropriate dieting: if you only need to lose a couple pounds for vanity reasons, skip all of this and go directly to "maintenance dieting." But if you have medical issues related to excess weight, a high BMI, and a larger-than-normal waist measurement, the drastic step of weight loss dieting is needed.

Losing weight requires you to get out of your comfort zone. You can't just choose lower-calorie options from the McDonald's menu board and expect results. Here's a guide for creating a self-directed weight loss plan that'll work nearly 100% of the time if you follow it closely.

## What's the Best Diet Style to Use?

The hardest part about self-directed dieting is picking a dieting style. There are thousands of books and websites vying for your attention. How do you choose? Sometimes it's best to avoid diet books altogether and just eat real food and count calories. There is nothing special about the paleo diet, keto, low-carb, or low-fat diets beyond eating less.

## Protein Requirements

A long-standing formula for protein needs is stated as 1g/kg of bodyweight for moderately active people (Phillips, 2016). This amount has proven satisfactory in preventing the loss of muscle and lean body mass during weight loss (Gibson, 2014) (Geisler, 2016).

In everyday terminology, here are protein requirements based on 1g/kg:

| Bodyweight (in pounds) | Protein Needed to Prevent Lean Body Mass Loss (grams) |
|---|---|
| 250–300 | 113–136 |
| 200–250 | 90–113 |
| 180–200 | 81–90 |
| 160–180 | 72–81 |
| 150 or less | 68–72 |

For reference, to visualize this amount of protein in meat and plant form:

- 1 pound of lean meat (raw weight) contains roughly 130g of protein.

- ½ pound of lean meat (raw weight) contains 65g of protein.
- 16 oz. of cooked pinto beans contains 21g of protein.
- 12 oz. of frozen black-eyed peas contains 32g of protein.

Therefore, the average (non-vegan) dieter should strive to eat roughly ½ to 1 pound of meat and numerous servings of high-protein vegetables such as beans and peas. You'll be surprised how quickly the protein in real, whole food adds up as you eat through the day.

When you set up your calorie-tracking tools, you'll be able to dial in your carb, fat, and protein intake. But you shouldn't obsess over it. The important thing here is to eat high-quality, nutritious food. If you get wrapped up in carbs, fat, and protein you'll quickly get sidetracked and derail your diet. Just be careful that you are getting enough protein to help prevent muscle loss.

## Hydration

Dieters are often told to drink more water to help with weight loss efforts. This may be more than just an old wives' tale. A 2010 study showed that drinking about 2 cups of water before meals led to a reduction in 225 calories eaten per day (Dennis, 2010). It's good advice to stay hydrated, drink when thirsty, and make sure your urine is clear. Beyond this, drinking an extra couple glasses of water before meals could have a really big impact on your weight loss efforts.

## Cheat Day

"Cheat days" can help reduce the lowering of your metabolism during prolonged dieting. I recommend overeating slightly one day a week during your diet. This would be like an extra 500–750 calories of a very healthy yet indulgent snack, or extra helpings of starchy carbs with a meal. Some good cheat foods are: rice, potatoes, beans, ice cream, whole wheat bread, sugary fruit. This is not an excuse to eat a whole deep-pan pizza, but rather to prime your metabolism in the hopes that it does not slow excessively from long-term calorie restriction (Trexler, 2014).

## Stall Busting

Once you've dialed in your eating and start losing weight, the worst thing to have happen is to *stop* losing weight unexpectedly. This is known as a *stall* or *plateau*, and it happens to most dieters around the two-month mark. If your weight does not change for two consecutive weeks, it's time to make some changes. The first thing you should do is to check the accuracy of your calorie-tracking methodology. Are you just guessing, or are you really tracking every food you eat? Poor diet adherence is the number one reason for stalls. If you are doing a good job counting calories, it's time to lower your calories by about 200–300 per day, this should get the weight dropping again. Don't be tempted to starve yourself, and don't freak out. Stalls are a normal part of dieting. If you don't believe me, just look at any diet forum; you'll see numerous threads titled, "Why aren't I *loosing* weight?"

## Have a Plan

Consider this: most people who try self-directed dieting don't have *any* plan. They attempt to lower their calorie intake by making better food choices based on calorie counts or other random qualities of food. They don't focus on food quality or any of the other factors that make diets work. This type of dieter rarely loses weight. Other self-directed dieters buy a popular diet book or search the internet for dieting tips. They loosely follow a diet (e.g., keto, paleo, or DASH) but never fully commit themselves. They see few results after weeks of following the diet, so they quit. Here's a much better way to do a self-directed diet:

## Putting It into Action

### Pre-Diet

**Prep Step 1:** Choose a start date, set goals, and get a physical examination including blood work. You don't have to start today, but soon. Give yourself time to buy what you might need, get to the doctor, and read some books on the subject. Your goals need to be realistic and trackable. It's reasonable to expect a weight loss of 10–15 pounds in the first month of dieting, but it will slow considerably after that. Some reasonable expectations:

| Weight Loss Goal | Time Needed |
|---|---|
| Over 100 pounds | 1+ years. Talk with your doctor. |
| 100 pounds | 1 year |
| 75 pounds | 9 months |
| 60 pounds | 8 months |
| 50 pounds | 7 months |
| 40 pounds | 6 months |
| 30 pounds | 5 months |
| 20 pounds | 1–3 months |
| 10 pounds | 1–2 months |

**Prep Step 2:** Purge your pantry. Get rid of all the junk food that tempts you. Dump the candy jar you keep on your desk at work. Take stock of what you've been eating, and plan on how you can make the big changes needed to start eating better. If you're used to fast-food lunches, devise a better way to eat. Stock up on fresh and frozen veggies and unprocessed food.

**Prep Step 3:** Stop drinking, smoking, cavorting, partying, and fighting. Simplify your life for the duration of your planned diet.

**Prep Step 4:** Start a food log. Use a pen and paper or an app. Examine your pre-diet food intake to learn your biggest weaknesses. Learn to count calories and macros (fat, protein, carbs). Download some apps.

**Prep Step 5:** Start a weight log. Weigh yourself daily or weekly and write it down. Take some "before" measurements of your waist (also thighs, arms, chest if you like). Take some "before" pictures of your minimally clothed body.

**Prep Step 6:** Start "lurking" in online weight loss forums (examples later). Create forum user accounts, make introductions.

**Prep Step 7:** Develop a plan to exercise (see Section 4). Join a gym, or buy equipment to exercise at home. At a minimum, prepare to start walking every day and doing some light bodyweight exercises.

**Prep Step 8:** Determine your weight loss calorie and protein needs. Here's a good start:

| Current Body Weight (shown in pounds) | Calories Needed for Weight Loss (Assuming a BMI over 27) | Protein Needed to Prevent Lean Body Mass Loss |
|---|---|---|
| 250–300 | 2,200–2,500 | 113–136 (grams per day) |
| 200–250 | 2,000–2,200 | 90–113 |
| 180–200 | 1,900–2,200 | 81–90 |
| 160–180 | 1,600–1,900 | 72–81 |
| 150 or less | 1,500–1,800 | 68–72 |

## Start Your Diet

**Day 1:** Reduce your daily food intake to an appropriate calorie level for your current bodyweight (see chart above). Cut back on processed food and eliminate ultra-processed food from your diet (NOVA Categories 3 and 4):

| NOVA Food Category | Examples |
|---|---|
| **Group 1— Unprocessed or Minimally Processed Foods** <br><br> Eat unlimited amounts on a weight loss diet. | Fruits, vegetables, grains, legumes/beans, starchy roots and tubers, fungi, red meat, poultry, fish and seafood, eggs, milk, fresh fruit or vegetable juices (without added sugar, sweeteners or flavors), pasta, couscous, polenta, tree and ground nuts, seeds, spices, herbs, plain yogurt with no added sugar or artificial sweeteners, tea, coffee, drinking water |
| **Group 2—Processed Ingredients** <br><br> Use as needed on a weight loss diet. | Salt, sugar, molasses, honey, syrup (e.g., maple), vegetable oils crushed from olives or seeds, butter and lard obtained from milk and pork, starches extracted from corn and other plants |
| **Group 3—Processed Foods** <br><br> *Eat sparingly* on a weight loss diet; 1–2 servings a day. | Canned or bottled vegetables, fruits and legumes/beans; <br> salted, oiled, or sugared nuts and seeds; salted, cured, or smoked meats; canned fish/meat/poultry; fruits in syrup; cheeses; unpackaged freshly made breads |
| **Group 4—Ultra-processed Foods** <br><br> *Eat rarely* on a weight loss diet; 1–2 servings a week max. Best to eat none of these during active weight loss. | Carbonated drinks; packaged snacks, potato chips, pretzels, corn chips; ice cream, chocolate, candies (confectionery); mass-produced packaged breads and buns; margarines and spreads; cookies, pastries, cakes, and cake mixes; breakfast cereals, energy bars; energy drinks; milk drinks, "fruit" yogurts and "fruit" drinks; cocoa drinks; meat and chicken extracts and "instant" sauces; protein bars and drinks; meal-replacement bars and drinks; ready to heat products including pre-prepared pies and pasta and pizza; poultry and fish "nuggets" and "sticks," sausages, fast-food burgers, hot dogs, and other reconstituted meat products, and powdered and packaged "instant" soups, noodles and desserts |

*Adapted from da Costa, 2018*

**Day 1 (cont.):** Start tracking your food intake with an app c logging method; use pen and paper if you must. Do not rely on your memory! Become an active member of a weight loss forum or community, or just continue lurking. Bear in mind that most people on these forums are dieting *wrong*. Don't argue, just observe and join in conversations when you are ready.

**Day 2:** Start your exercise program.

**Day 2–7:** Fight urges to snack between meals. Focus completely on your eating. Read all you can in books or online. Dig deep! The first week is the hardest.

**Day 7:** Weigh yourself if you haven't already. Write it down. If you did not lose weight, just stay the course for another week. If you lost a couple pounds, do a happy dance.

**Day 7–14:** Once you're fully committed to the plan, start telling people about it. Ask for help in avoiding off-plan food.

**Day 14:** If you haven't lost at least 4 pounds, something is wrong. Reevaluate your plan. Double-check your calories.

**Day 30:** If you haven't lost 5–10 pounds, something is wrong. Reevaluate your plan. Review your exercise program.

**Days 30–60:** Continue the plan, and fight the urge to change things if you are losing weight steadily. If weight loss slows down or stops, consider making some slight changes (e.g., lower calories by 250 per day or switch to a low-carb or low-fat diet). Keep reading. Keep talking.

**Day 60:** If you haven't lost 10–15 pounds, reevaluate your plan. Review your exercise program.

**Day 90:** If you haven't lost 15–20 pounds, reevaluate your plan.

If weight loss is steady, and you are taking meds for high blood pressure, high cholesterol, pre-diabetes, etc., talk to your doctor to ensure you still need them. Review your exercise program.

**Day 120:** If you haven't lost 20–25 pounds, reevaluate your plan. Review your exercise program.

**Day 150:** If you haven't lost 25–30 pounds, reevaluate your plan. Review your exercise program.

**Day 180 (6 months in):** Total weight loss should be around 30–40 pounds. If more weight loss is desired, keep on going. Make an appointment for follow-up bloodwork and discuss medications with your doctor. Examine your weight logs and activity. Begin planning for a transition to a maintenance diet. Review your exercise program.

## Transitory Stage

As you get close to your goal weight, you'll need to develop a maintenance plan. This is where most people mess up. See Part 3 for maintenance diet ideas.

**Transition Step 1:** Take some "after" pictures and measurements for your log.

**Transition Step 2:** Stop tracking calories, eat intuitively of foods from NOVA Categories 1, 2, and 3 mainly. Category 4 foods should only be considered occasional treats. (See NOVA chart [page 168].)

**Transition Step 3:** Continue weighing and checking your waist measurement for the rest of your life—daily, weekly, monthly, or yearly as desired. If weight starts to creep up a bit, don't be alarmed. If you are exercising and eating mainly from Categories 1, 2, and 3, you are doing things right; your weight will stabilize, and you can go about your life without focusing excessively on diet.

**Transition Step 4:** Shift completely to your new maintenance diet (see Part 3). Stick around the forums to help struggling dieters; your help will be appreciated.

## Conclusion

Forgive me if this section lacks concrete recommendations on specific diets to follow, but everyone is so different that this is impossible to do. Over 100 million Americans are on a self-directed diet; most will fail to lose weight. If you just can't stand the thought of signing up for a commercial weight loss program like WW, Slimming World, or Atkins, you'll have to develop you own plan, one that mirrors theirs. "Eating right" and "watching what you eat" won't work. The plan you develop needs goals, timelines, and support alongside a method to eat less and exercise. There are thousands of diet books, but they all boil down to three basic weight loss plans: low-carb, low-fat, or balanced meals. It's always best to start out eating well-balanced meals that contain ample fruit, vegetables, whole grains, dairy, and meat. The only "food groups" that should absolutely be eliminated are the ultra-processed foods of NOVA category 4. You'll need a way to log and track the food you eat. For this, there are several good apps available, but a pen and paper work in a pinch. Social support can come from the people around you or from virtual strangers you connect with over the internet in weight loss forums. Weight loss forums are an invaluable tool; you can learn a lot from successful losers as well as from those that can't lose no matter what.

# CHAPTER 17

# BEST WEIGHT LOSS WEBSITES AND APPS

**TL;DR:** *SparkPeople, MyFitnessPal, Fitbit, LoseIt, FatSecret, and FitDay: Check them out.*

If you want your self-directed weight loss diet to stand any chance of working, you'll need to carefully track the food you eat. When you are following a plan like WW or Slimming World, they take the guesswork out by assigning point values to food, and you simply track the points, or you follow a strict food list, as provided by the Atkins plan. Everything else you need is neatly packaged on the website of the commercial diet program. They don't want you looking elsewhere for help; they want to keep you firmly in their grasp.

When you're on your own, you'll have to count calories, track your weight, learn about exercise, and meet other people all by yourself. Guessing at it is no good; we just can't be trusted to eyeball our food and try to remember what we've eaten. It won't work. The only way to count calories is to meticulously log each food eaten into a calorie tracker. Or you could just jot down what you eat on a piece of paper and look up the calorie values at the end of each day. Besides counting calories, you'll also need a place for social support, education, exercise logs, and weight tracking. Sounds hard? Never fear, there's an app for that!

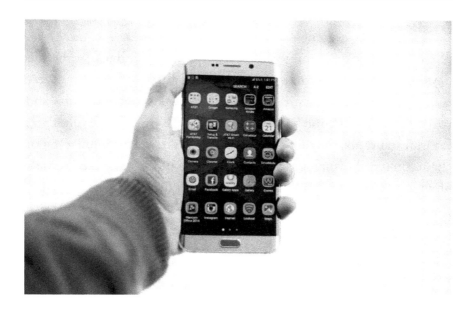

## Best Apps

Two apps have taken the dieting world by storm: SparkPeople and MyFitnessPal. Both can be used as smartphone apps or through their websites.

## www.SparkPeople.com

SparkPeople.com was founded in 2000 as a health and fitness website. By 2012, they had over 10 million users. In 2019, there were over 16 million registered users. SparkPeople is free but offers a "premium" membership for $5 a month. Using the free option, you'll get a private account and access to numerous food, fitness, and lifestyle trackers as well as thousands of articles on health and wellness. The premium option gives you access to a weekly meeting with a health coach, advanced reports, an ad-free browsing experience, and some other perks not available to the general membership. I'd recommend using the free version for a couple weeks before deciding to pay for the premium upgrade.

## **Trackers**

The calorie trackers are incredibly comprehensive. Back in the old days of food trackers, you had to kind of guess at what you were eating and create a custom entry for most foods beyond fruits and vegetables. SparkPeople's database of foods is immense. Even if you eat in restaurants, they'll have specific menu items from most major chains on file. As you log your food throughout the day, it keeps track of what you've eaten and how you are doing with your daily goal.

| | CALORIES | CARBS | FAT | PROTEIN | FIBER |
|---|---|---|---|---|---|
| | 0 | 0 | 0 | 0 | 0 |
| Totals: | 1,100 | 115 | 39 | 69 | 18 |
| Your Daily Goal: | 2,480 - 2,830 | 279 - 460 | 55 - 110 | 75 - 248 | 25 - 35 |
| Remaining Today: | 1,380 - 1,730 | 164 - 345 | 16 - 71 | 6 - 179 | 7 - 17 |

*SparkPeople Calorie Tracker*

The fitness tracker is just as impressive. It allows you to set custom goals and track them throughout the week. There's a workout generator to help keep your workouts fresh and an extensive video library and resource center, all free for the looking. The fitness tracker has a feature to make custom reports and will sync up with Fitbits and other devices. Premium membership unlocks a data tab and a premium workout tab.

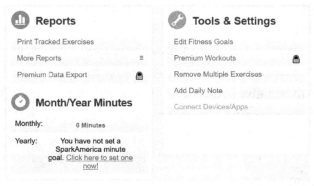

*SparkPeople Fitness Tracker*

The weight tracker is amazing, too. They've thought of everything—right down to the Wi-Fi-enabled scale. It doesn't get any easier!

## Weight / Measurements

**Weigh yourself**

Measure your Waist

Measure your Hips

Measure your Thigh

Measure your Upper Arm

## Wellness

Energy Level

Stress Level

## Fitness Tests

**No Measurements Selected** Add Measurements

## Health Measurements

**No Measurements Selected** Add Measurements

**Save Measurements**

*SparkPeople Weight Tracker*

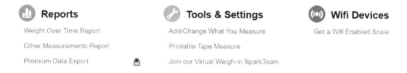

**Reports**

Weight Over Time Report

Other Measurements Report

Premium Data Export

**Tools & Settings**

Add/Change What You Measure

Printable Tape Measure

Join our Virtual Weigh-In SparkTeam

**Wifi Devices**

Get a Wifi Enabled Scale

*SparkPeople Weight Tracker Reports and Tools*

## Message Boards

The SparkPeople message boards are very active, and there are five boards to choose from:

- Community Contact
- Get Help Here

- Results
- Support Groups
- Recipe Suggestions

Each message board contains 3–5 sub-boards with thousands of posts in each.

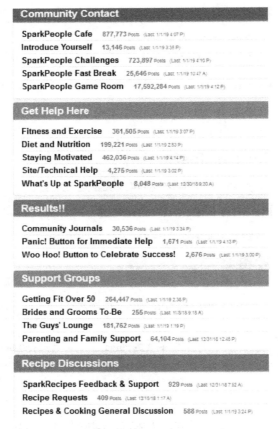

*SparkPeople Message Boards*

There's a search function to help you look through all these discussions. Anything you can think of has been discussed here; just look. But feel free to ask anything.

## Bottom Line

SparkPeople has everything you'll need to make your self-directed weight loss plan a success. Check to make sure it works with the phone or computer you use before going all in. From what I've seen, it's fast and glitch-free. The community and message boards could mean the difference between failure and success in your weight loss attempt. If you like it, pay the $5 for the premium experience: it's *always* worth it if it means dealing with fewer ads.

## www.MyFitnessPal.com

If you looked at SparkPeople and thought it was a bit too hectic for you, you'll love MyFitnessPal—affectionately referred to as MFP. It has all of the elements of SparkPeople but in a much more laid-back style. The food-logging feature of MFP works much better on a PC than SparkPeople's logging system, but it doesn't have as many features. If you just want to see your daily calorie count and don't care for fancy reports, MFP is probably the tracker for you.

MFP is totally free, and they also offer a premium upgrade for $9.99 a month, or $49.99 if you pay for a year. The premium experience gives you access to more content, logs, and reports—and it hides all the ads. Play with the free site first. You probably won't need to upgrade, but if you are really getting into it, it might be worth it. Sometimes simpler is better.

MFP has over 150 million user accounts and about 25 million active users.

## Trackers

The calorie tracker on MFP is super-easy to use and has a comprehensive database of foods. You'll find the exact brands of the food you commonly eat. In fact, I don't think I've ever struggled to find a food in the MFP food log.

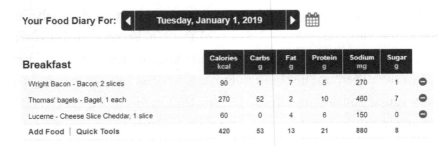

| Breakfast | Calories kcal | Carbs g | Fat g | Protein g | Sodium mg | Sugar g | |
|---|---|---|---|---|---|---|---|
| Wright Bacon - Bacon, 2 slices | 90 | 1 | 7 | 5 | 270 | 1 | ⊖ |
| Thomas' bagels - Bagel, 1 each | 270 | 52 | 2 | 10 | 460 | 7 | ⊖ |
| Lucerne - Cheese Slice Cheddar, 1 slice | 60 | 0 | 4 | 6 | 150 | 0 | ⊖ |
| Add Food │ Quick Tools | 420 | 53 | 13 | 21 | 880 | 8 | |

The fitness tracker is completely adequate for a self-directed weight loss program and perfect for a long-term maintenance diet. It will let you track all the elements of a well-rounded fitness program. I really couldn't ask for more. I don't like that they combine "calories burned" during exercise with the "calorie goal" on your food log. I think it gives a false sense of being able to eat more than you should. Ignore it and you'll be fine.

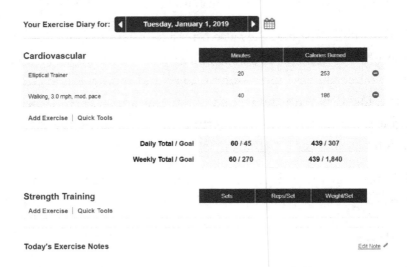

The MFP weight tracker is also great. It's very simple and has all you could ask for. It's accessed through the "Check-in" tab at the top of the home page. You can get a graph showing long-term weight changes under the "Reports" tab. This is a great tool to track your daily or weekly weigh-ins during a weight loss diet and less-frequent weigh-ins during maintenance.

### Check-In

Measurements updated

**Enter today's weight:**      **lbs**

Last recorded weight: 178 lbs on 1/01/2019

| Other Measurements | Last Entry | Today's Entry |
|---|---|---|
| Neck | None | |
| Waist | None | |
| Hips | None | |

## Message Boards

With over 25 million users on this site, you can imagine how active the message board is! The MFP message board is laid out in forum fashion just like the forums I grew up in. There are 15 forums on the message board:

- Introduce Yourself
- Getting Started
- General Health, Fitness, and Diet
- Goal: Maintaining Weight
- Goal: Gaining Weight and Body Building
- Success Stories
- Food and Nutrition
- Fitness and Exercise
- Motivation and Support
- Recipes
- Challenges

- Debate: Health and Fitness
- Chit-Chat
- Fun & Games

Every single forum gets numerous new posts every day. This makes for a very fun experience. The tone of the forums is just as laid-back as the entire MFP website. Every dieter can get invaluable insight by perusing the forums. You'll see a recurring theme that weight loss is a real struggle for most people, and failure is common. The problem is that most people simply don't have a good plan for weight loss; they try what's popular and don't follow through.

## Bottom Line

MyFitnessPal is an outstanding portal for tracking weight, food intake, and exercise and for getting support while you lose weight. You'll need to make sure your devices are compatible, but it seems like MFP is designed for all smartphones (i.e., iOS and Android) as well as computers (e.g., Mac and PC). Get comfortable with the trackers and forums and you'll be well on your way to successful weight loss and maintenance. I doubt you'll be disappointed.

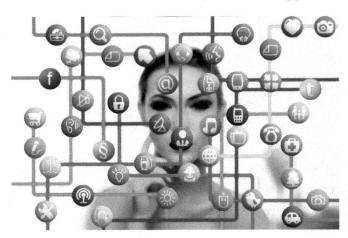

## Runners Up

In case you don't like SparkPeople or MyFitnessPal, there are a couple other weight loss apps worth taking a look at.

- FatSecret.com has been around for over 10 years. It's available for computers and devices. FatSecret has great calorie-counting tools as well as weight and fitness trackers, community support, and lots of free information. FatSecret is the number one choice of calorie counting apps for industrial hygienists (Moore, 2019).

- FitDay.com is one of the older calorie calculators. I've used it since 2010. It has everything you need, but the forums lack participation, and the website is a bit clunky. It's totally free and adequate for what we need. Check it out; maybe there's something you like better than the others.

- Fitbit.com is predominately used for tracking fitness (e.g., steps and heart rate), but it also provides apps for scanning food barcodes, taking pictures of food for logging purposes, and calorie and weight trackers. If you already have an account and you're comfortable with it, use it. The social aspect of Fitbit is done by connecting on Facebook. I'd recommend joining the forums at SparkPeople or MFP if you use a Fitbit to get the full experience of community support.

- Loseit.com is only available for smartphones (Android and iOS). It's a simpler version of MyFitnessPal with fewer options, but many people like its food tracking system that uses barcodes, pictures, or manual entries. It has a feature that lets you search for nearby restaurants as well. LoseIt has a forum, but it has much less activity compared to SparkPeople and MyFitnessPal. As this app is relatively new, you can expect glitches and changes, many of the tabs throughout the app say, "Coming soon." If you are looking for a phone-based calorie-tracking app only, have a look.

## Conclusion

These websites/apps will complement your self-directed weight loss diet very well. They fill in the blanks you miss when you merely read a book or try to watch what you eat. I'm not kidding you on this: your diet stands a 95% chance of failing if you don't carefully track what you eat, weigh yourself, and connect with other dieters. Using apps designed exactly for this purpose will give you the best chance of losing weight. This is not a suggestion—this is a *requirement* for weight loss. If you still aren't convinced, write down the food you eat in a day, take a guess at the calorie count, and then plug the foods into a calorie tracker and compare the results. Hardly anyone can guess at calories within a 30% accuracy. A difference of 500 calories per day will mean the difference in weight loss or gain over a week's time when you are on a diet.

# CHAPTER 18

# OFF-THE-GRID WEIGHT LOSS DIETS

**TL;DR:** *If you want to lose weight without using the internet or a smartphone, read a couple good books first. Have a plan. Good luck.*

Let's say you hate computers and still use a flip phone. How in the world will you lose weight if you can't get online? It will be hard, but you can probably do it. Back in the day, before the internet, it was all done by the book. The "original gangsters" of diet, Weight Watchers and Slimming World, both realized that dieters also needed support and devised programs where members met weekly to discuss their progress. But countless millions of people just read diet books to lose weight without using a support network. Did it work? Not very well. But maybe *you* can make it work.

## Pick a Diet, Any Diet!

In the '60s, '70s, and '80s, dieters were *desperate* for help. This was the era that brought us aspartame, fenfluramine, and Ayds—the appetite suppressing candy. Diet books made their authors millionaires. Anyone over 50 will recognize most of these popular diets:

- *The Drinking Man's Diet* (1965), 2.4 million sold
- *The Stillman Diet* (1967), 2 million sold
- *The Pritikin Program* (1975), 10 million sold
- *The Complete Scarsdale Medical Diet* (1978), 21 million sold
- *Dr. Atkins' Diet Revolution* (1981), 10 million sold
- *Fit for Life* (1986), 12 million sold

Those diets are still probably just as good as today's top-selling diets:

- *Food Rules: An Eater's Manual* (2010)
- *Perfect Health Diet* (2013)
- *Wheat Belly* (2014)
- *Whole30* (2015)
- *The Complete Ketogenic Diet for Beginners* (2016)
- *The Setpoint Diet* (2018)

People are suckers for new diets. Everyone wants to lose weight without trying *too* hard, even though we all know down deep that all you really need to do is eat less. But that's not quite true either, is it?

As we've already discussed, diets need to follow a pattern that involves decreasing calories, providing support and education, increasing physical fitness, and providing personalized advice. Diet books generally just describe a way to eat that results in fewer calories than the Western diet provides. When designed to change the foods most people eat—Big Macs, deep-pan pizza, Big Gulps, and M&M's—it's incredibly easy to craft a diet that will result in quick weight loss. Any diet that gets people away from ultra-processed food will result in weight loss without much effort. The problem is keeping people away from Western foods after the diet becomes a bore.

Book-reading dieters who don't want to use the internet for support and education will have a difficult time trying to make a diet work. You'll still need to set goals, track calories, log your weight, and create a social network to discuss problems and garner support. If you're fiercely independent and don't need much human interaction, perhaps you have what it takes to go it alone.

## Book Reviews

Here are a couple of standalone diet books that will have all you need to create a weight loss diet without once having to log in to the worldwide web.

### *Live Young Forever: 12 Steps to Optimum Health, Fitness and Longevity* by Jack LaLanne

Jack LaLanne (1914–2011) was one of the fittest men ever to walk the earth. He passed away at age 96 of complications related to pneumonia. As far back as the 1950s, LaLanne was warning about the dangers of eating processed food. LaLanne's book *Live Young Forever* gives numerous life lessons on living, eating, and exercising. It has an extensive section on calories found in whole foods.

> I believe that most foods that have been tampered with or manufactured by man, or even foods that have undergone man's attempt at improvement ... are less than perfect. And, I hasten to say, these foods are in all likelihood bad for our long-term health. What am I talking about? I'm talking about food coloring, preservatives, thickeners, thinners, so-called taste enhancers and the zillion other chemicals thrown into the food we are buying and ingesting every day, week after week, year after year. (LaLanne, 2009)

*Live Young Forever* is a must-read for anyone who wants to develop their own weight loss protocol and maintenance diet. You'll get real-world advice from a 94-year-old titan of health and fitness. No bull, just proven methods.

### *The Primal Blueprint: Reprogram your genes for effortless weight loss, vibrant health, and boundless energy,* by Mark Sisson

Mark Sisson's *The Primal Blueprint* has helped thousands of people escape the dangers of the modern diet. This comprehensive diet book lays out a plan for losing weight and keeping it off through healthy eating, exercise, and lifestyle changes.

> All the answers are found in a set of 10 simple, logical Primal Blueprint diet, exercise, and lifestyle behaviors. Modeling your 21$^{st}$-century life after our primal hunter-gatherer ancestors will help you greatly reduce or eliminate almost all of the disease risk factors that you may falsely blame on genes you inherited from your parents. (Sisson, 2013)

*The Primal Blueprint* will set you on a path for life-long weight stability. After reading this book, you'll not only look forward to eating right and exercising, you'll crave it.

### *Daily Dash for Weight Loss: A Day-By-Day Dash Diet Weight Loss Plan* by Rockford Press

The DASH (Dietary Approaches to Stop Hypertension) diet consistently gets high ratings from diet experts, but there really is no official DASH program, it's mostly done by reading books and following advice. This diet relies on evidence-based dietary guidelines and can help you break free from modern eating patterns.

The DASH diet is promoted by the US National Heart, Lung, and Blood Institute of the National Institutes of Health to prevent and control hypertension. The origin of the DASH diet was a medical research study, described in the Annals of Epidemiology in an article titled, *Rationale and design of the Dietary Approaches to Stop*

*Hypertension trial (DASH): A multicenter controlled-feeding study of dietary patterns to lower blood pressure* (1995).

> By developing dietary habits that promote long-term and slow but steady weight loss, the DASH diet can help you lose weight and keep it off while also helping you reduce your blood pressure. (Rockford Press, 2014)

A wonderful side effect of the DASH diet is controlled weight loss. You'll find dozens of books that describe the DASH diet, but the one I've recommended here is the best I've seen. It details the exercise you need, includes food and exercise logs, and has a massive recipe section for healthy eating.

### *The 20/20 Diet: Turn Your Weight Loss Vision into Reality* by Phil McGraw

Yes, *I'm* recommending a Dr. Phil book. He's a smart guy who's helping millions of people every day—his diet book is no exception. You'll quickly realize this ain't Dr. Phil's first rodeo when you read his advice on eating, exercising, and living.

> You've got to stop being a sucker! People can tell you, "Eat everything you want and lose weight!" Come on, really?! Or they'll tell you about the new fad "kumquat soup diet" or "cabbage and cardboard diet." If you believe all of that, then you are a "Double D": dumb and desperate. That is the wrong kind of Double D. You know better (McGraw, 2015).

The *20/20 Diet* is more than silly Dr. Phil-isms, it has shopping lists, exercise programs, and real-world advice for losing weight and keeping it off. If you like Dr. Phil, you'll love this book. If you don't like him, you'll be rolling your eyes on nearly every page. Dr. Phil says, "never miss a good chance to shut up." I think I'll do just that.

### *The Mayo Clinic Diet, 2nd Edition* **by Donald Hensrud**

The first edition of The Mayo Clinic Diet was published in 1949, written by a group of doctors from the Mayo Clinic. Over the last 60 years, numerous unofficial knockoffs have been written, but in 2017, a second edition was released along with a companion book, *The Mayo Clinic Diet Journal.* The diet promises a 6–10-pound weight loss in the first two weeks by changing your eating and lifestyle habits. This Mayo Clinic Diet is designed for people to safely lose up to 100 pounds in a year through diet, exercise, and lifestyle.

Before you start, take these steps (Hensrud, 2017):

- Know the plan.
- Pick a start date.
- Ready your kitchen.
- Line up your gear.
- Set up a tracking system.
- Get mentally prepared.

Sound familiar? The Mayo Clinic Diet is a tried-and-true weight loss method that uses most of the elements I describe throughout this book. It will never be as popular as keto, but it works.

## Make a Plan and Stick to It

Get all five books or just one. The secrets to weight loss and lifelong weight stability are hidden within the covers. But don't think you can just read a book and pull this off without a hitch. You'll need a good plan.

Most of these books will urge you to take some action before starting the diet. Take their advice. If you want to lose weight on your own, you'll need to work harder than people who are doing this through a guided program.

At a minimum:

- Start weighing yourself and keep a log.
- Come up with some reasonable goals.
- Discuss your plan with your doctor.
- Keep a food log and track your calories, at least for a while.
- Start an exercise program.

While this looks like a recipe for weight loss disaster, if you aren't willing to get online to track calories or meet with other people, you'll *have* to do it this way. Reading some or all the aforementioned books will greatly improve your odds of success.

## Conclusion

Old-school weight loss is tough. Many millions try to lose weight by watching what they eat, exercising, or attempting to diet in a certain way without really understanding the basics of dieting. This method works rarely if ever. If for some reason you don't have access to the internet, you'll have to find a way to track calories, make logs, meet people, and get support on your own. Perhaps you can find a local weight loss support group. Start your diet by reading some good diet books. The five I reviewed above are all excellent choices. If you can't be bothered to at least get a couple books to read, then as Dr. Phil would say, "How's that working for you?"

# CHAPTER 19

# THE ART OF COUNTING CALORIES

**TL;DR:** *Counting calories is a lost art form among dieters. Learn to do it the correct way to reap the rewards.*

Losing weight requires a hypocaloric diet (Nackers, 2013). This means eating less food so that your body must tap into its own fat stores for energy. Any diet that promises you will lose weight without counting calories relies on the *hope* that you will eat less *spontaneously*. Most people who are eating the standard Western diet will ingest fewer calories when they stop eating things like cake, ice cream, cookies, and fast food. Whole, unprocessed food is more filling than ultra-processed food. Many dieters find they can, indeed, lose weight without counting calories. But many dieters also find that their weight loss stalls ("plateaus") after a couple months and long before they are at their desired weight. When this happens, it pays to start counting calories to ensure continued weight loss.

## Why Calories Get Such a Bad Rap

No diet plan currently on the market discusses "calories." They talk instead in terms of points, portions, carbs, fats, or allowable foods. This is all just a ruse to make calorie counting easier. The calorie content of a given food is a terrible way to judge its healthfulness. For example, 100 calories of ice cream in no way equals the nutritional value of 100 calories worth of baked salmon.

Here's a striking comparison between a small potato, 6 teaspoons of sugar, and 1 tablespoon of olive oil. Each contains very close to 100 calories.

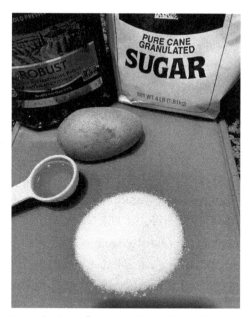

*100 calories of sugar, olive oil, and potato*

The small potato weighs 98 grams (3.5 ounces); it's quite small. Nutritionally, it looks like this:

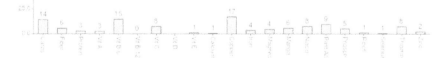

*Nutritional Value of 100 Calories of Potato (FitDay.com)*

This tiny potato contains small amounts of the vitamins, minerals, and fiber we need to be healthy humans. Contrast this to 100 calories worth of sugar:

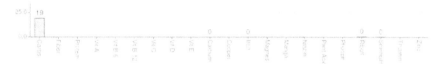

*Nutritional Value of 100 Calories of White Sugar (FitDay.com)*

As you see, sugar contains virtually zero nutritional value, similar to olive oil:

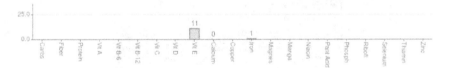

*Nutritional Value of 100 Calories of Olive Oil*

Most restaurants now display the calorie contents of their food on the menu to help people make "*healthier*" choices. But as you see, calories are not indicative of the *healthfulness* of a food item. However, once you've successfully weaned yourself from suckling at the teat of Big Food, you can use calories as a guide to eating just the right amount of food for a successful weight loss diet.

Counting calories and eating Big Macs, shakes, and fries is not a diet that *I* want to be associated with. People who eat healthy food and track calories are all but guaranteed success in weight loss (Nackers, 2013). Therefore, I highly encourage you to learn to count calories to ensure you are eating just the right amount of food for your weight loss needs.

## What Is a Calorie?

The energy available in food is measured in calories. A calorie is the amount of energy contained within a food item that when burned, will raise the temperature of 1 kilogram of water 1°C. Originally, calories were measured by surrounding encapsulated food with water and lighting the food on fire then measuring the temperature of the water. This device, called a bomb-calorimeter, was quite accurate, but cumbersome to use. Today, calories are not measured but estimated using the average values of calories based on standardized charts. This is called the Atwater method, and it's subject to vast interpretation (Zou, 2007). The calories listed in charts and on labels can be off by 5–20%, making it even harder to use calories for weight loss. But the studious dieter can still count calories with great success if they focus more on their weight and on food quality than on calories.

## Counting Calories Correctly

Counting calories 10–20 years ago was incredibly more difficult than it is today. Smartphones and computer programs have taken most of the guesswork out of calorie counting. There are apps that let you take a picture of your plate of food and will calculate the calories for you. There are many calorie-tracking apps and programs that will keep a running tab of calories and help you to choose the best foods to keep from exceeding your calorie goals. We discussed several of these apps and programs in Chapter 8, so please review.

Once you've decided on a method for counting calories, you must be diligent to accurately weigh the food you eat. Here are some "tools of the trade" for calorie counters:

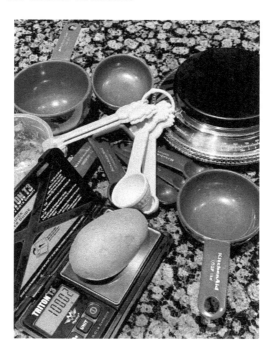

Most calorie counting apps will ask for the weight or amount of food in standard measurements such as cups, spoons, grams, etc. Having a digital scale and some measuring devices will help you learn portion sizes and calorie contents of the food you eat. At the very least, doing these calorie measurements will open your eyes to why you may have gained weight in the first place!

*Pro Tip: Round UP when measuring food and calories.*

Yes, counting calories is an extreme inconvenience. It's no way to live. But counting calories is the only *true* way to ensure you are eating a hypocaloric diet *required* for weight loss. Even diets that don't officially ask you to count calories (e.g., WW, Slimming World, Atkins, keto) can stop working if you are eating too many of the allowable "unlimited" food selections available. Just visit any weight loss forum and you'll see, people will overeat on any diet when they are not counting calories.

Humans cannot look at a food and guess its calorie content without practice. Just like guessing your speed when driving or knowing what time it is without looking at a clock, there is no way to tell how many calories you eat unless you measure the food and tally the amounts. After many months of practice, it will be easier to limit your food intake by estimation, but savvy weight loss maintainers will always track intake by measuring their food and looking up the calories.

## Putting It All Together

Since the calories found in food are just an estimation, it doesn't pay to design a diet around a calorie chart. And since every person has a unique metabolism and starting point, it doesn't pay to blindly follow advice on calorie needs. Broadly speaking, most people will lose weight if they eat between 1,500 and 2,000 calories per day (Nackers, 2013). Most people will not feel overly deprived eating 2,000 calories per day, especially if they are eating lots of fruit, vegetables, and lean meats. Daily intakes of 1,000–1,200 calories per day will leave most people feeling hungry (even *hangry*!).

My recommendations: *Obese* dieters (based on the BMI chart) should start out at 1,800 calories per day, and *overweight* dieters should start out at 1,500 calories per day. No one should eat less than 1,000 calories per day unless supervised by a doctor.

Since the calories you will be tracking are just an estimation, expect the need for adjustments. Carefully measure your food, and log calories each day using an app of your choice. You should be able to accurately predict a weight loss rate of 1–2 pounds per week. If you are feeling exceptionally hungry and losing more than 3 pounds per week, consider adding 300–500 calories per day. Eating too little can be detrimental to long-term weight loss success (Soeliman, 2014).

If you are losing 1–2 pounds a week at the caloric level you picked, stay this course until weight loss slows or stalls. Reduce daily calorie allowance by 100–200 calories per day to restart stalled weight loss. Remember, most stalls are caused by either eating too much or a slowing metabolism, or both. As you approach your goal weight, you can stop counting calories and just eat intuitively again. If weight starts to creep back up, get out the scales and measuring spoons and get back on track.

## Conclusion

I know I'm going to catch a lot of flak in dieting circles for recommending calorie counting, but this is the only way to create a sustainable hypocaloric diet. If you can find a diet plan that allows you to lose weight by food choice alone, use that method until it stops working. Please don't be lulled into a false sense of security by counting calories without also considering food quality. While you might lose weight eating 1,500 calories worth of double cheeseburgers and Kix cereal, your health will suffer, and you'll quickly become a statistic in the 95% failure rate. In our age of great technology, counting calories has never been easier, especially if you understand that calories are only an estimation and that everyone will react differently. The result we must strive for is sustained weight loss on a true hypocaloric diet.

# CHAPTER 20

# TIM STEELE'S SOW DIET

**TL;DR:** *Try Tim Steele's SOW Diet: eliminate sugar, oil, and wheat (SOW) for effortless weight loss and lifelong weight stability.*

What would a book called *The Diet Hack* be without a brand-new diet? Well, here's a little something I've been playing with for a couple years. This diet was hatched one afternoon while I was camping with an old friend who was struggling with his weight. He wasn't big on computers or organized dieting. I said to him, "Mac, if you'd just avoid sugar, oil, and wheat you would probably lose weight." We then spent several days discussing it and came up with the acronym "SOW" as a quick reminder of what not to eat. When I saw Mac a year later, he'd lost a good 50 pounds and looked great. He gave me a thumbs-up and said one word, "SOW." Since then, I've put dozens of people on a similar trajectory, and they all lose weight.

If you need to lose weight, give this a try. Like I warn throughout the book, don't diet if you don't *have to*. If your BMI, waist measurement, and lab results (cholesterol, glucose, etc.) are in a healthy range, but you still want to drop a few pounds, then start at Month 3.

The SOW Diet provides adequate protein to prevent loss of muscle and lean body mass. There's also a once-a-week "cheat meal" to keep the metabolism from slowing down during the caloric restriction phase. This diet incorporates exercise proven to aid weight loss. Additionally, the calorie allowances are based on your weight and results. Calories never get so low that your metabolism suffers. Support and tracking of key items are included as well. This diet has everything that the most effective diets have, with no membership fees. If you are totally lost in picking a plan, try my SOW Diet.

## Tim Steele's SOW Diet: Lose 20 pounds in the 1st 30 Days!⁶

| Tim Steele's SOW Diet | | | | | |
|---|---|---|---|---|---|
| Phase | Avoid | Calories/ Day | Fiber/ Protein | Cheat Day | Exercise |
| Month 1 Sowing the seeds of successful weight loss | **No:** Added sugar, added oil, or wheat | 1,500–1,800 (based on starting weight) | **Fiber:** 20g+ daily / **Protein:** 80–100g/ day | +500–750 cal. Consisting of: Meat, potatoes, brown rice, beans, bananas | Walk 30 minutes every day |
| Month 2 Active weight loss | **No:** Processed food with added sugar, oil, *or* wheat **OK:** Natural sugar Olive oil Whole wheat | 1,500–1,800 (based on weight) | **Fiber:** 30g+ daily / **Protein:** 80–100g/ day | +500–750 cal. Consisting of: Meat, dairy, potatoes, rice, beans, fruit, beer/ wine | Walk 60 minutes 3–6 days per week |

---

6   **Maybe, maybe not … it sounds good!**

| Tim Steele's SOW Diet | | | | | |
|---|---|---|---|---|---|
| **Phase** | **Avoid** | **Calories/ Day** | **Fiber/ Protein** | **Cheat Day** | **Exercise** |
| **Month 3 Active weight loss** | **No:** Processed foods with added sugar, oil, *or* wheat **OK:** Natural sugar Olive oil Whole wheat | 1,500– 2,200 (based on weight and progress) | **Fiber:** 30g+ daily <br><br> **Protein:** 80–100g/ day | +500–750 cal. Consisting of: Meat, dairy, potatoes, rice, beans, fruit, pasta, whole-grain bread, beer/wine | Walk 30–60 minutes each day One strength training session per week |
| **Month 4 Transition month** | **No:** Processed foods with added sugar, oil, *and* wheat **Avoid:** Artificial colors, flavors, or sweeteners | 1,500– 2,500 (based on weight and progress) | **Fiber:** 20–40g daily <br><br> **Protein:** 50–100g/ day | May be used if desired Whole foods only! | Daily walking. One strength training session per week One vigorous aerobic session per week |
| **Month 5 Lifelong maintenance diet** | **Limit:** Processed foods with added sugar, oil, *and* wheat **Avoid:** Artificial colors, flavors, or sweeteners | 1,500– 3,000 (based on weight and goals) | **Fiber:** 20–40g daily <br><br> **Protein:** 50–100g/ day | As desired | Daily walking 1–3 times weekly strength training 1–3 times weekly aerobic training |

## Sleep and Stress

On the SOW Diet, you're encouraged to:

- Sleep at least 8 hours a night in a sleep-friendly environment.
- Omit alcohol/cannabis completely during the first three months.
- Worry less.

## Keep Some Logs

### Daily Logs

- Using MyFitnessPal's free trackers, log your *daily* food intake, exercise, and weight.
- Optional: Using a large wall calendar, place an X on every day that you exercised and ate according to plan.

**Monthly Logs** (Using a piece of paper and pencil or computer spreadsheet.)

- Record your waist measurement.
- Record your weight. Indicate change from previous month.
- Make notes of weights used in strength training and speed/duration of aerobics workouts, average walking, etc.
- Optional: Record the number of X's from your calendar.
- Optional: Record your average hours of sleep for the month.

### Yearly Logs

- Record weight and waist measurement.
- Keep records of medications, blood lab reports, doctor visits, and any illnesses through the year.
- Develop a plan for the following year.

**Get Support**

- Join the forum at MyFitnessPal, SparkPeople, FitDay, or any you prefer.
- Start a thread called "Tim Steele's SOW Diet Results."
- Discuss your amazing weight loss and fitness gains.
- Help others to lose weight by *SOW*ing the seeds of weight loss success.
- Optional: If you are anti-computer, find some other people to join you on this journey. Spouse, girlfriend, boyfriend, coworkers are all good support options.

Wouldn't this make an awesome book? The free infographics write themselves. I can already see a need for calendars, weight logs, fitness logs, apps, shirts, cookbooks, and maybe even home-delivered SOW-free Chow. Until then, just enjoy this free preview.

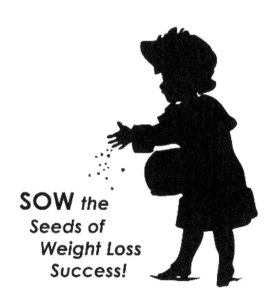

**SOW** *the* Seeds of Weight Loss Success!

## Sugar, Oil, Wheat

Avoiding SOW will help you *sow* the seeds of successful weight loss. SOW stands for sugar, oil, and wheat. The SOW Diet doesn't limit real food, just processed foods that contain SOW. Avoiding these easily identifiable ingredients is easier than trying to adhere to a list of *allowable* foods. Eat what you want with the SOW Diet; just don't eat SOW.

Ultra-processed foods *nearly all* contain a mixture of SOW. These three cheap ingredients form the basis of 90% of the *worst* foods in the world (Kearny, 2010). If you are eating the Western diet, undoubtedly most of what you eat contains sugar, oil, and/or wheat. To make *food* out of SOW, all the tricks of ultra-processing are used. These foods also contain artificial colors, flavors, preservatives, emulsifiers, and other chemicals used to turn tasteless ingredients into addictive, shelf-stable food. This processing destroys any nutritive qualities of the food and destroys gut integrity of those who eat the food (Aguayo-Patrón, 2017).

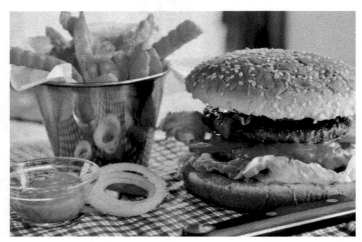

*SOW Foods*

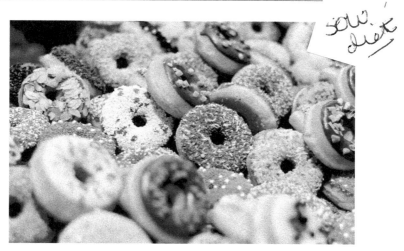

*SOW Foods*

Compared to the Western diet, the SOW Diet is filled with vegetables, fruits, fungi, fermented food, whole grains, potatoes, legumes, fish, poultry, eggs, honey, and contains moderate amounts of red meat, healthy oils, bread, and alcoholic beverages. What you won't find is ultra-processed food that contains a mixture of SOW. Exercise and a healthy lifestyle are intertwined with the SOW Diet.

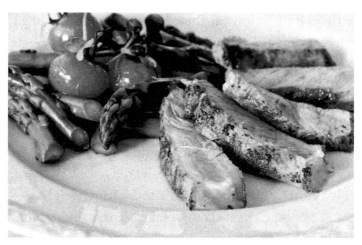

*SOW Diet Approved*

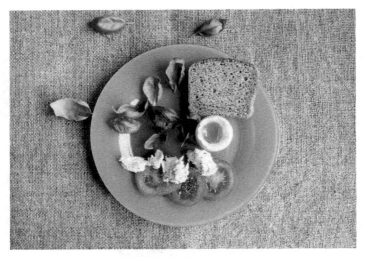

*SOW Diet Approved*

## Conclusion

The SOW Diet is as real as any diet, and it's better than most. Try it as outlined. It combines elements of *Wheat Belly*, *McDougall's Starch Solution*, *The Case Against Sugar*, and the *Mediterranean Diet*. This diet removes the three worst offenders of the Western diet but lets you add them back as long as they don't contain SOW (e.g., Krispy Kreme donuts, Wonder bread, and thousands of other Western diet staples). Avoiding this *specific combination* will help you avoid 90% of the worst foods on earth. This combination, especially when prepared with emulsifiers, chemicals, and refined beyond recognition, is highly inflammatory and damages the immune system and gut. Removing this unholy trio will result in rapid weight loss as the body rids itself of excess water and fat. A long-term diet devoid of Western staples will result in a return to good health and lasting weight loss. Extra protein and periodic cheat days will ensure metabolic success. You have my money-back guarantee! It's even keto-compatible.

# CONCLUSION TO PART 2

That was a lot to take in, I know. I hope I entertained and informed you on the current state of dieting, how to lose weight safely and efficiently, and how to create your own diet should you not want to try a commercial program.

The Diet Industry is a real mess. You don't know who to believe. You don't *want* to think they are intentionally misleading you, either. But, oh, they are. Big Diet's number one concern is attracting new customers. With 150 million potential clients, commercial diet programs have less than 8% of the market share. They want all 150 million and will do whatever it takes to get them. Some diet giants, like WW, spend billions to rebrand and keep up with the technology to attract new dieters. Others, like Slimming World and Atkins, are still around after nearly half a century because they get results. The rest spend millions on viral advertising to attract people to a program that won't work.

Then there are the books and websites. Thousands and thousands of them. Every single one is just a rehashing of three basic diets (low-carb, low-fat, balanced). The good ones also discuss exercise and lifestyle modifications. The really good ones focus on eating healthy foods, keeping logs, and creating a social network. Without all these elements, a diet will fail quickly. And beware the fads. Watch how quickly "keto" fades away after the next diet boom hits. But never fear, it'll be back!

Weight loss does not need to be a career, just a summer job. Lose weight, then transition to a healthier way of eating. Never, ever go back to eating the Western diet. You can get away with eating a handful of Oreos now and then, but you can't get away with eating KFC or Wendy's for lunch every day. Hamburger Helper isn't helping anybody. Learn to feed yourself from a list of unprocessed foods—you'll never look back.

# PART 3

# WEIGHT MAINTENANCE, THE LONGEST ~~MILE~~ POUND

# INTRODUCTION TO PART 3

Perhaps you've jumped to this section in the book because you've already lost weight but are now having trouble keeping it off. Or maybe you are taking my advice to skip weight loss dieting altogether if you don't need to lose very much. I've written this section as a standalone resource, so reading the entire book is not required. It would be helpful, though, since much of the advice builds upon the descriptions used in Part 1 and the efforts used to lose weight in Part 2.

Researchers have long noted that weight *loss* and weight *maintenance* are two separate issues, and both have unique needs. Maintaining your weight after dieting is a struggle with an extremely high failure rate ... more than 95% of dieters will regain most or all the weight they've lost within five years. Many will gain even *more* than they lost (Fildes, 2015). This has not gone unnoticed. Big Pharma loves it; they are busily developing drugs to aid in weight stability. Big Diet loves it because it makes you a repeat customer. Big Food loves that you hungrily purchase anything with a healthy label on it. Your doctor doesn't like it, but you'd never know it.

Several landmark studies have examined thousands of dieters who managed to keep their weight off for longer than five years. They found several commonalities. Successful maintainers have used the following tactics (alone or in combination) to keep their weight off long-term (Turk, 2009) (Soeliman, 2014) (Champagne, 2011) (Montesi, 2016) (Astrup, 2017):

- Consuming healthier food
- Drinking fewer sugar-sweetened beverages
- Exercising
- Getting more sleep

- Increasing fiber intake
- Increasing protein intake
- Low-carb diets
- Low-fat diets
- Low intake of fast food
- Intensive dieting therapy
- Self-monitoring weight
- Participating in support groups

Five common themes are noted as reasons for *failure* to maintain weight loss after dieting (Turk, 2009) (Soeliman, 2014) (Champagne, 2011) (Montesi, 2016) (Astrup, 2017):

- Excessive calorie restriction
- Using meal-replacement drinks/bars
- Continuing to use weight loss programs or protocols
- Loss of willpower
- Loss of social support

We'll be discussing these and more in this section. Each chapter will end with an "R for weight maintenance." I've put all the prescriptions together at the end for your convenience. I figured most of the reading audience is used to getting new prescriptions, so here are some you can look forward to for a change.

# CHAPTER 21

# WEIGHT MAINTENANCE/EATING STYLES: TALES OF WOE

**TL;DR:** *Maintaining your weight requires a completely different set of rules. There are many proven eating styles well-suited to lifelong weight stability. Try them all!*

For lifelong weight maintenance, a person needs to get as far away from the Western diet as possible. This means your dietary staples should be real whole foods minimally processed and not filled with stabilizers, colorants, artificial flavors, chemicals, etc. Dieters often refer to these alternate eating styles as WOEs, or ways of eating.

When we hacked into the weight loss programs in Part 2, we explored three different diets (low-carb, low-fat, and balanced meals). During *active weight loss*, it's best to stick with one plan if it's working for you. During *maintenance*, it can benefit you to switch things up periodically. Keep your body guessing. For example, switching between eating lots of carbs then lots of fat ensures you are metabolically flexible. Metabolic flexibility refers to the body's ability to switch between burning fat and carbs with ease. Eating a high-fat/high-carb diet, such as the Western diet, leads to metabolic *inflexibility* and is associated with poor health, insulin resistance, and metabolic syndrome (Galgani, 2008). When transitioning from the Western diet to a weight loss diet and finally a maintenance diet, it's important that you regain metabolic flexibility by including varying amounts of fat and carbs (Grandl et al., 2018).

I am diet-agnostic. I don't know all there is to know, and I don't think anyone else does either. We know more about the universe than we know about the inner workings of our body and nutrition. What I *do* know is that there *are* diets that work great for some and terrible for others. I also know that everyone can find a diet that works for them if they keep an open mind. As Roman poet Lucretius said, "One man's meat is another man's poison."

---

**Weight Loss Industry Insider Secret:** *Throughout the medical literature, a figure of "95%" is widely circulated as the number of diets that fail. Failure in this case means a person isn't "losing weight and keeping it off for more than 5 years." This percentage has been hotly debated for decades since it first appeared in a medical journal in 1959 (Fritsch, 1999). One expert in weight loss claims the number could actually be a bit higher since many diet studies fail to keep long-term records on subjects (Wolpert, 2007). Whether "95%" is the right percentage or not, there's one thing researchers agree on: diets do not normally work to treat obesity (Mann, 2007).*

---

Thousands of studies have been conducted to understand the physics of successful weight loss. A key finding is that to keep the weight off, it's important to switch from a "diet plan" to an "eating style." An oft-cited reason for failure to maintain is, "continued adherence to a strict diet" (Turk, 2009).

Therefore, I think everyone should be encouraged to try any manner of dietary intervention that's proven successful for others. Somewhere in this moveable feast you just might find the perfect diet for *you*. Perhaps it will be due to the food choices, the community of people eating *that* way, or because it *just works*.

This doesn't have to be *and is not supposed to be* hard. It will only be as hard as you make it. Just remember: Don't eat too much and stay away from Western diet, meaning ultra-processed food. But do it with a purpose. "Watching what I eat" is not a valid weight *loss* plan, but it's a perfectly acceptable weight *maintenance* plan. There needs to be balance between obsessing over what you eat and enjoying the way you eat. And don't make yourself a social pariah. No one will fault you for avoiding fried foods, high-sugar desserts, and candy, but you'll not be invited to many parties if you refuse to eat most *normal* food. Find that balance and you'll have it made.

**Eating styles worth exploring for weight maintenance:**

- Carnivore
- Counting calories
- DASH
- High-carb/low-fat
- High-carb/high-fat
- High-protein
- Keto
- Low-carb
- Low-fat
- Mediterranean
- Mostly-plant
- Paleo
- Peasant Diet
- Potato Diet
- Vegan/Vegetarian
- Misc

I'm going to quickly recap each of these eating styles in case you want to try to wing it on your own. I'll also give you a link or two if you'd like to check out a good example. Don't be a fool and spend a lot of money to eat in these styles. These WOEs can all easily be hacked by just surfing the net for a few minutes. Buy a book, sure. But if they ask you to join a special club or buy strange gadgets, then move on. Beware of Facebook ads that tempt you with, "This week I'm giving away a FREE COPY of my [insert diet plan]!"

*Note: I receive zero compensation for the recommendations I've made here.*

**Carnivore:** All you eat is *meat*. This approach is followed by several famous practitioners, including Steve Cooksey, who was taken to court by the North Carolina Board of Dietetics and Nutrition in 2012 for giving advice to diabetics without a license. The courts ruled in Cooksey's favor, and he now dispenses advice for diabetics freely. He recommends ditching all carbs and just eating meat. Watch for the Carnivore Diet to take center stage as the keto movement matures. Steve is one of the nicest people I know—I even pulled him from a raging river in the middle of Alaska one time! Steve cured his own diabetes over ten years ago and regularly updates his blog and stays active on Facebook. Read about his exploits and see his carnivore plan at: www.diabetes-warrior.net.

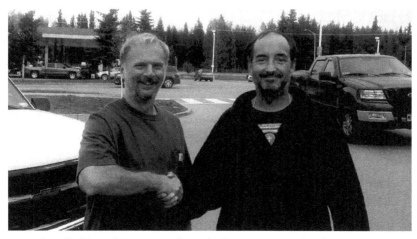

*Author (left) and Steve Cooksey before Steve embarks on his epic Alaskan trip of a lifetime.*

**Counting Calories:** Counting calories, especially when focused on eating healthier food, is one of the best maintenance plans ever devised. It lets you eat whatever you want while limiting how much you eat. SparkPeople has cornered the market in calorie counting for weight maintenance. With their extensive database containing every food imaginable, you'll easily keep within your personalized calorie target each day. Mega-popular message boards, numerous online help features, and apps make SparkPeople a real win for calorie counters. Visit their website at www.sparkpeople.com. There are numerous calorie counting apps available. Find one you like, and start tracking your food for accurate accountability.

**DASH:** DASH stands for Dietary Approaches to Stop Hypertension. This diet was developed by the National Heart, Lung, and Blood Institute, a part of the National Institutes of Health. The DASH diet is designed to be heart-healthy and gets high rankings every year by numerous watchdog groups that rank diets. Since it started as a governmental program, it's hard to access the "real" DASH diet. Instead, there are many *official-looking* descriptions and books found all over the internet. The basis of the DASH diet is eating fruits, vegetables, whole grains, and low-fat dairy foods. It includes meat, fish, poultry, nuts, and beans but is limited in sugar-sweetened foods and beverages, red meat, and added fats. You can read more about the DASH diet at www.dashdiet.org.

**High-Carb/Low-Fat:** Though not in widespread use, HCLF is the traditional diet of many indigenous groups who ate mainly starchy tubers and little meat. The inhabitants of the Ryukyu Islands in Japan ate this way until the 1960s and were noted to live extremely long lives with almost no instances of heart disease or cancer. This is sometimes referred to as the Okinawan diet. Rusty Moore of Visual Impact Fitness teamed up with elite athlete and Olympic trainer Mark Kislich to create a course called High Carb Fat Loss, which outlines a program of eating a diet that is high in starchy carbs and very low in fat. The athletes they train profit from this dieting philosophy and thrive eating this way. This diet is also lower in protein than most dieting approaches. Rusty takes good care of his members and sends tons of free stuff to anyone who buys one of his courses. You'll really feel Rusty is your own personal trainer. Rusty and Mark are very active on Facebook. This "beer and bread friendly" course can be accessed at www.visualimpactfitness.com/high-carb-fat-loss/ and is well worth the $40 or so it will cost to download.

**High-Carb/High-Fat:** Ha! Tricked you. This is the Western diet that got you in trouble in the first place. You can try maintaining your weight on Big Macs and supersized fries, thick chocolate shakes, Pringles, and Ho Hos, but don't come crying to me when it doesn't work. That said, there are millions of people eating this way and not getting fat. What's their secret? No one knows. Maybe it's the special sauce.

**High-Protein:** High-protein diets are very similar to low-carb diets, but they focus more on meat and beans or tofu. Most high-protein diet plans have a "protein needs calculator" to help you determine how much protein you need to eat. The Mayo Clinic says that a high-protein diet "Generally isn't harmful, particularly when followed for a short time. Such diets may help with weight loss by making you feel fuller" (Mayo Clinic, 2018). I recommend you buy a book or research this WOE well before trying to do it on your own. One such plan has been promoted heavily by Drs. Michael and Mary Dan Eades, authors of *Protein Power: The High-Protein/Low Carbohydrate Way to Lose Weight, Feel Fit, and Boost Your Health–in Just Weeks!* (1997). Their book is available wherever books are sold or at www.proteinpower.com.

for ketogenic diet, keto is a fat-centric diet that has seen ...cess when used as a weight loss diet. Most keto programs start as a very strict low-carb diet and then transition to eating more carbs for weight maintenance. Keto is the latest diet craze to hit the internet. There are hundreds of keto diet websites and books. The Atkins Diet is the longest-running and probably the best example of using ketogenic principals for weight loss (www.atkins.com). However, Atkins seems to be distancing themselves from a "keto" label. Beware: keto is the hottest thing at the moment thanks to internet marketers. For the most part, it's all hype. Keto is just a low-carb diet no matter how you slice it. The only thing "special" about the slew of new keto diets is the zealotry by which faddists protect this WOE. Check out www.ketogains.com to see one of the older keto programs.

**Low-Carb:** Low-carb diets work well for weight maintenance. The most effective low-carb maintenance plans allow ample grains, potatoes, fruit, and even alcoholic beverages if the total daily carb count does not exceed a certain amount. Low-carb maintenance diets allow a range of carbs between 50–200g per day. A great example of a long-term maintenance diet using low-carb principals is *The Primal Blueprint* by Mark Sisson (2016), available wherever books are sold. Mark Sisson is a pioneer in clean eating and living. His "carb curve" has been widely copied by other diet programs and can be considered the gold-standard for carb counters. Find loads of free content on healthy eating and low-carb living at www.marksdailyapple.com.

# The Primal Blueprint Carbohydrate Curve

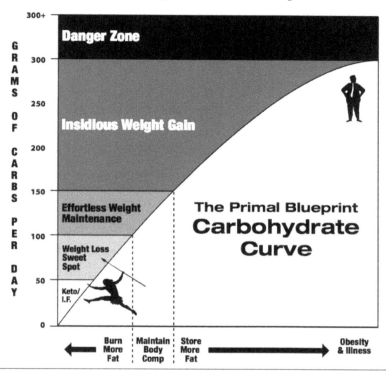

*From www.Marksdailyapple.com*

**Low-Fat:** Low-fat diets had their heyday in the 1970s. This led to an explosion of low-fat cookbooks, diet plans, and foods labeled "low-fat." The expansion of low-carb diets in the '80s and '90s pushed low-fat diets to the sideline, and now you rarely see much mention of low-fat diets. However, reducing dietary fat to below 25% of daily calories can be an extremely effective way to maintain weight loss, especially when there's a focus on eating whole, minimally processed foods. A great example of a healthy low-fat diet for weight maintenance is the Zone Diet® created more than 30 years ago by Dr. Barry Sears. Learn more about the Zone Diet® at www.zonediet.com.

**Mediterranean:** This diet is modeled after the eating styles of people from Greece, Italy, and Spain who enjoy vibrant health eating staples such as pasta, seafood, beans, fruit, vegetables, and olive oil. There aren't many Mediterranean diet "plans," mostly just cookbooks. Most diets (e.g., low-carb, paleo, etc.) can easily be adapted to Mediterranean principals by using the ingredients found in Mediterranean cooking. A bestselling Mediterranean diet cookbook was written by America's Test Kitchen and can be found wherever books are sold: *The Complete Mediterranean Cookbook: 500 Vibrant, Kitchen-Tested Recipes for Living and Eating Well Every Day* (2016).

**Mostly-plant:** A diet of mostly plants with small servings of meat and animal products is well-tolerated by nearly everyone and makes weight maintenance much easier. Many diets (e.g., DASH, Mediterranean, and High-carb/Low-fat) are "mostly-plant" by default. Angelo Coppola of *Humans are not Broken* is developing a Mostly Plant® diet program on his website www.mostlyplant.com. Check it out while it's still free. You can access recipes, the diet rationale, and lots of pictures to make eating mostly-plant a breeze.

**Paleo:** The Paleo Diet© was pioneered by Loren Cordain, author of several books on the subject of Paleolithic cavemen. However, this was a very difficult copyright to protect, and now the term "paleo" is freely used in many diet plans that focus on eating whole, minimally processed foods. Paleo diets can be taken to extremes, asking people to walk barefoot and shun food that was not available 10,000 years ago such as dairy products, grains, or certain plants such as rice and potatoes. Most paleo diets are low-carb by default, since they ban most starchy foods. An effective use of the paleo theme is used by Chris Kresser of the California Center for Functional Medicine. His take on the Paleo Diet is very open-minded and not overly restrictive. He's easily approachable on his wildly popular blog or on Facebook; Kresser also offers clinical services. He has written several books, such as NY Times best seller, *The Paleo Cure*. See Kresser's work at www.chriskresser.com.

**Peasant Diet:** The Peasant Diet recommends eating like a poor person before the Industrial Revolution. Shun Western diet foods and instead fill up on staples that would have been readily available to peasants. Beans, potatoes, whole grains, and other traditional staple foods are both filling and highly nutritious. Make these the base of your food intake for lasting weight loss and great health. A pioneer of the Peasant Diet is Michael Allen Smith, who writes about his dieting adventures at www.criticalmas.org.

**Potato Diet:** Diets that focus on potatoes have blossomed recently. You all know about my book, *The Potato Hack: Weight Loss Simplified*, but there's another famous spuddy who's been really making headway—Andrew "Spudfit" Taylor. Andrew famously spent an entire year eating nothing but potatoes. Go check him out at www.spudfit.com. He's written two great books, *The DIY Spudfit Challenge* and the *Spudfit Cookbook*. WOEs that use potatoes as staples are almost guaranteed to result in lasting weight stability.

**Vegan:** Veganism started in England in the 1940s as a protest of the exploitation of farm animals. Veganism is still a popular diet but is not known as a weight loss or weight maintenance diet unless principals of calorie restriction or certain food avoidance (e.g., refined oils) are applied. There are low-carb, low-fat, paleo, Mediterranean, etc. versions of the vegan diet suitable for long-term weight loss. You can easily find many books and websites devoted to vegan eating. One immensely popular and effective vegan weight maintenance plan was written by Dr. John McDougall. McDougall has trained thousands of health coaches using the methods he outlines in his NY Times best seller, *The Starch Solution* (2013). His program books can be found on his website: www.drmcdougall.com.

**Miscellaneous:** There are dozens of variations of all of these diets you might find useful. For instance, whole-food diets are quite popular, as are plant-based diets. There are diets that advocate eating just one type of meat—such as the pescatarian diet, where only fish is consumed. Lacto-ovo vegetarian diets allow dairy and eggs, but no other animal products. The only diets I advise *against* are diets that are extremely restrictive in food choices. These usually do not make good long-term eating plans but can be fun to try for short periods. A program such as Jenny Craig where all your food is delivered to your house, doesn't work out in the long-term because it gets too expensive, or you get bored with the choices. Also, any diet that uses meal-replacement shakes, drinks, or bars is not a viable long-term solution.

## Woe Is Me

Let me tell you about all the different styles of eating I tried in *my* weight loss journey. During my active weight loss, I started out using an unstructured low-carb approach ("watched what I ate"), but I realized I was eating really bad Western diet foods, so I switched to low-carb paleo. After a few months, I hit a weight plateau and went even lower in carbs, adopting a keto diet approach. The keto diet helped to restart my weight loss again, but it left me feeling cold and drained. My workouts suffered, so I switched to a higher-carb Mediterranean diet and counted my calories. On the Mediterranean diet, I finally achieved my goal weight. I continued eating this way for several years. The past two years I have been eating a high-carb low-fat diet with periods of eating in the spirit of the DASH diet and the Mediterranean diet. I don't think it pays to eat one way forever, I like the olive oil, grains, and seafood of the Mediterranean diet, but I also like to eat lower fat, too.

The only diet I will NOT try again is the Western diet. I can count on one hand the number of fast-food meals I've eaten over the last five years. I've not had a soda pop in years, nor do I eat anything that's been breaded and deep-fried. I'll eat a cookie on occasion, a handful of potato chips, and even a couple slices of pizza now and then, but I like my food to be whole and minimally processed. It makes me feel great, and I don't worry that I'm eating too much. It feels amazing to be a long-term weight loss maintainer. I hope you get the chance as well.

## Case Study #1: Former Vegan and Low-Carber Finds Her Groove with a High-Carb Low-Fat Pescatarian Diet ... and Potatoes

Kate Ann is a popular figure in Facebook diet and fitness circles. She's a critical thinker who loves to discuss diet and fitness tips and strategies with others. Kate Ann was a vegetarian for many years, thinking it was the healthiest approach to eating. Eventually she found herself weak and didn't like looking "skinny fat." Kate Ann thereafter became a zealous proponent of very low-carb dieting after reading Gary Taubes' *Good Calories, Bad Calories* and vociferously defended that WOE for several years. She ultimately found after two and a half years of adherence that the long-term outcome of a very-low-carb diet was not what she expected.

Kate Ann's goal was achieving a lean, athletic physique and having constant satiety and energy; both vegetarianism and zero carb have failed her in those regards. In typical Kate Ann fashion, she did a complete 180 and has for the past several years been eating a high-carb low-fat (HCLF) diet that contains roughly 75% carbs, 20% protein, and 5–6% fat. One interesting twist on Kate Ann's diet is that she eats nearly the same thing day after day, using an intermittent fasting approach by eating in an eight-hour window. This allows her to effortlessly track calories and macronutrient ratios. Kate Ann avoids metabolic inflexibility by including weekly to bi-monthly sushi feasts, her favorite "cheat day" food.

She enjoys lifting heavy in the gym and performs low-intensity steady-state (LISS) cardio. She has finally achieved her goal physique along with easy satiety and energy on HCLF. She is renowned on Facebook for her love of boiled potatoes, which form the largest part of her diet. We can learn a lot from Kate Ann's daily meals. Berries, potatoes, Cream of Rice, cinnamon, and fish provide Kate Ann with nutrient density and ample fiber:

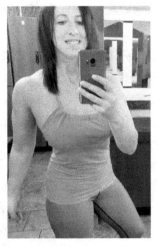

*Kate Ann's High-Carb Physique*

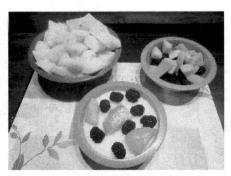

*Kate Ann's Typical Dinner: Boiled Potatoes, Cream of Rice, Berries, and Melon*

## Case Study #2: Michael Allen Smith's Peasant Diet

Michael Allen Smith is a successful weight loss maintainer. He's also very successful in other parts of his life. As a web developer, "MAS" operates five or six different websites at any one time and still has time to keep up with current trends in the diet and fitness industries. MAS has tried every diet in the world, it seems. He has maintained his weight over many years using proven techniques such as intermittent fasting, low-carb, high-carb, and others. He documents his weight loss and maintenance journey on his Critical MAS blog (www.criticalmas.org) and is never afraid to tell people when he gets something wrong or tries something new.

Switching between eating styles seems to be discouraged in dieting circles, especially by diet gurus who will have you believe there is no other way than theirs. MAS is a totally different kind of guru. He'll lead you to a diet plan and let you decide whether it's for you or not. MAS' current diet is what he calls a Peasant Diet:

- No processed foods. A peasant is not the same thing as a modern poor person. A peasant chooses to consume boiled potatoes and black coffee, where a poor person might eat French fries and drink Mountain Dew.

- High-volume, low-calorie food. Foods with high volume and fiber reduce hunger at a lower calorie level.

- Missing meals. Since willpower is not unlimited, many find it easier to skip breakfast or dinner rather than reduce calories at every meal. Plus, being exposed to missing the occasional meal teaches you how to respond better to hunger and make better decisions. This is why so many people have success with intermittent fasting.

- No snacking. A peasant isn't sitting around snacking. Snacking can make you heavy or reduce the odds you are able to lose weight.

- Very little flavor novelty. Reducing flavor novelty reduces the entertainment value of eating, which lowers appetite.

- Financially rewarding. My waist gets smaller, and I have more money left over at the end of the week. It is like I'm being paid to lose weight. I win twice.

Visit MAS on his blog to learn more. We can learn a lot about successful weight maintenance by looking at what he typically eats:

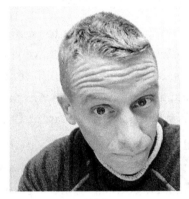

*MAS*

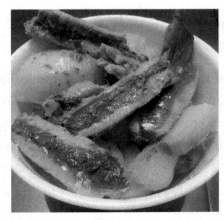

*Critical MAS' Peasant Breakfast: Plain Boiled Potatoes and Sardines*

R for weight maintenance #1: Research, then try several different ways of eating during your first year of maintenance. This will help you find an eating style that is right for you and will ensure metabolic flexibility.

# CHAPTER 22

# WEIGHT MAINTENANCE TIPS AND TRICKS

**TL;DR:** *Track your weight, count calories, and play around with meal frequency and size of meals.*

*Maintaining* your weight long-term is much harder than *losing* weight. Statistically, 95% of people who lose 10 pounds or more will gain it all back within 1–5 years (Poulimeneas, 2018). I guess I'm an oddball. I lost about 90 pounds in 2011 and have kept most of it off ever since. I started that diet at 250 lbs and ended at 160 lbs. Then I started exercising and lifting weights and now maintain my weight around 180 lbs (I'm 5'11", if you wondered). But this isn't about *me*, it's about *you*. And *you* need to have a plan. Most people don't. Once they lose some weight, they return to their old patterns of eating, and the cycle repeats.

Let's talk about exercise, sleep, stress, and some other things that help with long-term weight control. In "Part 1" I described how all these different inputs affect your weight and health; now I'll be shifting to more practical ideas on how you can leverage this insider information to your advantage.

First, I want to show you a chart that examines the obesity epidemic. You'll notice that the number of overweight people has remained fairly constant over the last 54 years, but the number of *obese* people has skyrocketed. This didn't come about because people simply started eating too much, it was a combination of factors, many of them completely out of our control. I shudder to think what this graph will look like 50 years from now, but quite possibly people are starting to catch on and the number of obese people will sink back to pre-1976 levels.

In this chapter, I'm going to discuss the "low-hanging fruit" of weight maintenance.

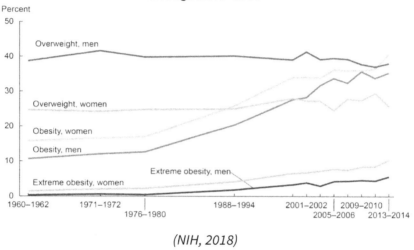

**Trends in adult overweight, obesity, and extreme obesity among men and women aged 20–74: United States, 1960–1962 through 2013–2014**

*(NIH, 2018)*

## Weigh-ins

After losing body fat, one of the best ways to keep your new, lower weight is to periodically weigh yourself. During your weight loss phase, you came up with a target weight. Hopefully you hit it. Many people find their target weight was too easy and go on to lose even more. Conversely, it's easy to diet down to a weight that's unsustainable and you gain some back. Wherever you ended up, you'll find it's nearly impossible to stay at the bottom. Strict weight loss diets usually also cause you to lose some muscle, or maybe you didn't have much lean body mass to begin with. Either way, you'll find that once you lose considerable weight, you'll be more active and if you are doing this right, you'll gain strength, endurance, and muscle. Muscle weighs more than fat, so don't be shocked to see the scale creeping back up over the first couple years as you gain muscle. Muscle builds slowly, though, so be careful … maybe it's not all muscle-weight you're gaining. A good sign that you are doing everything right is revealed when you gain weight but your clothes get looser. This is a sure sign you've lost fat but gained muscle.

If you've struggled with your weight for a long time or you've been a yo-yo dieter in the past, there's nothing wrong with weighing yourself daily. So often I see diet gurus telling people to "ditch the scale!" or "forget the numbers!" I think they are saying this because they want to keep you as a faithful follower as long as they can, and they know that if you see the scale moving upward, you'll abandon their flock. I think the best plan is to fully understand your weight fluctuations. It's rare that a person's weight doesn't fluctuate normally through the course of a day, week, month, and year. To ignore your weight is a recipe for disaster.

Weighing yourself periodically is a feature of some of the best diet programs. Weight Watchers (now WW) gives its members perks if they come to meetings (or online) for periodic weigh-ins. If they maintain the weight loss, they become a "Lifetime Member," and may even get a little trinket to help celebrate the occasion. The prerequisite for becoming a coveted Lifetime Member is keeping your weight within a four-pound band or not straying from your target weight by more than two pounds. I suspect that many people slide out of range and give up on WW after a few years. They don't publicize how many Lifetime Members there are or give statistics to show how many people maintain this elite status for several years. But the fact is, the weigh-ins of WW are a very effective tool for the weight maintenance phase of dieters choosing this plan. If you aren't an official weight watcher, you can still weigh yourself to track your progress.

Here are some proven techniques for implementing a successful weigh-in program:

- Get a good scale.
- Weigh yourself first thing in the morning, wearing minimal clothing.
- Keep a log.
- Weigh yourself periodically (daily, weekly, monthly).
- Note trends.
- Take action if your weight trends upward.

Most people have a morning routine of getting up, visiting the loo, brushing their teeth, showering, shaving, etc. Just insert "weighing yourself" in there someplace, too easy! Keep a notebook; better yet, there are now Wi-Fi-enabled scales that will send your weight straight to your phone for later analysis. A tech geek's dream.

At a minimum, have a maximum weight in mind, and if you ever see this weight, act on it. By weighing yourself daily, you'll get a good feel for what is normal. If it drives you crazy, then by all means stop weighing daily and do it less frequently. Some people just tend to stress out more than others with constant weigh-ins. Stress causes weight gain, remember. Aside from the scale, also track your waist measurement. The BMI chart we looked at in Part 2 also had a waist-circumference chart. This is also a good metric to track. You don't have to measure your waist daily, by any means, but it's good to know and to keep it where it should be.

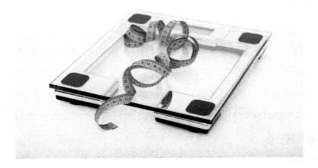

## Weight Regain

You *will* regain some of the weight you lost. That's what they call a "truth-bomb" in the fold of many a diet cult. Once you get the hang of losing weight, it's a blast watching your scale move lower and lower every day. It gets addictive, I know. But all good things must end. Once you've transitioned from dieting to maintaining, the trick is to keep your weight in a healthy band and only fret when it starts climbing uncontrollably.

Some of us will never be done dieting, it will be a lifelong struggle. Usually what causes the end of dieting is a return to bad habits. Exercise gets to be too much. French fries and ice cream become too tempting. You change jobs or get divorced. BAM, next thing you know you're back on the internet Googling, "How to *loose* weight," or starting a diet forum thread titled, "I'm baaaack!"

Daily weigh-ins can be a tremendous boost to your psyche during the weight maintenance phase. You'll make unconscious choices when you see your weight has increased a bit. Perhaps you'll walk a bit faster, eat a bit better, or get to bed a bit earlier. But you still need a bit of flexibility.

## Be Flexible

Your ideal weight needs to be a *range* not a firm number. This number will help guide you through the years. Your weight range also needs to be on a sliding scale, increasing as you get stronger or decreasing as you find your target weight was too high. Your body wants to get into a comfortable groove and find its perfect weight. It will do this if you eat right, exercise, get good sleep, and control stressful situations.

Everyone should have a weight in mind that will prompt them to action. When you see this weight during a couple of consecutive weigh-ins, you'll know it's time to batten down the hatches and get serious about bringing those numbers back down.

Your preferred weight should be effortless to maintain, but life sometimes gets in the way of best intentions and we gain weight. Here's the thing: if you are eating right, *and you know what that means*, and you are adhering to a well-executed exercise program, you are doing good. *Real good.* If you are sleeping soundly and your life is smooth, you are doing great. *Really great.* In this case, don't worry about a few extra pounds. Remember, stress causes weight gain. Focus on your life, not the weight. But use your weight to easily judge how well you are living.

If you just simply *cannot and will not* step on a scale, then come up with your own scale of measurements. Are your shirts too tight? Can you pinch more than an inch? Can't wear your skinny jeans? Getting a muffin top? You know *you* better than I do.

## Counting Calories

During your weight loss phase, you learned to count calories. For an effective *weight loss* program, creating a hypocaloric (low calorie) diet is paramount. But for *weight maintenance*, it's best to focus more on the quality of the food than the calorie content. It pays quite well to know how many calories you eat in any given day. It's very easy to overeat when you get lax and comfortable with your weight.

Calories can be a valuable commodity in your diet ledger, but they only work on paper. Eating to a specific calorie goal is a surefire way to get a surplus of calories. One way to accurately count calories is to eat *processed* food that has a food label, but this is most likely 10–20% off. The FDA even *allows* a 20% underreporting of calories on packaged foods (Jumpertz, 2013). Weighing *unprocessed, whole food* doesn't consider ripeness, sugar content, fat, or fiber differences. Attempting to count calories in real food is likely to be up to 20% off from the published calorie charts as well. Bananas, for instance, range from 80–110 calories for a medium depending on ripeness. Apples can vary widely in sugar content and calories depending upon the type of apple and even the weather where it was grown, though most charts list them all as 95 calories (Le Bourvellec et al., 2015).

According to the experts, men require about 2,200–3,000 calories per day and women 1,800–2,400 (HHS, 2010). You'll have a hard time finding a calorie chart showing that anyone should ever eat over 3,000 calories a day, except for athletes in training. There are a couple of very good calorie requirement calculators found online—play around with them. Just search the internet for "calorie calculator" and you'll see what I mean. And you'll see it's not *me* who decided to separate calorie needs by gender (in case that was starting to get annoying). I love charts, so:

| | | Activity Level (Assuming Normal BMI) | | | |
|---|---|---|---|---|---|
| Sex | Age | Sedentary | Moderate | Active | Very Active |
| Male | 19–30 | 2,400cal/day | 2,800cal/day | 3,000cal/day | 3,300cal/day |
| Male | 31–50 | 2,200 | 2,600 | 3,000 | 3,300 |
| Male | 51+ | 2,000 | 2,400 | 2,800 | 3,200 |

| Sex | Age | Activity Level (Assuming Normal BMI) | | | |
| | | Sedentary | Moderate | Active | Very Active |
|---|---|---|---|---|---|
| Female | 19–30 | 2,000 | 2,200 | 2,400 | 2,700 |
| Female | 31–50 | 1,800 | 2,000 | 2,200 | 2,500 |
| Female | 51+ | 1,600 | 1,800 | 2,200 | 2,500 |

*Adapted from (HHS, 2005)*

Moderate: Walking 1.5–3 miles per day, light physical activity

Active: 60 minutes of moderate activity such as walking/jogging at 3–4 mph, or 30 minutes vigorous activity such as jogging at 5.5 mph

Very Active: 45–60 minutes of vigorous activity daily

When I first started counting *my* calories, I was amazed how *little* food was in 1,500 calories. I think it's very important that dieters see what 1,500 and 3,000 calories look like, so they don't overeat or undereat, even if it's just an estimation that might be 10–20% off.

## Calories In

Diets that promise you can eat as much as you want have a common side effect: weight gain. I always laugh when I see the diet gurus snarkily tell their followers they need to cut calories if they are gaining weight after repeatedly saying calories don't matter. But it happens. You can simply eat too much, even of the best whole unprocessed foods.

If you eat mostly real foods without a food label, it's nearly impossible to count calories, so just eat. Don't worry about calories, but know they exist, and know they might be responsible for your failure to maintain weight. There are some amazingly accurate apps for counting calories if you are into that sort of thing. Some apps even let you take a picture of your plate of food and will recognize the items and give you a detailed calorie count, complete with fat-protein-carb breakdown and key nutrients.

Where calories get us in the most trouble are restaurants, coffee shops, and bars. Fast-food joints have started listing calories on their menus, and it's shocking to read how many calories are in some of those super-value meals. But the calories in coffee drinks and mixed alcohol drinks are *really* crazy. If you eat out a lot, get smart: Order salads with no dressing. Get a coffee instead of a double venti caramel macchiato. Have beer or wine instead of a Long Island iced tea.

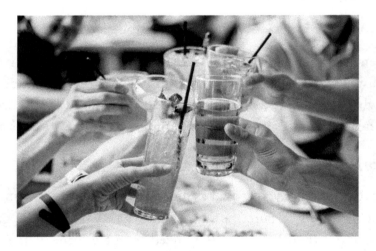

It's perfectly fine to overeat on occasion, possibly even good to do so. Your metabolism will ramp up to burn off the extra calories. No need to strictly eat X number of calories each and every day. Confusing? You bet. Eventually you'll just eat intuitively, but it doesn't hurt to reassess your diet every now and then.

## Calories Out

Never, ever count calories burned during exercise to give you an excuse to eat more. It doesn't work like that. Sure, exercise can be measured in calories, but it's a slippery slope when you exercise for the reward of food. Keep eating and exercising separate in your mind. They're two different things. I can't tell you how many times I've heard someone loudly proclaim it's "okay" to eat some extravagant piece of junk food because "they exercised." Or after noshing down a giant dessert they promise to "hit it really hard" tomorrow. You're just tricking yourself if you are guilty of this.

You've most likely heard that weight is all about "calories in versus calories out." While this is true on a very basic level, it's not the whole story. Ever wonder where all those "calories out" go? It looks something like this:

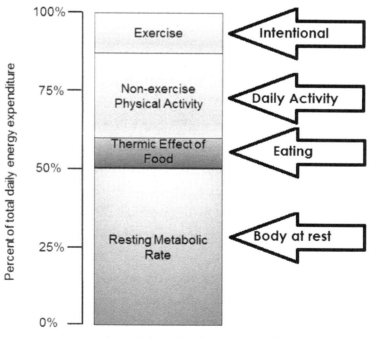

*Adapted from (Melanson, 2017)*

There are several calculations for determining your calorie burn rates, but they are just estimates (Gerrior, 2006). Each person has a unique energy signature based on their metabolism, the food they eat, how much and how hard they exercise, how much movement they do in their daily activity—even fidgeting (Melanson, 2017). To make matters even more confusing, these four factors are very fluid, changing by the minute in response to each other (Melanson, 2017). For example, after performing a vigorous bout of exercise, your resting metabolic rate may increase for a couple hours, but then you may not "fidget" as much so your non-exercise calorie requirement decreases (Herrmann, 2015).

> **Weight Loss Industry Insider Secret:** *"Calories out" and how humans regulate energy are highly dynamic processes that are very poorly understood by anyone in any field.*

## Bottom Line on Calories

A lowered metabolism caused by restricting calories is a function of the "resting metabolic rate." While this effect is hardly understood, it is real. It can be measured, and it must be dealt with by dieters. For long-term weight stability, it's best to focus more on food quality than calories. *Each person* will need to determine how much *they* can eat in a given day based completely on how *they* respond. It's good to get your diet dialed in and get to know what 1,500 and 3,000 calories of your normal food looks like. Most humans will need to eat in the 1,500–3,000 calorie range to maintain their weight. If you regain at a fast pace on 3,000 calories, then try reducing your intake to an average of 2,500 calories per day. But be careful! Reducing too much can affect how you burn calories, and it might lead to a reduction in metabolism. Sound entirely too confusing? It's not. Just eat *good* food *in a controlled manner*, exercise, sleep well, remove stress from your life, and take care of your health and all of this will work out … like magic.

## Protein Requirements for Maintenance

During active weight loss when calories are cut very low, there is a tendency to lose lean body mass and muscle. Great care must be taken to eat the recommended amounts of protein while dieting. During maintenance, most people find they don't need to track protein intake closely. If a person eats 40–100 grams of protein per day, they will be "in the zone" for protein needs. This is enough to keep your muscles healthy and fuel your exercise program (Gibson, 2016) (Leidy, 2015) (Geisler, 2016).

If you eat ¼–½ pound of meat and lots of vegetables every day, your protein needs are more than covered. Vegans will have to do what they do to fill their protein needs. Beware of diets that call for 150–200g or more of protein per day; this level is not needed nor recommended (Geisler, 2016).

## Bottom Line on Protein

Beware of any advice that you need more protein than can easily be eaten in a day. Eating some meat and/or protein-rich plants with every meal will be perfectly adequate. However, you also don't want to shortchange yourself on protein, either, so attempt to get at least the minimum recommended amount.

## Fat and Carb Requirements

There is no official recommendation on either fat or carbs, other than to "limit" fat intake (Liu, 2017). Generally speaking, carbs should be kept between 50–400g per day and fat between 10–50g per day. As you get into the specifics of the diet you choose for maintenance, this will become clearer. Diets that focus on nutritious food will be easier than diets that focus on strictly controlling the absolute number of fat or carbs.

## Water Requirements

While it seems like a no-brainer, most people are under-hydrated. We are advised to drink a little more than a quart of water daily, but this also includes water used in cooking, coffee, etc. There is no daily recommendation other than to drink when thirsty (Riebl, 2013). Studies show that hydration has positive effects on weight loss and maintenance and that drinking about 2 cups of water before a meal will lead to a reduction in food intake (Dennis, 2010) (Davy, 2008). Therefore, it's a good practice to go out of your way to drink a bit more prior to meals.

## Meal Size, Frequency, and Skipping Meals

How *often* you eat is a big part of weight loss. For weight maintenance it pays to experiment with what works best for *your* long-term eating style. The style of eating that helped you lose weight might not be the best style for weight maintenance. No matter if you settle into a low- carb, calorie counting, or low-fat type of diet, meal frequency and size are worth considering.

The research here is all over the place and not even worth mentioning. If I wanted to find studies to *support* skipping certain meals, eating many small meals, or eating only every other day, it'd be very easy to find dozens of papers to support *those patterns*. How *you* eat is completely an *individual* decision, and *whether* it works depends solely on *you*.

## Meal Size

In general, it's best to eat most of your food during pre-established meals. If you find you're always hungry an hour after eating, make it a point to eat more during meals. Eating only during meals allows the body to recover between meals. After a meal, insulin and hunger hormones (e.g., leptin, ghrelin) increase or decrease in response to caloric load. In a normal eating pattern, these hormones ebb and flow as nature intended to put the food where it belongs in your body. Insulin causes glucose to enter cells throughout your body, others cause fat to go where it belongs, etc. When you snack between meals, these chemicals are kept artificially elevated (or lowered) and create resistance to proper signaling (Yildiz, 2004).

*Diet Industry Insider Secret: "Hara hachi bu" is a Japanese Confucian saying that literally means, "Eat until you are 80% full." What a concept! I wish this were taught to children everywhere, it would start a lifelong pattern of eating just the right amount of food. Stuffing yourself is just silly. Perhaps a periodic food-fest is okay—on Thanksgiving or the Fourth of July. But not during your daily meals.*

Many researchers have spent their entire careers studying meal size and frequency. There are thousands of published papers on the different factors involved with meals and digestion. This research all points to two key concepts:

- Don't eat too much at any one time.
- Don't snack often.

In other words, no gorging and no grazing.

## Meal Frequency

Going hand-in-hand with meal *size* is the frequency of meals. In previous decades we were told to eat 5–6 small meals throughout the day for weight maintenance. Now we are seeing advice to skip meals and just eat once or twice per day. The truth is, any of these tactics will work well if you tolerate them.

## Intermittent Fasting (IF)

IF is mostly done for weight loss, but IF can also be a great strategy for weight *maintenance* (Patterson, 2015). There are numerous IF plans out there, but they all basically just play on three themes:

- Skipping meals
- Eating just once a day
- Occasionally skipping a whole day of eating

These IF patterns are great for people who tend to overeat at meals and/or snack uncontrollably. Mentally, some find that being strict with meal timing makes life easier while others find it to be unimaginably cruel. Preoccupation with eating is a huge stressor, and stress leads to weight gain. If you constantly think about food, try IF. No need to buy any programs or books on the subject, it really is as easy as just skipping meals, being careful not to overeat at meal times. The daily calorie recommendations don't change, so you can eat a bit bigger meal—another plus for some. Some even argue that IF can lead to losing fat while sparing muscle. Studies show that IF also helps with insulin sensitivity, hunger, etc. making it a very wise choice to at least try (Gotthardt, 2016).

## Alternate Day Fasting (ADF)

ADF has a proven track record in weight maintenance. It's just as it sounds, you eat every other day. This cuts your weekly calorie intake by approximately 50% if done correctly, but many tend to overeat immensely on their eating days, so sometimes it's a wash. In a year-long weight maintenance study, one group of people practiced ADF and another group ate every day but kept their calories fairly low (Headland, 2018). The ADF group performed just as well as the daily calorie trackers. The dropout rate, however, was higher in the ADF group mainly from "dissatisfaction with the diet." Cheating was a big problem with both groups, showing that it doesn't pay to be too strict with your diet. ADF just might be for you, but play with it. Skip full days once a week or a couple times a month if you like. If nothing else, this type of calorie restriction has several quantifiable benefits such as lowering inflammation, improving cardiovascular health, and burning fat (Longo, 2016).

## Fasting

Some have popularized the use of multi-day fasting for better health. Fasting is not generally recognized as a weight loss diet technique. Periodic, short fasts are not harmful, many religions have fasting as a central theme. But long periods without food, five days or more, requires serious forethought. Longer-term fasting, a week or more, has shown incredible promise as a treatment for diabetes and brain disorders. Fasting can be dangerous to some people, so please consult with a doctor if you want to try fasting (Longo, 2014).

## Several Small Meals

If the thought of periodic fasting or skipping meals just feels *wrong*, try the standard advice from the fitness industry and eat 5–6 small meals throughout the day. This eating pattern takes a lot of planning. You'll be the person bringing a sack full of labeled Tupperware to work. Many people find this is a much better way to eat, as it prevents mindless snacking and helps you to control hunger and overeating.

Normally, each small meal is carefully planned, weighed, and tracked for calorie purposes.

The research indicates that eating 5–6 small meals throughout the day works well for weight maintenance *if* it helps you to keep hunger in check and avoid overeating. There's no problem with eating this way except for the time it takes to do it properly. If three of your five meals are Otis Spunkmeyer Blueberry Muffins, this plan is not going to go well for you.

## Three Squares

The habit of eating three structured meals a day began with the Industrial Revolution. Even today, schools indoctrinate kids into adult eating patterns with a set lunch schedule. The military runs on three meals a day, as do prisons. This is the most common eating pattern for those on the Western diet, and maybe that should give us pause.

There's an old saying, "Eat breakfast like a king, lunch like a prince, and dinner like a pauper." If we ate in this way—a big breakfast, smaller lunch, and a snack for dinner—it would probably be ideal. The Western diet is more commonly eaten as:

- A fatty/sugary ultra-processed snack for breakfast (1,000 cal)
- Candy snacks (250 cal)
- Lunch on the go (1,000 cal)
- Processed meat snacks (250 cal)
- A gorging dinner followed by dessert and alcoholic drinks (1,500 cal)
- After-dinner sugary/salty/dairy snack (500 cal)

Just seeing that in writing should raise the hackles on your neck. This eating pattern belongs in a museum of horrors. But eating three solid meals with a healthy snack or two is okay if that's what you like.

Just focus on the best-quality food, with calories spread equally, staggered to your desire. A better meal plan based on three squares meals a day would be:

- Whole-wheat buttered toast, eggs, banana, and "overnight" oats (800 cal)
- Handful of nuts for a snack (100 cal)
- Fish, steamed broccoli, rice, and large salad for lunch (700 cal)
- Chicken breast, mushrooms, baked potato with butter, and a salad for dinner (700 cal)
- Piece of cheese for a snack (100 cal)

These three meals can be any real food you like. Enjoy low-carb or vegan? Go for it. Just make sure you are getting plenty of whole, unprocessed food. You don't *have* to eat meat, but if you don't, make sure you are getting a lot of high-protein produce.

To maintain your weight, you'll need to find a way of spreading your food intake throughout the day in a way that keeps you satisfied on the calorie limit you've imposed upon yourself. A guideline is just that, a guide. Please don't ever assume you *need* to eat 2,500 or 3,000 calories, it will only serve to confuse. The holy grail of weight maintenance is never needing to count calories, also called *eating intuitively*. This is stress-free eating at its best but requires practice, trial runs, and false starts. You'll get there if you try.

## The Potato Hack for Weight Maintenance

In case you hadn't heard, I wrote a book in 2016 called *The Potato Hack: Weight Loss Simplified*. In this book, I outlined a weight loss method devised in 1849. The rules are simple:

1. Plan on eating just potatoes for 3–5 days.
2. Eat 2–5 pounds of potatoes each day.

3. No other foods allowed.

4. Salt, pepper, and vinegar allowed, but not encouraged.

5. Drink when thirsty; coffee, tea, and water only.

6. Heavy exercise is discouraged; light exercise and walking are encouraged.

7. Take your normal medications, but dietary supplements will not be needed.

Following these seven easy steps, most find they can lose 3–5 pounds in 3–5 days. By doing this once a week, or even just once a month, you can lose a considerable amount of weight over the course of several months.

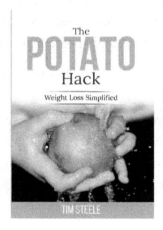

The Potato Hack also works well for weight maintenance. I've been toying with this for many years. I like to do the Potato Hack in early November and again after Christmas to keep my holiday weight down. Winter weight gain is a very common phenomenon and can sneak up on you if you aren't careful. Other people I know eat potatoes several days each week so that they can enjoy heartier meals on the weekend. Try this simple plan if your weight creeps up. There's no danger, and it's kind of fun.

## A Warning about Undereating during Maintenance

Not eating *enough* can also lead to problems. Very often dieters learn to ignore hunger signals and intentionally eat very little food. This is fine during the active weight loss phase of dieting, but eventually there must be a shift toward maintenance levels of food intake.

According to Chris Kresser of the California Center for Functional Medicine, many dieters end up eating too few calories and should consider upping their calorie level if they notice any of these six warning signs (Kresser, 2018):

- Feeling cold
- Hair loss
- Low energy
- Mood swings
- Poor sleep
- Preoccupation with food

Additionally, Kresser says that eating too few calories for too long leads to loss of muscle and lowers your metabolism, conditions that are incompatible with good health. Better, Kresser says, to eat within the range that keeps you feeling good and keeps your metabolism high.

### Case Study in Undereating: Professional Bodybuilders

Bodybuilders go through a rigorous pre-competition phase known as "cutting." During this phase of training they reduce calories by approximately 15% for 6–12 weeks to "cut" all traces of visible body fat so they appear sculpted and the judges can see their muscles. According to surveys of male and female bodybuilders, cutting is very hard on bodybuilders psychologically (Andersen, 1995 and 1998).

46% report binge-eating after competitions

60% report being unhappy with their weight on the day of competition

80% report psychological distress (fatigue, short temper, anxiety, depression, anger) while cutting

82% report being preoccupied with food while cutting

Most dieters don't consider a 15% reduction in calories "extreme," but you can see here that a 15% reduction leads to significant mental distress in well-trained athletes. Eating at your lower level of maintenance calories is quite important to the success of your weight maintenance efforts.

## Good Luck!

Long-term weight maintenance is the hardest part of dieting. In case you hadn't noticed, the deck is stacked against you. By following the advice I've laid out, you should have a much better chance at succeeding than the 95% who fail at weight maintenance. Becoming a successful long-term maintainer requires that you dig deep and work hard. Play around with meal frequency and meal size, and watch your calorie intake. Expect some setbacks and readjustment of your goals. You must be flexible, but above all, don't give up and don't return to eating Western ultra-processed food for every meal. Next, we'll discuss some other factors that most people overlook, but all have sound backing in science and the experiences of thousands of successful maintainers.

℞ for weight maintenance #2: Weigh yourself daily. If it causes stress, weigh less frequently. Measure your waist once a month.

℞ for weight maintenance #3: Strive to keep your weight within a range that makes you feel good.

℞ for weight maintenance #4: Know your weight, but focus on your life.

℞ for weight maintenance #5: Track your calories for a couple days especially if you are having trouble maintaining your weight. Are they in the correct range?

℞ for weight maintenance #6: Learn what 3,000 calories of food looks like, and only rarely exceed that amount in a single day.

℞ for weight maintenance #7: Practice *hara hachi bu*. No gorging, no grazing.

℞ for weight maintenance #8: Try intermittent fasting for two weeks. If it stresses you, stop.

℞ for weight maintenance #9: Try eating several small meals per day for two weeks. If it stresses you, stop.

℞ for weight maintenance #10: If you eat three meals a day, pack them with whole, unprocessed food and balance the calories to your pleasure.

℞ for weight maintenance #11: If you experience symptoms of undereating (feeling cold, sleeplessness, hair loss, low energy, mood swings, or binge-eating), examine your calorie intake to ensure you are eating enough food.

℞ for weight maintenance #12: Take two potatoes and call me in the morning.

# CHAPTER 23

# LIFESTYLE CHOICES THAT
# ENCOURAGE WEIGHT STABILITY

**TL;DR:** *Get lots of exercise, sleep well, and reduce stress. Also, be careful with nicotine, weed, and booze.*

Thanks to influences of the Western diet and Big Food, *eating* is usually what gets us in the most trouble with our weight. Most diets focus mainly on the food portion of this melodrama when we should be taking a wider-angle shot of the scene. Food and exercise are major players, but equally important is how we are living our life. Now we'll look at lifestyle factors that influence weight maintenance and give some tips for overcoming some hurdles.

- Exercise
- Stress
- Sleep
- Nicotine
- Recreational Drugs/Alcohol

## Exercise

Just a paragraph here so you don't try to skip over this step. There is a *whole section* devoted to exercise and weight maintenance because it's *that important*. Please read Part 4.

Depending on how much weight you lost during your weight loss diet, you undoubtedly also lost substantial muscle/lean body mass. Exercise is of vital importance to rebuilding lost muscle and bone as well as building up aerobic capacity of the heart and lungs. Hopefully, your weight loss program included an exercise component. If not, it is very important to begin if there is to be any hope of maintaining your weight loss.

Aside from eating, exercise will be your number one ally in maintaining your weight. You simply *must* start an exercise program. If you still are wanting to fight me on this, let me try to convince you with some case studies.

The National Weight Control Registry (NWCR) was started in 1994. This registry currently tracks over 10,000 people who have lost at least 30 pounds by dieting and have kept it off for more than a year. The participants are surveyed annually to check their progress and share weight maintenance strategies with the program admins. Here are some successful weight maintainers the registry tracks (NWCR, 2019):

- **Anthony** has maintained an 88-pound weight loss for over 11 years. Anthony was a stress eater who learned to deal with his stress. Now instead of eating in response to stress, Anthony walks or goes to the gym.

- **Emily** has maintained an 85-pound weight loss for over four years. Emily learned to eat better and walks every morning before school and in the evening, in addition to hiking and practicing yoga.

- **Pat** has maintained her 114-pound weight loss for almost two years. Pat eats a low-carb diet and exercises 6–7 times a week.

- **Lynn** has maintained a 50-pound weight loss for nearly ten years. She started by cutting out sugary drinks and fast food. Lynn walks three miles every morning and works out three times a week. Her workouts include yoga, Zumba, and strength training.

- **Pamela** has maintained a 178-pound weight loss for over seven years. She joined Weight Watchers and walks for exercise.

- **Sue** has maintained a 52-pound weight loss for five years. Sue limits sugar and walks at least 60 minutes each day.

- **Jessica** has maintained a 60-pound weight loss for four years by walking four miles a day and working out, including an hour on a stair-stepper machine.

- **Fran** has maintained a weight loss of over 100 pounds after joining Weight Watchers and working out. Fran now runs 10Ks and half-marathons and trains daily for endurance running.

The exercise program you develop needs to become a part of you. I've written a detailed exercise program that anyone can use (see Part 4). It contains all the elements that successful maintainers use. The science is clear on this, exercise benefits every part of our body and leads to a metabolism that won't allow you to become obese. It's not about burning more calories; exercise keeps your heart, lungs, and bones strong as well as keeping *you* young inside.

## Stress and Sleep for Weight Management

Besides eating right and exercising, the biggest cause of failure to maintain weight loss is related to experiencing stress and sleeping poorly. Sleep deprivation is a form of stress, so I've placed them together in this discussion. Most of us, and that includes doctors and nutritionists, don't realize how stress and lack of sleep affect our weight.

Consider the following from the research paper "Does stress influence sleep patterns, food intake, weight gain, abdominal obesity and weight loss interventions and vice versa?" (Geiker, 2018):

- Despite over 50 years of research, there are only "weak associations" between food intake and weight gain.

- Researchers have noted for many years that abdominal obesity and the metabolic syndrome are connected to stress and an unhealthy lifestyle (e.g., poor diet, smoking, alcohol, and lack of exercise).

- Stress is a "negative emotional experience" involving "biochemical, physiological, and behavioral changes."

- Lack of sleep causes many of the same chemical imbalances as stress.

- Stress can come from "insecurity in personal, social and professional life" and also from "insufficient sleep"; 80% of Americans report stressful lives and poor sleep habits.

- Certain vitamin deficiencies are associated with stress: "Vitamin D, Vitamin B3 (niacin), Vitamin B9 (folate), Vitamin B6, Vitamin B12, and omega-3."

- Both stress and lack of sleep cause cravings for high-fat/high-carb "comfort" foods.

- Today's researchers are completely missing the connection between stress, sleep, and bodyweight even though there is ample evidence showing the connection.

Are you connecting the dots like I did? This is quite alarming, really.

## Is Weight Gain Even about the Food?

There appears to be overlooked evidence that the obesity epidemic is more about stress and poor sleep than bad food. But it's a circular pattern. The Western diet lacks nutrients that keep us resilient in the face of stress (Anderson, 2017) (Costa, 2018). When deprived of certain nutrients we are more prone to stress (Geiker, 2018):

| Vitamins Associated with Stress | Where Found |
| --- | --- |
| Vitamin D | Sunlight, mushrooms |
| Vitamin B3 (Niacin) | Liver, chicken, tuna, peanuts |
| Vitamin B9 (Folate) | Legumes, asparagus, eggs |
| Vitamin B6 | Potatoes, bananas, liver, fish |
| Vitamin B12 | Meat |
| Omega-3 | Fatty fish, fish oil |

It's a vicious cycle. Stress and lack of sleep cause chemical imbalances that can make us crave bad food. The Western diet lacks key nutrients and causes chemical imbalances. Stress, sleep deprivation, *and* poor eating cause weight gain. Eating our standard Western diet causes stress just like a bad marriage or a job you hate. Lack of sleep makes us eat more and causes even more stress. A triple-whammy.

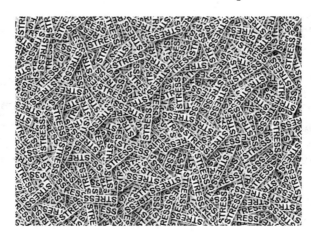

## De-stressing Your Life

Some stress cannot be avoided; it's simply the human way. But it pays to de-stress your life as much as possible. Sometimes we cause ourselves stress without even realizing it. Over-dieting and over-exercising can also be stressful.

*Healthcare Industry Insider Secret:* Noise pollution is a part of modern life we all wish didn't exist. Nearly 4,000 adults took part in a study to examine the effects of noise pollution in their metabolism. It was discovered that for every 10 dB increase in background noise there was a 17% increase in obesity and people that were exposed to the most noise were more obese (Foraster, 2018).

## Gimmicks

Humans are keen to turn any big problem into an industry. Stress is a big enough problem it would appear judging by the number of stress-management products now on the market:

- Adult coloring books
- Body wraps
- Essential oils
- Herbs
- Lights
- Massagers
- Punching bags
- Soaps
- Squeeze balls
- Teas
- Zen gardens

And don't think the marketers have overlooked sleep! Sleep-aid is now a multimillion-dollar industry in the United States. After a couple nights without sleep, people aren't thinking right and the manufacturers know this. A quick perusal of sleep-aid ads on Amazon turns up the following:

- Biofeedback devices
- Blue-light blocking glasses
- Chin straps
- Drugs
- Ear plugs
- Electrical grounding devices
- Gels
- Herbs
- High-tech pillows
- Metronomes
- Mouth guards
- Nasal strips
- Night lights
- Nose vent plugs
- Oils
- Skin patches
- Tongue patches
- Weighted blankets
- White noise generators
- Window covers

Whatever happened to counting sheep?

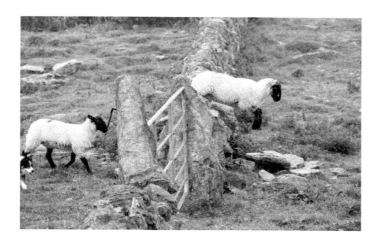

## Sleeping Better

While sleep-aid devices might work, don't be duped into spending money. Better advice would be to simply practice good sleep hygiene.

- Adhere to a strict bedtime/waking schedule.
- Mellow out the hour before you go to bed.
- Limit computer use in the 2–3 hours before bedtime.
- Avoid eating meals 2–3 hours before bed.
- Avoid alcohol before bed.
- Stop drinking caffeinated drinks eight hours before bed.
- Be physically active during the day.
- Keep your bedroom quiet, cool, and dark.
- Take a bath or shower before bed.
- Keep pets off the bed.

Shift workers have an extremely tough time with sleep hygiene, and shift workers tend to be 29% more obese than day-shifters (Sun, 2018). Some tips for shift workers:

- Set your sleep schedule in concrete.
- Keep lights bright at work.
- Try to get on a set schedule rather than rotating schedules.

- Limit caffeine to the early part of your shift.
- Ensure your bedroom is highly conducive to sleep (dark, cool, quiet).
- Change jobs.

If you have chronic insomnia. Please see a doctor. You may need a sleep study to rule out sleep apnea, narcolepsy, or other physical or mental problems preventing sleep. Do not be tempted to take over-the-counter sleeping pills or recreational drugs, and don't try to "nightcap" your way to a good night's sleep. Alcohol, especially, is counterproductive to sleep, as it disturbs sleep patterns despite making you drowsy (Stein, 2006). Your waistline, mental state, and health will all benefit if you get adequate sleep.

## Is Eight Hours Enough?

The older we get the less sleep we need, but every person is different. The table below shows the recommended amounts of sleep for each age group (Hirshkowitz et al., 2015):

| Age | Minimum Recommended | Recommended | Maximum Recommended |
|---|---|---|---|
| Newborn (0–3 mos.) | 11–13 hrs. | 14–17 hrs. | 18–19 hrs. |
| Infant (4–12 mos.) | 10–11 | 12–15 | 16–18 |
| Toddler (1–2 yrs.) | 9–10 | 11–14 | 15–16 |
| Preschool (3–5) | 8–9 | 10–13 | 14 |
| School Age (6–13) | 7–8 | 9–11 | 12 |
| Teen (14–17) | 7 | 8–10 | 11 |

| Age | Minimum Recommended | Recommended | Maximum Recommended |
|---|---|---|---|
| Young Adult (18–25) | 6 | 7–9 | 10–11 |
| Adult (26–64) | 6 | 7–9 | 10 |
| Older Adult (65+) | 6 | 7–8 | 9 |

Too much sleep also has its problems, but too little sleep is the biggest culprit for health-related concerns. The human body attempts to regulate itself to the sleep required for each individual, but very often tight schedules and our hectic lifestyle keep us from getting enough sleep.

## Case Studies on Sleep

Athletes learned a long time ago that sleep is vital to performance.

### NBA Performance and Late-Night Tweeting

Sleep researchers examined basketball game stats between 2009 and 2016 for 112 NBA players with Twitter accounts. They discovered that Tweeting during sleeping hours caused the players' shooting percentage to drop 1.7%, and they had 1.1 fewer points and less rebounds in the next day's game (Healthday, 2018).

### Sleep-Deprived Elite Swimmers

Eight Olympic swimmers were deprived of two and a half hours of sleep for four nights. Mood states were "significantly altered" with increased confusion, depression, tension, anger, and fatigue noted. There was a significant effect on bench press, leg press, and deadlift maximum weights. The biggest changes were found later in the study, suggesting a cumulative effect of sleep deprivation (Halson, 2014).

## Nicotine

I'm not going to lie: quitting nicotine usually causes weight gain. A large study placed the average weight gain at 12 pounds (Courtemanche, 2018). Is it worth it, quitting? I think the answer is clear: you must give up nicotine—and that means smoking, chewing, vaping, and using patches or gum or however else the cool kids are doing it today.

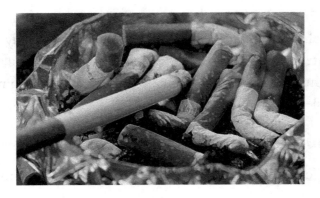

If you smoke or chew, shame on you. It's a nasty habit, so unhealthy that each pack must be labeled with the diseases it will cause. In some countries they even put pictures of the diseases, yet people still smoke. Smoker-friendly places are becoming rare. Restaurants, businesses, and public gathering places are nearly all smoke-free now, and smokers must sneak off somewhere to get a fix. I remember feeling so *alive* as a kid sneaking a smoke behind the school cafeteria's dumpsters. Do adults feel that way now?

While smoke damages lungs and tissue, nicotine is the real problem. Nicotine is kind of cool. Many studies show that nicotine has anti-inflammatory effects. Humans have receptors for nicotine throughout our body (nicotinic acetylcholine receptors). When activated, these receptors signal to our immune system that all is well, lowering inflammation and stabilizing our metabolism. Nicotine has been studied as a drug to treat multiple sclerosis, type 1 diabetes, rheumatoid arthritis, sarcoidosis, and inflammatory bowel diseases among other autoimmune conditions (Gomes, 2017).

The amazing anti-inflammatory properties of nicotine have a downside, though. All this immune signaling stuff? Turns out it's not so great after all. By turning down the immune system, it lowers our natural defenses against cancer and bacterial invaders. Normally, your body senses and destroys new cancer cells (apoptosis) and foreign bodies that don't belong. An immune system clouded by nicotine operates at a fraction of its efficiency and allows tumors to invade and spread (Widysanto, 2018). Nicotine users are more susceptible to viruses and bacterial infections (Qiu, 2017).

Nicotine is highly addictive, and the methods of ingestion can cause grave damage to the human body, especially smoking (Levy, 2018). E-cigs, or vaping, is a newer form of nicotine delivery that may or may not be any healthier than smoking, depending on who you talk to (Gomes, 2017). The biggest dangers from tobacco are the carcinogens delivered to the lungs from smoking, cancers of the mouth from chewing, and the immune system effects of nicotine. Vaping has been touted as a safe alternative but still gets new users addicted in short order and affects the immune system in harmful ways.

## Recreational Cannabis Use

There are very few studies on how cannabis affects weight gain or weight maintenance due to the illegal nature and lack of federal funding. However, there has been some new research that shows long-term cannabis use leads to lower weight and better health outcomes (Scheffler et al., 2018).

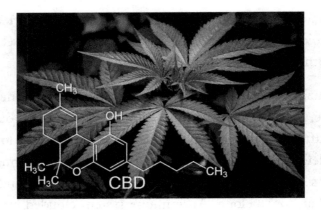

I must urge caution if you want to try newly legalized weed in your state. The legal cannabis industry is still in its infancy. The pharmaceutical-grade extractions now legally being sold are extremely powerful, and local authorities are unprepared to analyze them. Even cannabis flowers (buds) can be contaminated with mold and chemicals that go undetected by mandatory inspections. Smoking cannabis regularly can lead to lung irritation and laziness, making exercise difficult. Cannabis in all forms causes "the munchies," and leads people to make extremely poor food selections in their uninhibited search for food.

## Alcohol

Drinking is a hard one. A few drinks a day have shown to be a healthy habit. A glass or two of wine or a beer does not seem to hamper weight maintenance at all, and in fact seems to be protective of weight stability (Traversy, 2015). Still, the principals of getting adequate sleep and exercise apply.

### Women Will Love This One!

Almost 20,000 women aged 39–89 were watched for 13 years to see what drinking did to their weight. Over the study period, the women who drank the most (more than three drinks per day) gained the least amount of weight; the women who did not drink at all gained the most. The happy medium for drinking and weight stability was around two drinks per day.

> Our study results suggest that women who have normal body weight and consume light-to-moderate alcohol could maintain their drinking habits without gaining excessive weight. (Wang, 2010)

Studies in men did not have the same outcome, with even moderate drinking leading to long-term weight gain (Suter, 2005). And in all people, men and women, lifestyle played the biggest part. Weight gain was highest in people who overate, didn't exercise, and slept poorly among some other factors.

**R for weight maintenance #13: Don't fall for scams or bad science. If it seems too good to be true, it probably is. Gadgets, clothing, pills, or teas for magical weight loss don't work.**

**R for weight maintenance #14: Start an aerobic and strength training exercise program.**

**R for weight maintenance #15: Get as far away from stressful situations as you can. Seek professional help if you need it.**

**R for weight maintenance #16: Clean up your diet, and eat lots of food high in B-Vitamins and omega-3 oils.**

**R for weight maintenance #17: Consider supplementing Vitamin D3, especially in the winter. Take a B12 supplement if you're vegan.**

**R for weight maintenance #18: Parents, make sure your kids are happy, well-fed, and well-rested.**

℞ for weight maintenance #19: Get a good night's sleep, meaning 7–9 hours a night.

℞ for weight maintenance #20: If you smoke, switch to vaping or patches. Then quit.

℞ for weight maintenance #21: If you are a cannabis user and cannot control your weight, consider giving it up for a year. If you want to try legalized cannabis for the first time, be aware that what you are buying may not be safe or adequately tested.

℞ for weight maintenance #22: Ladies, take two glasses of merlot and call me in the morning. Guys, lay off the booze.

# CHAPTER 24

# SOCIAL SUPPORT

**TL;DR:** *Getting others involved and tracking your ongoing progress will help ensure weight stability.*

Support systems are a critical part of weight maintenance. Losing weight is easy compared to keeping it off. Indeed, millions of people regularly lose 10–15% of their bodyweight doing various diet programs, but within a year most have gained nearly all of the weight back, and fewer than 5–10% manage to maintain a 10% weight loss for more than five years.

To examine this effect, researchers in Providence, Rhode Island, set up an experiment (Ross, 2018). The team recruited 75 obese men and women to go on a diet and then track their weight for a year. The 75 "guinea pigs" were all employees of a large healthcare organization; the weight loss portion of the experiment was designed as a workplace challenge with modest monetary rewards ($1–$10/week) and other small perks.

The dieters were given specific instructions on how to eat, calorie and fat limits, exercise requirements, and details about how to track their weight using a "smart" Wi-Fi-enabled scale that reported directly to the research team.

The weight loss diet was an intensive lifestyle intervention. Each dieter was given a tailored diet specific to their starting weight and health, taught to eat specific foods, and given instructions on exercise. The participants engaged in walking, jogging, swimming, and strength training. As the diet progressed, each person logged into a website for 12 weeks and tracked calories, exercise, and weight loss and were given feedback and help with challenges encountered from a team of dieticians.

The dieters all did great! The average weight loss was about one pound per week as expected. After the 12-week weight loss phase, the dieters were instructed to maintain the healthy habits they learned but were given no further incentives, support, encouragement, or instructions. As the dieters continued to log their weekly weights for nine more months, they regained the weight they had lost at a near linear rate of ½ pound per week until nearly all of them ended at or near their starting weight.

This experiment showed that without a support network, weight maintenance is nearly impossible. This quite clearly mirrors the experience of the 150 million dieters each year who regain their weight upon completion of a diet. Why can't people help themselves? Why do we require a support network to maintain our weight?

## Creating Your Own Support Network

When you're dieting aggressively like we discussed in Part 2, it's imperative to develop a support network. During our weight loss diet, we used support networks provided by commercial diet programs like Atkins, WW, or Slimming World. Some of us also used forums and message boards from around the web. While these worked great for losing weight, you'll find that you won't need the intensity of daily discussions for weight maintenance. Still, these communities would love to have you stick around and help others to lose weight. You'll find no end of "return customers" on these same forums looking for help in keeping their weight off. Becoming a mentor to those having trouble is a very rewarding way to keep a support network going.

It's no secret that weight loss occurs much more easily when the dieter is on display and has announced his or her weight loss intentions to friends, family, and coworkers. The people around a dieter are an important part of the weight loss effort, giving encouragement and compliments, and removing tempting treats from the dieter's reach.

Another way to create a social network is to join a gym, yoga class, or other fitness program and make new friends who are interested in health and fitness. Surrounding yourself with successful weight maintainers will keep you motivated, small as that club might be.

For the most part, your weight maintenance phase is going to be a lifelong struggle. At some point you'll need to stop focusing on your weight and just live your life. This part, the support network, needs to just be in the background. It gives me immense pleasure knowing I've kept my weight off nearly ten years now. That's enough to keep me motivated.

## Weight Maintenance Accountability

Here are some tips and tricks I've learned from reading research studies on weight maintenance, watching hundreds of dieters, and living my own experiences. I've witnessed many successful weight loss and maintenance journeys by joining and participating in online dieting forums. I've also watched as coworkers and friends lost and regained weight over a 40-year timeframe. Aside from adherence to a good diet and exercise, installing an accountability system is a huge factor in keeping weight off.

### Take Before-and-After Pictures

Most overweight people don't want to take pictures of their minimally clothed body, so "before" pictures usually come in the form of old digital pics or scanned Polaroids taken at family picnics.

It's invaluable to capture your weight loss and maintenance journey with pictures. Nobody needs to see them, they are your reminder of what you looked like and how you compare at various stages along the way. Posting these pictures on Facebook or dieting forums is also quite empowering and adds a layer of accountability that cannot be matched.

Here's a picture of me before I got serious about my weight:

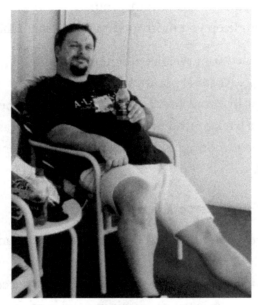

*Author at 240 pounds (2009)*

Keep in mind that most before-and-after pictures you see on dieting websites are actors or professionally remastered images that give the best effect. Some are laughable. In the before picture, the person is invariably sad-looking with poor posture, belly poked out, and standing in dark shadows. The after is always well-lit, showing the person looking happy, sucking in their gut, and flexing their muscles. Some of the sets are taken in the same photo shoot with only minutes between the poses.

But there are also many examples of real people posing for their own before-and-after photos. Search for "before and after weight loss pics" on Pinterest.com, and you'll see hundreds of pictures of real dieters.

Here's me after a year of steady dieting:

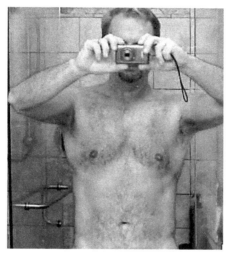

*Author at 160 pounds (2012)*

## What about Loners?

If the thought of taking before-and-after pictures and joining online support forums totally goes against every fiber of your being, you'll have to dig deep and come up with some ways to keep yourself motivated. Keeping a log is a great way to start. Track your weight, waist measurements, etc. But you'll have a much harder time doing it on your own. Failure to keep good records and involve others is a top reason for the 95% of dieters who regain the weight. Organizations that track successful weight maintainers indicate that people do well with self-directed eating programs for weight maintenance, but careful tracking is key.

## Keep a Log

I'm a real numbers geek. I track and trend hundreds of different measurements in my daily job as administrator of the environmental control system in a large hospital. I track room temperatures, pressures, pump speeds, motor loads, and many other items of interest. When I first embarked on a serious diet in 2011, I started logging my weight weekly on an Excel spreadsheet, and I've kept the log ever since, but I switched to a monthly weigh-in after about five years because I kept forgetting to weigh in, and I was quite confident I was "over the hump." Here are some of the logs I kept on my weight loss journey:

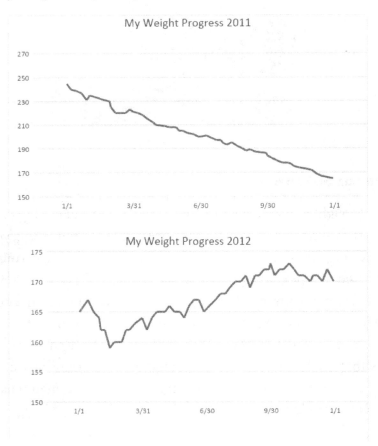

There are now apps that do this automatically. If I were to do this all over again, I'd get a "smart" scale and an app that automatically tracks my daily weight. There is no better tool for the prediction of future problem than an extensive trend of past performance. Check out MyFitnessPal.com or SparkPeople.com for excellent free weight tracking tools.

Trending your weight loss journey is always a mandatory feature of commercial weight loss programs, but most people stop this critical step when they switch to a maintenance diet, which is unfortunate.

## What Else to Track?

I showed you my weight charts, but over this same period I've tracked several other health markers because I knew this was going to be a lifelong journey. Some other things you might want to track to gauge your health progress through the years:

- Blood pressure
- Waist Circumference
- Fasting Glucose
- Triglycerides
- HDL Cholesterol
- LDL Cholesterol
- Medications and Dosage

Hopefully, everyone is on a medical plan that takes yearly blood labs. You can request a copy of your paperwork to get this data. Sometimes it takes years after you regain a healthy weight for these markers to fall into a healthy range, but it's such an amazing feeling to have everything in the normal ranges, and the look on your doctor's face will be priceless. With a 90% dieting failure rate, it's very rare for a doctor to see someone *improve* as they age. Most of my annual physical is usually spent giving diet advice to the doctor or physician's assistant and nurses.

## "Daily Win" Calendar

Here's an idea I came up with. Get a nice wall calendar, and every night before bed, you get a \ if you ate really well, and a / if you exercised that day. If you ate well and exercised, you get an **X**. As the month progresses, you want to see more **X**s than slashes or blank spots. It will give you a daily visual level of accountability that can't be matched by apps or your memory.

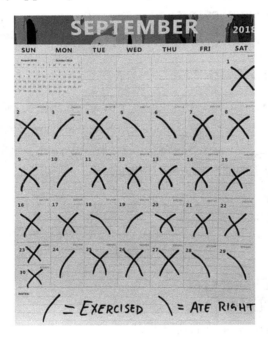

**R for weight maintenance #23: Build a social network for weight maintenance using online resources or personal friends, family, or coworkers.**

**R for weight maintenance #24: Take pictures of yourself to help gauge your progress.**

**R for weight maintenance #25: Keep a log to track your weight and other health markers.**

# CHAPTER 25

# GUT HEALTH AND WEIGHT STABILITY

> **TL;DR:** *Take good care of your gut. Eat real food. Gut testing is a waste of money.*

### The Gut Hack

One day I'll write a book about the human gut, but I'm afraid that today we don't know enough about our guts to make many recommendations past trying to eat well and live right. There are several companies that offer gut testing services. I jumped on this a couple years ago when affordable gut flora testing was a brand-new thing. I was very impressed back then, but over the years the promises failed to materialize. Today these companies are making millions of dollars testing gullible people's poo. These services offer tailored dietary advice based on the bacteria they detect in your stool sample, but the advice they are giving is beyond disappointing.

Gut testing services will promise that you can avoid obesity and lose weight if you let them analyze a sample of your feces, but the only advice that a gut testing service can really give is, "Eat more high-fiber plants." They'll frame it around the questionnaire you filled out beforehand and try to convince you they are doing you a distinct, personalized service, but, by God, who shouldn't be eating more high-fiber plants (Brandsma, 2019)? I'd die laughing if I ever saw a report that said, "Lay off the fiber, man. Eat a cheeseburger!" Consider that probably 95% of the tests they run are done on people eating a Western diet; advice to eat some beans and broccoli is probably the best advice most people *can* get.

## Probiotics

Probiotics are living microorganisms that convey health upon anyone that eats them. They live happily in your gut and help create an environment that promotes good health. Gut health is of *vital* importance for long-term weight stability (Thomas, 2017). If the gut balance is upset, your weight will suffer. So, let's all take probiotics, right?

The probiotics most often used in clinical trials and recommended by physicians and pharmacists are those that contain (Ciorba, 2012):

- *Lactobacillus*
- *Bifidobacterium*

It's easy to find probiotics that contain these two bacteria. Probably 90% of all the probiotics at Walgreens or on Amazon have them. I recommend only taking probiotics if you have been prescribed antibiotics for an infection or if you need a boost after a bout of bad food choices resulting in dyspepsia. Antibiotics will do damage to the delicate balance in your gut, and probiotics can quickly restore the balance, making recovery quicker (Tsai, 2019). Otherwise it's best to simply eat foods that contain probiotics (Homayoni, 2016).

### Grow Your Own

*Supplement Industry Insider Secret: Probiotics are found naturally in food.*

Unless you need a very high dose of probiotics, for example to prevent antibiotic associated diarrhea, it's best to simply eat foods that contain high levels of naturally occurring probiotics:

- Buttermilk

- Cottage cheese
- Kefir
- Kimchi
- Kombucha
- Kvass
- Miso
- Natto
- Pickles
- Raw cheese
- Sauerkraut
- Sourdough bread
- Tempeh
- Yogurt

Several of these food items are still quite unheard of in the US but are gaining popularity. Kombucha, for instance, is starting to become a popular fixture at farmer's markets and food festivals. Some of the foods listed (e.g., pickles and sauerkraut) can be made in a way that destroys all of the probiotics, so be sure you are only buying products that retain their probiotic properties (Fan, 2017).

All naturally fermented vegetables contain a multitude of lactobacillus species. You will get more probiotics in naturally fermented vegetables than in a purchased pill. It's simple to make your own pickles, sauerkraut, kimchi, and other types of tasty fermented condiments. A great book to get you started on a journey of flavor and probiotic discovery is *Fermented Vegetables: Creative Recipes for Fermenting 64 Vegetables & Herbs in Krauts, Kimchis, Brined Pickles, Chutneys, Relishes & Pastes* by Kirsten K. Shockey and Christopher Shockey (2014). You can get started with just a jar, fresh vegetables, a bit of salt, and time. Warning: Growing your own probiotics is addictive.

## Prebiotics

For the purpose of weight maintenance, you ought to be getting all your prebiotics from plants instead of supplements. Prebiotics are different from what we normally think of as "fiber." Prebiotics are special types of plant fiber that are eaten by the bacteria in your gut; when well-fed, these bacteria produce thousands of chemicals that signal wellness and keep the immune system humming along as it should. There is a well-proven and distinct connection between eating prebiotic foods and maintaining a lean weight (Yoo, 2016).

Taking a prebiotic supplement while eating a low-fiber, low-plant diet could cause gut damage (Dreher, 2018). Conversely, anyone eating a lot of plants is also getting a lot of prebiotics and likely has healthy a gut (Requena, 2018). Extracted prebiotics are not as effective as whole plant foods in conveying gut health (Macfarlane, 2006).

If you want to remove all doubt that you are eating enough prebiotics without resorting to purchasing them in a powdered form, eat these very-high-fiber foods regularly:

- Berries
- Dark chocolate
- Garlic
- Green Bananas (as green as you can tolerate)
- Leeks
- Legumes (pulses, beans, peas)
- Nuts (tree nuts and ground nuts)
- Oatmeal (groats or steel-cut are best)
- Onions
- Raw potato (1–2 slices)
- Seeds (e.g., flax, chia, sunflower, etc.)
- Whole grains

If you decide you want to take a prebiotic supplement, look for these in the ingredients:

- Inulin
- FOS
- Resistant starch
- Beta-glucan
- Glucomannan

When taking supplements, it's best to mix them in smoothies that contain several other real foods (e.g., berries, seeds, or fruit). These supplements are also good to mix with yogurt or milk.

It starts to get confusing, discussing the gut. The gut is the center of our health universe, anything that upsets the balance of your gut is quite likely to keep you from becoming a successful weight loss achiever. Most eating styles (WOEs) will advise you to eat plenty of plants. *Wink wink.* But we all know that you probably don't want to eat lots of veggies, but they also know if you don't, you'll end up with digestive issues. A person with a healthy gut can eat just about any way they like for a while, but it will eventually catch up with them. To keep your gut happy and engaged in helping you to maintain vigorous health and lower weight, follow these advisements:

**R for weight maintenance #26: Avoid diets that restrict starchy tubers, grains, seeds, vegetables, and fruit.**

**R for weight maintenance #27: Eat several servings of fruit and vegetables each day.**

**R for weight maintenance #28: Regularly consume fermented foods such as sauerkraut, pickles, and kombucha.**

**R for weight maintenance #29: Take a probiotic that contains "lacto" and "bifido" if you need to take antibiotics for an infection.**

# CHAPTER 26

# HEALTH MANAGEMENT

> **TL;DR:** *Strive for perfection in your blood pressure, waist size, blood sugar, triglycerides, and cholesterol. Stay away from supplements. Antibiotics suck—probiotics rock.*

When you first embarked on your weight loss journey, you most likely had some medical conditions that precipitated the desire to lose weight. Perhaps your doctor urged you to lose weight and make some lifestyle changes or you were just fed up with all the new pills that came with a diagnosis of metabolic syndrome. At any rate, it's urgent that you regain your health and manage any problems that might linger.

*Healthcare Industry Insider Secret:* Only about 12% of adults in the US are metabolically healthy based on six markers (Araújo, 2018):

- *Blood pressure: Close to 120/80*
- *Waist Circumference: Under 40" for men, 35" for women*
- *Fasting Glucose <100 mg/dL and HbA1c <5.7%*
- *Triglycerides <150 mg/dL*
- *HDL-C ≥40/50 mg/dL in men/women*
- *Not taking medications for blood pressure, diabetes, and cholesterol*

*According to the researchers who gathered this data, the numbers are "alarmingly low," and the large number of metabolically unhealthy people has "serious implications for public health."*

## Let's Change Things

People who lose and maintain a significant amount of weight are very rare. Doctors hardly ever see people who maintain their weight for long after dieting, and only about 1 in 9 of the people who doctors see are metabolically healthy. It must be frustrating.

To get all this right, you need to do four things first: Eat right, exercise, sleep well, and remove as much stress from your life as you can. I'll bet you knew I was going to say that, didn't you?

Once you have the "big four" covered, here are some more tips to becoming metabolically healthy:

### Blood Pressure:

- Cut back on salt, but this isn't usually a problem unless you are on the Western diet.
- Walk more. Start with 30 minutes a day.
- Cut back on the caffeine. Stick to 1–2 caffeinated drinks per day.
- Stop drinking alcohol to excess. Limit yourself to 1–2 alcoholic drinks per day.
- Stop smoking.

### Waist Circumference:

Hopefully you beat the battle of the bulge when you met your goal weight. If your waist circumference is still above the guidelines (35" or 40"), please make an appointment with your doctor. Unless you are over 6'5", a waist that's over the recommended limit indicates a problem with your internal organs or accumulation of visceral fat related to a serious medical condition. Get evaluated.

### Fasting Glucose a bit high (100–130 mg/dL):

- Perform more strength training exercises.
- Cut back on carbs, especially sugar and flour.
- Eat more fiber, such as resistant starch as found in potatoes, beans, and green bananas.

### Fasting Glucose Quite High (130 mg/dL or higher):

See your doctor for an HbA1C test and counseling on how to lower your blood glucose levels. Something's wrong.

### High Triglycerides:

- Eat less sugar.
- Eat less refined grain (e.g., white bread and pasta).
- Stop eating fried food.
- Eat more whole grains, especially oats.
- Try eating a low-carb diet for a year.
- Try eating a high-carb diet for a year.

### Low HDL-C, the good cholesterol:

- Eat more healthy oil (olive oil, coconut oil).
- Eliminate fried foods.
- Eat more fish, especially salmon, sardines, and herring.
- Eat lots of berries, especially blueberries.

- Stop smoking and drinking.
- Try eating a low-carb diet for a year.
- Try eating a high-carb diet for a year.
- Get serious about exercise.

## Getting Off Medications:

Hopefully, your doctor has been on board with your weight loss efforts and will let you know when to get off your meds or lower your dosage. Don't try this on your own! Sometimes you'll still be on meds even after losing weight. Don't be discouraged; stay the course of healthy eating, exercising, etc. It will pay off in the long-run. Luckily, medications for type 2 diabetes, high blood pressure, and cholesterol can be stopped eventually after following a sound diet plan and avoiding Western diet foods like the plague. To become weight-stable with none of the health markers that indicate an unhealthy metabolism should be everyone's goal.

*Pro Tip: If you are a control freak like me, buy a blood pressure machine and a blood glucose test kit. Both are under 40 bucks.*

## Antibiotic Use

If you end up getting sick (e.g., upper respiratory infection, toothache) or need surgery, you'll be prescribed antibiotics. Take them. But first ask the doctor or prescribing pharmacist to double check to be very certain this is the correct course of treatment. The CDC estimates that 30% of antibiotics are prescribed needlessly—to treat viral infections, for instance. There is a very good chance that your doctor is getting it wrong.

It's a good practice to begin a course of probiotics at the same time you start with antibiotics, and continue the probiotics for a week or two afterward. Also make sure your diet is impeccable and contains many high-fiber vegetables.

*Healthcare Industry Insider Secret:* Up to one-fourth of patients taking antibiotics develop antibiotic associated diarrhea (AAD). AAD can be fatal. Taking a probiotic alongside antibiotics has shown that approximately 66% of cases of AAD can be avoided (Rodgers, 2013) (Agamennone, 2018).

What do antibiotics have to do with weight maintenance, you ask? Well, the likelihood of anyone needing antibiotics in any given year is quite high. Antibiotics can destroy a healthy gut in a matter of days while helping to cure your bacterial infection. A healthy gut, as we all know, is paramount to health and weight stability. It can take years to recover your gut from antibiotic use unless your diet and health were impeccable to begin with.

## Supplements

Dietary supplements are a $120-billion-dollar industry in the US. Supplements generally fit these categories:

- Amino acids
- Enzymes
- Fiber/Prebiotics
- Herbs and botanicals
- Minerals
- Oils
- Probiotics
- Vitamins

The following are the top 10 highest selling supplements on Amazon in 2018:

- CoQ10
- Creatine

- Digestive Enzymes
- Fish Oil
- Gelatin
- Hemp Oil
- L. Arginine
- Probiotics
- Vitamin D
- Vitamin E

There are an estimated 85,000 supplement products in the US marketplace (Dwyer, 2018). How does one choose? Simple … choose none. You most likely don't need *any* supplements.

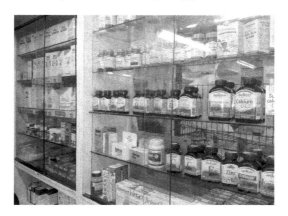

*Supplement Industry Insider Secret:* The FDA does not have enough people or facilities to inspect and analyze even a portion of the supplements being sold in the US today. When checked, many supplements contain very little of the advertised active ingredients and also many contaminants.

Nearly 100% of supplement purchases are impulse buys. You read an article or see a shiny bottle and realize that this one single thing is what has been keeping you from reaching perfection, so you buy it. But how do you really know what's in that shiny bottle? You don't, and neither does the Food and Drug Administration. All the government cares about is if the labeling is correct and the packaging plant passes inspection.

## Which Supplements Should We Take for Weight Maintenance?

Unless your doctor draws blood and tells you that you're low in something and recommends a supplement, *don't take anything*. All of your vitamins and minerals should come from the food you eat. Many are produced by the bacteria in your guts.

> *Supplement Industry Insider Secret:* In 2008, over 200 people were poisoned after taking Total Body Mega Formula, a multivitamin sold in health stores across the United States. The liquid was supposed to contain 200 micrograms of selenium but actually contained 40,800 micrograms ... enough to cause hair loss, fingernails to fall off, nausea, vomiting, and diarrhea (MacFarquhar, 2010).

If you decide you need a supplement, such as creatine or fish oil, first ask yourself, "Can I get this from real food?" The answer is almost always yes. Let's hack the top 10:

| Supplement | Used for ... | Found in ... |
| --- | --- | --- |
| CoQ10 | Energy production | Organ meats such as animal liver and heart. Beef, pork, chicken, and fatty fish such as tuna, with beef having the highest amounts |
| Creatine | Athletic performance | Red meat, pork, poultry, and fish |

| Supplement | Used for ... | Found in ... |
|---|---|---|
| Digestive Enzymes | Aids digestions | Bananas, papayas, avocados, soy sauce, sauerkraut |
| Fish Oil | Prevents heart disease | Salmon, cod, sardines, and most other saltwater fish |
| Gelatin | Skin, joints, bones | Gelatin, cartilage/bone broth |
| Hemp Oil | Skin care, pain | Pass the hemp seeds, man |
| L. Arginine | Heart health | Meat |
| Probiotics | Digestive aid | Sauerkraut, kimchi, pickles, yogurt |
| Vitamin D | Bone health | Sunlight, mushrooms, fish |
| Vitamin E | Eye health, immunity | Nuts, seeds, oils |

There really is no excuse for buying supplements on impulse. There are some regularly prescribed by doctors that can't be easily found in food, such as folic acid for pregnant women and vitamin B12 for elderly patients. But beyond a specific need for a valid medical concern, just eat good food.

Rx **for weight maintenance #30: Focus on your metabolic health; strive for normal blood pressure, waist measurement, blood glucose, triglycerides, and cholesterol.**

Rx **for weight maintenance #31: Talk to your doctor about getting off medications.**

Rx **for weight maintenance #32: Take probiotics if you are prescribed antibiotics. This will help preserve your gut health.**

Rx **for weight maintenance #33: Don't waste your money on supplements. Eat real food.**

# CONCLUSION TO PART 3

**TL;DR**: *Weight maintenance after losing weight is d\*mn hard!*

One researcher describes weight maintenance for formerly obese patients as "uneven combat."

> Weight loss is not a milestone, but rather part of a dynamic process. Following weight loss, the weight-reduced individual enters an uneven combat, commonly resulting in weight regain. (Poulimeneas, 2018)

In fact, people that maintain over 10 pounds of weight loss for more than five years are so rare that the governments of several countries have started tracking these people to learn how they do it. The bar is low. It's a rare person who maintains more than a 5-pound weight loss for over a year; and even rarer is the person who maintains a loss of 15 pounds or more, no matter what the starting weight was. To go from obese to a healthy weight and stay there for longer than five years is virtually unheard of. *But it happens.*

I've done it. Eight years and counting. *You can, too.*

It's not that people fail at dieting, it's that diets fail people. To be a weight loss success story, you don't need to have a six-pack or a cute little butt; success can be measured in many ways. If you avoid Western ultra-processed food 90% of the time and your meals consist of whole, healthy foods from every food group, then you are eating like a human should be eating. If you are exercising several days a week, then you are doing better than about 90% of your peers. If you are sleeping 7–9 hours a night and feel rested most days, then you are doing better than about two-thirds of the adults in the world. If you are trying to avoid stressful situations, you are going to reduce your chances of weight regain several times over.

Underlying everything you do should be a focus on your gut health. Don't fall for quick-fixes, powders, pills, or gadgets. You don't have to be perfect in everything you do, but you *do* need to give this the "old college try." If you need support, come visit me at my blog, www.thediethack.com, and tell me what's going on. I'd love to hear from you!

# FULL LIST OF PRESCRIPTIONS FOR WEIGHT MAINTENANCE

1.  Research, then try several different ways of eating during your first year of maintenance. This will help you find an eating style that is right for you and ensure metabolic flexibility.
2.  Weigh yourself daily. If it causes stress, weigh less frequently. Measure your waist once a month.
3.  Strive to keep your weight within a range that makes you feel good.
4.  Know your weight, but focus on your life.
5.  Track your calories for a couple days, especially if you are having trouble maintaining your weight. Are they in the correct range?
6.  Learn what 3,000 calories of food looks like, and only rarely exceed that amount in a single day.
7.  Practice *hara hachi bu*. No gorging, no grazing.
8.  Try intermittent fasting for two weeks. If it stresses you, stop.
9.  Try eating several small meals per day for two weeks. If it stresses you, stop.
10. If you eat three meals a day, pack them with whole, unprocessed food and balance the calories to your pleasure.
11. If you experience symptoms of undereating (feeling cold, sleeplessness, hair loss, low energy, mood swings, or binge-eating), examine your calorie intake to ensure you are eating enough food.
12. Take two potatoes and call me in the morning.
13. Don't fall for scams or bad science. If it seems too good to be true, it probably is. Gadgets, clothing, pills, or teas for magical weight loss don't work.
14. Start an aerobic and strength training exercise program.
15. Get as far away from stressful situations as you can. Seek professional help if you need it.

16. Clean up your diet, and eat lots of food high in B-Vitamins and omega-3 oils.

17. Consider supplementing Vitamin D3, especially in the winter. Take a B12 supplement if you're vegan.

18. Parents, make sure your kids are happy, well-fed, and well-rested.

19. Get a good night's sleep, meaning 7–9 hours a night.

20. If you smoke, switch to vaping or patches. Then quit.

21. If you are a cannabis user and cannot control your weight, consider giving it up for a year. If you want to try legalized cannabis for the first time, be aware that what you are buying may not be safe or adequately tested.

22. Ladies, take two glasses of merlot and call me in the morning. Guys, lay off the booze.

23. Build a social network for weight maintenance using online resources or personal friends, family, or coworkers.

24. Take pictures of yourself to help gauge your progress.

25. Keep a log to track your weight and other health markers.

26. Avoid diets that restrict starchy tubers, grains, seeds, vegetables, and fruit.

27. Eat several servings of fruit and vegetables each day.

28. Regularly consume fermented foods such as sauerkraut, pickles, and kombucha.

29. Take a probiotic that contains "lacto" and "bifido" if you need to take antibiotics for an infection.

30. Focus on your metabolic health; strive for normal blood pressure, waist measurement, blood glucose, triglycerides, and cholesterol.

31. Talk to your doctor about getting off medications.

32. Take probiotics if you are prescribed antibiotics. This will help preserve your gut health.

33. Don't waste your money on supplements. Eat real food.

# PART 4

# EXERCISE FOR WEIGHT LOSS AND MAINTENANCE

# INTRODUCTION TO PART 4

I felt compelled to have a section dedicated to exercise. I tried writing this into the other sections, but they quickly became too long and convoluted. This isn't your normal "Exercise for Dummies" type of essay, rather I'll try to convince you with sound science why each movement is needed, and then I'll show you how to perform the basic exercise movements and what to expect from each exercise. Maybe I'll also make you chuckle. My target audience is people who do not currently exercise, or people looking to revamp their boring old routine. If you're a pro on the squat rack with a 1RM of 320, you're better off looking somewhere else for advice. If you have no idea what that means, read on!

I'm not a natural exerciser. I had to force myself to start exercising when I realized how important exercising is for health and weight stability. I hate going to gyms—I'd rather get a tooth pulled. If there's a gym at a hotel or resort I'm staying at, I'll check it out, but I'm not about to become a life member of Planet Fitness any time soon. I have great respect for people who do frequent gyms, though.

Each chapter in this section will begin with a TL;DR summary so you don't waste time reading, and each ends with a "non-negotiable" exercise requirement. I'm big on minimum effective doses, just don't try to out-minimum me, please. Consider my exercise outline a starting point for your new program. Please know, this is NOT about burning more calories or trying to tell you you've been too lazy. This is about very compelling research that suggests the only way to become metabolically healthy is to exercise in a very specific way, and that way is a simple combination of aerobic and strength training exercises. The programs I am about to outline for you are *not that hard*. You'll see.

# CHAPTER 27

## WHY EXERCISE?

**TL;DR:** *80–90% of adults don't engage in regular exercise. The health benefits of exercise are many and far outweigh any excuses you could have not to exercise. Start an exercise program today if you haven't already.*

So far, we've discussed the Western diet, eating better, sleeping, de-stressing your life, how to lose weight by hacking industry secrets, and maintaining your weight loss. All along, I kept mentioning exercise. If you take all the other advice, you could probably skip this whole "exercise" thing and be okay. But I'll give you about a 30% chance of keeping your weight off for more than a year. If you want to be one of the 3–5% of dieters who maintain a weight loss for over five years—and you do—you'll want to keep reading (Spring, 2018) (Wing, 2005).

Aerobic and strength training exercise are of *vital importance* to keeping your weight in check and staying healthy. Without exercise, your heart becomes complacent and your muscles weak; it makes your genes work against you. Look at exercise to hedge your bets on living a long, healthy life free of heart disease and the host of debilitating illnesses that inflict nearly everyone as they age. Exercise isn't about losing weight—it's about having a body that's resistant to weight gain and aging (Swift, 2014). It works. It *really* works. But maybe you have to see it to believe it.

The exercises I'm about to discuss can be done alongside a weight loss diet to prevent loss of muscle and lowered aerobic capacity

(Schwarz, 2011). These programs should also be improved upon and kept up *after* weight loss to ensure weight stability for the long run (Booth, 2012) (Spring, 2018).

## Exercise Recommendations

You'll recall from a previous discussion that the "official" recommendations for exercise are (World Health Organization, 2010):

- Moderate aerobic exercise: 2 ½ hours per week, and/or
- Vigorous aerobic exercise: 1 hour 15 minutes per week, and
- Strength training: 2–3 times per week

The moderate and vigorous aerobic exercises may be combined for 2 ½ hours per week. Also acceptable is 1 hour and 15 minutes of vigorous activity alone. Best practice is a minimum of 30–60 minutes per day of some type of aerobic exercise with a couple days focused on strength training.

These aren't just arbitrary numbers. These recommendations are backed not only by the World Health Organization but also by the US Centers for Disease Control, the American College of Sports Medicine, the American Heart Association, and Department of Health and Human Services (Oja, 2011). Nearly every exercise program in existence uses these guidelines as a basis for "enough" exercise.

## Insulin Sensitivity

Insulin sensitivity, that is the body's ability to sense and store glucose, is the holy grail of metabolic health. Resistance to insulin is the start of a long, slow decline into poor health (Freeman, 2018). Along with diet, exercise is the best method to increase insulin sensitivity and stave off disease (Buresh, 2018). The recommended amounts of exercise almost guarantee increased insulin sensitivity. The problem is, nobody wants to exercise.

## How Many People Exercise?

According to a large survey, less than 20% of Americans get the recommended level of exercise. When you look at people older than 24, the number drops even further to about 15% (Jaslow, 2013).

Let's do some math: 50% of adults are on a diet, 80–85% don't exercise, and 95% of diets fail. I'm not a statistician, but those numbers don't look surprising. Why don't more people exercise? When people were surveyed, these are the most cited reasons they gave (The Heart Foundation, 2018):

- Can't afford it.
- Don't like to exercise alone.
- Don't like to sweat.
- Embarrassed around opposite sex.
- No motivation.
- Too boring.
- Too busy.
- Too old or unfit.
- Too tired.
- Tried and quit.

I get it. Exercise takes a very low priority for most people. Plus, people seem to think that they move around enough in their life and don't need to go out and intentionally move more. But I think the underlying theme is that people just don't see *why* they need to. None of the respondents answered, "Don't care about insulin sensitivity," or "My bones are strong enough." They just gave excuses. This tells me most people don't *know* what benefits we get from exercise. So, I'll tell you.

*Healthcare Industry Insider Secret: If people exercised to the minimum recommendations, they would (Warburton, 2006):*

- *Enjoy longer life.*
- *Delay the onset of 40 chronic conditions/diseases (e.g., cardiovascular disease, diabetes, cancer, hypertension, obesity, depression, and osteoporosis).*
- *Enjoy better cardiovascular fitness.*
- *Have stronger bones.*
- *Sleep better.*
- *Have less stress.*
- *Maintain their weight.*

## Minimum Effective Dose

Scientists have established that burning an extra 500 calories, or getting about an hour of exercise, weekly is effective for health benefits associated with exercise.

> A volume of exercise that is about half of what is currently recommended may be sufficient, particularly for people who are extremely deconditioned or are frail and elderly (Warburton, 2006).

Getting started with an exercise program is like planting an oak tree: The best time was 30 years ago; the second-best time is today.

*Non-negotiable: Start an exercise routine today, anything, just get started.*

# CHAPTER 28

# YES, YOU HAVE TIME TO EXERCISE

**TL;DR:** *Truly, 30–60 minutes a day is plenty of time for aerobic exercise and strength training.*

There's not a legitimate diet program in the universe that doesn't advise you to exercise in conjunction with the plan. If you do find one, it's a scam. Unfortunately, this is the part most often overlooked or ignored. Why? Exercising takes time, and most people have no idea how to exercise effectively.

Before we discuss the movements involved in a good exercise program, I want to show you what a good routine looks like.

## Three exercise requirements
- Aerobic movement (moderate)
- Aerobic movement (vigorous)
- Strength training (all muscle groups)

## Optimal time required
- 5–10 minutes for warm-up and stretching (Andersen, 2005)
- Combination of moderate and vigorous aerobics, 30–60 minutes per day
- Strength training, 20–30 minutes 2–3 times a week

## Minimum time required
- 30 minutes, 3 times a week of aerobic exercise, like walking
- 10 minutes, twice a week for strength training

- 15 minutes, once a week of vigorous aerobics, like cycling, swimming, jogging, fast walking

## How Vigorous?

Most people get the *moderate* aerobic requirement. Walking, light cycling, yoga, etc. but what exactly does "vigorous" mean? And what does "combined" mean?

It is a bit confusing. The intent of the aerobic requirement is to get people moving for 30 minutes most days of the week. Walking is fine. More is better. If you walk 30 minutes every day at lunch, that's enough. If you can't walk every day, you'll need to get in a more "vigorous" activity to make up for it. For example, if you can only walk three days a week for 30 minutes each day, it would be best if you jogged those 30 minutes. If you hate jogging, just jog for 30 seconds every couple of minutes as you walk. The goal of vigorous exercise is to work up a sweat, to really get your heart pumping.

## Stretching

It's always a good idea to stretch before doing any type of exercise (Andersen, 2005). In fact, stretching along with balance is equal in importance to aerobic exercise and strength training. Please watch some videos on stretching prior to setting up your fitness routine. Everyone needs something a little different, but stretching is just hyping up the muscles. A couple jumping jacks and push-ups plus running in place is a good start. Start the exercise set slowly with lower weight before you get into it. Just don't hurt yourself!

## Problems

Many people make the mistake of jumping into an exercise program without thinking. They end up hurting themselves or not seeing any results, so they quit. Or they join a gym only to find out the people there are big sweaty jerks, and they feel intimidated. Or you find it gets to be too expensive, there's not enough equipment, or it's too crowded, inconvenient, etc.

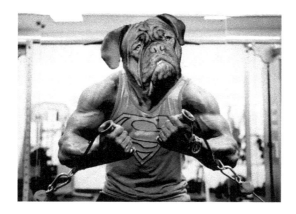

## <u>Some Solutions</u>

There are many people who simply refuse to exercise. No one really cares because the vast majority of people don't exercise, either. If you want to be a shining example for others, be one of the few who exercise regularly. If family and work commitments are a problem, become *militant* with your schedule. Create and adhere to a strict exercise schedule. Soon, everyone will know not to bother you when you are in "exercise mode." Your health depends on it, so why not? Some other solutions that might get you over the hump to keep you motivated:

- Download the latest fitness apps for walking, and go for a walk.
- Join an online forum for people who share similar struggles.
- Keep a calendar. Put an X on every day that you exercised.

- Pay yourself. Put $5 in a jar every time you exercise, and spend the money on yourself at the end of the month.
- Start an exercise club. Social support is a massively good way to stay motivated.
- Start listening to audiobooks while you walk.

*Non-negotiable: Take dedicated 30-minute walks at least three days a week. Do some strength training (e.g., push-ups/squats) 1–2 days a week. Learn to stretch.*

# CHAPTER 29

## AEROBIC EXERCISE

> **TL;DR:** *Walk, run, skip, hop, or ride a bike. Create a program that gets your heart rate up a bit for 30–60 minutes on most days. Sex doesn't count!*

Aerobic exercise is done for cardiovascular conditioning. Also called "cardio" or "endurance training." Aerobic means "with oxygen." Your breathing and heart rate will increase during aerobic activities, leading to numerous health benefits including weight loss and weight stability.

Aerobic exercise is NOT a punishment for eating too much. It's not a way to justify bad eating habits. Don't pay any attention to calculators or digital displays that show how many calories you burned during your workout. It's very important that you completely separate exercise from eating: *the two have nothing to do with each other*.

The best exercise program is the one you will do, week after week, year after year. Looking at aerobic exercise specifically, it takes no special equipment other than comfortable clothes and good shoes. The movements are not difficult. You can buy DVDs and follow along at home or join an organized aerobics class. Yoga studios are really popular now, and even yoga is easy to do at home. The hardest part is just getting started.

Aerobic exercise is the foundation of your fitness program. This will ensure a healthy heart and lungs. If you can continue with a well-planned, meaningful aerobic program into old age, you'll be so far ahead of your peers that you won't even recognize them. You'll be the envy of the old folks' home (because you won't be there). I can't stress enough how important it is to do aerobic exercise as simple as just walking. As you get more fit, you'll feel like doing more. Let your body guide you in this endeavor, it won't let you down ... even if you've let *it* down.

## More Than Just Classes

One of the best aerobic workouts you can do is walking. It's free, and you can do it just about anywhere. Treadmills are cheap enough to buy for your home. Bicycling and exercise bikes also fit the bill for cheap, easy aerobic workouts. It doesn't have to be an organized class. Here are some ideas:

- Bicycling
- Calisthenics
- Cardio machines
- Cross-country skiing
- Dancing
- Hiking
- Kickboxing
- Pilates
- Running
- Snowshoeing
- Swimming
- Tai chi
- Walking
- Yoga

An excellent plan is to be able to do several of these workouts on a whim, with a backup plan in case you run out of time. A nightly walk after dinner is perfect. Some would rather get up early and do it before work. However, you do it, *just keep doing it.*

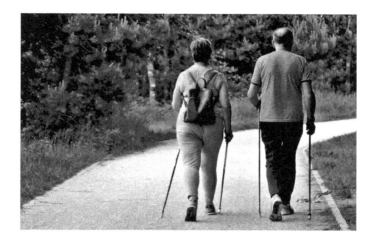

## How Much/How Often?

The ideal amount of aerobic exercise is 30–60 minutes a day of low-level exercise (e.g., walking), with some "more vigorous" exercise thrown in 3–4 days per week. This amount of aerobic exercise is optimal for human health (Mann, 2014). You can develop a great routine based on exercising five or six days a week. If you miss a day, you can play catch-up on the weekend.

## Do Gardening, Shopping, and Chasing Kids Count?

Moms with young'uns will argue, but the short answer is no (Ceria-Ulep, 2011).

There is a big difference between "physical activity" and "exercise." While it's great to get lots of physical activity, it's not considered exercise. Sure, vacuuming a house, taking laundry up and down the stairs, mowing the lawn, and having sex burn calories, but you can't count this as your aerobic exercise requirement unless it can fit a specific pattern. Think of it this way: the *exercise* you do enables you to perform *physical activity* better.

## No Days Off?

I'm sure I lost a couple of you with this seemingly aggressive routine. It's okay to take some breaks from your normally scheduled program—just don't make a habit of it. If you're sick or you've overdone it, take it easy for a week or so. You'll soon be back on your game. What I love about a six-day exercise schedule is that if you miss a day, you can pick it up on your off-day, and if you miss a couple days it's no big deal. Aerobic exercise is not physically demanding, and it's not supposed to be.

## Catch Me Outside. How 'bout Dat?

Try to do much of your aerobic program *outside,* if you can. Breathing fresh air and getting sunshine while you exercise is one of the best stress-relievers there is and helps you sleep better (Lee, 2014). It's important for humans to get a good dose of sunshine, while being careful not to burn. Lack of sunlight has been implicated in many modern diseases such as cancer, auto-immune conditions, multiple sclerosis (MS), high blood pressure, metabolic syndrome, and more (Mead, 2008). You'll need a back-up plan for inclement weather.

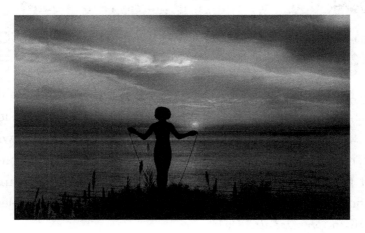

## Developing Your Aerobic Exercise Program

To separate exercise from physical activity, we can look at it like this: Physical activity is what your normal life is all about—work, hobbies, family, leisure, *lurrrve*. Exercise needs to be *intentional, timed, controlled, and meaningful.*

**Intentional:** You cannot count daily movement unless you are a foot patrolman or a mail carrier (many of whom are also overweight, by the way). Look at how the military does it; they line up every morning for physical training (PT) and do an hour or so of jumping jacks, push-ups, squats, and sprints followed by several miles of marching or running. Then they go about their day of marching to and fro, carrying heavy packs, jumping out of airplanes, or any number of physically demanding tasks. They exercise so they can better perform their daily movements. They never say, "Let's skip PT this morning, guys. We have a big day ahead of us." Daily activity doesn't count. You can only count it as aerobic exercise if it is done intentionally, above and beyond your normal daily life. Normal activities are great (mowing, gardening, etc.) but they are rife with problems (e.g., frequent breaks, gaps between activity, and poor form). Better to mow your lawn, hoe your garden, vacuum your floor, then go for a jog or a fast walk.

**Timed:** You need to time your aerobic exercise session. Plan on 30 minutes a day as a minimum. One hour is better. Much more is not needed (Mann, 2014).

*Pro Tip: Buy an inexpensive "interval timer." With this you can time your fast and slow aerobic sessions with a loud buzzer to tell you when to switch. Once you get your routine down, timing becomes easy.*

**Controlled:** You should tightly control your aerobic workouts. Everyone around you needs to know when you are in "exercise mode." Perhaps you need to go to bed at 8 p.m. and get up at 4 a.m. to make this work. So be it. If you miss a session, you should perform it at the next available time. Sure, it's hard, but priorities people, *priorities*! The gym stays open till 9, right? Maybe instead, go for a fast walk around your neighborhood. Live in a crappy part of town? Do jumping jacks and run in place for 30 minutes. Don't want to miss *Survivor*? *I don't want to hear it.* If this just doesn't sound like you, if your life is in shambles and there's no way you can control your aerobic exercise schedule, then maybe it's time to reevaluate what's going on in your life. Stress is also bad, remember?

**Meaningful:** The 2000 Fitbit steps you get from brushing your teeth don't count. Yes, I wore one for a while. I know the tricks. Your aerobic exercise routine must be meaningful. Here are some good guidelines:

> *Moderate Aerobics:* Brisk walking. This just means walking at a pace like you want to get somewhere fast, but not quite so fast you are out of breath. About 3–4 miles per hour (Slaght, 2017).

> *Vigorous Aerobics:* Work up a good sweat. Do this in conjunction with your daily walks, or in addition to the walking. This can be done in repeated short bursts that last just 30 seconds or so with a minute or two of rest in between, or a steady jog/run/speedwalk. This portion does not need to be based on running. You can do anything that makes you sweat: Sports, step aerobics, bike riding, stationary bike, elliptical machines, stair-stepper, running up and down real steps, flipping tires, or whatever you like. Join an aerobics class if you so desire, but it's not necessary. It can be fun to do this with some friends, or alone. The goal is to get your heart rate up a bit more. Since tracking heart rate is quite cumbersome and confusing, just go until you start to get sweaty or out of breath (Patel, 2017).

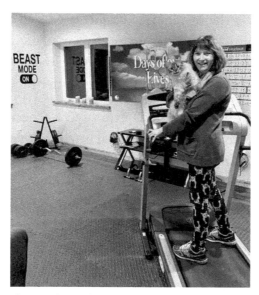

*Jackie and Hemingway gettin' their cardio on.*

## Some Cool Aerobic Exercise Terms

*HIIT*: High Intensity Interval Training (Boutcher, 2010). This is basically what "running sprints" was all about in high school. With HIIT, you perform short (30 second) powerful bursts of speed broken up by longer periods (1–3 minutes) of low-intensity walking. Times of the intervals can vary, some recommend doing 40 seconds of high intensity with a 20-second rest. The key is very powerful bursts of speed interspersed with a rest cycle. HIIT lends itself well to walk/jog routines, bicycling, hill-climbing, or many machines designed to maximize HIIT (ellipticals, stair-climbers, rowing machines, etc).

*LISS:* Low-Intensity Steady State (Fisher, 2015). LISS is basically walking for a long time. With LISS, you want to get your heart rate up a bit, but not to the point where you're out of breath or sweating. This is the "moderate" activity that everyone recommends. LISS should be performed 30–60 minutes a day, 3–7 days a week.

*VO₂ Max:* This is the maximum volume of oxygen that your body can efficiently utilize during exercise. This measurement is used by doctors to assess cardiorespiratory (aerobic) fitness. As you exercise more, your $VO_2$ max increases, indicating better fitness.

*MHR:* Maximum Heart Rate is expressed in "beats per minute." When doing aerobic exercises, the goal is to make your heart pump harder, but not too hard. Most experts agree that getting your heart pumping to about 50–60% of your MHR is just right for LISS (moderate intensity) aerobics, and 70–90% for HIIT. To calculate your MHR, simply take 220 minus your age. For example, a 50-year-old person: 220 − 50 = 170 beats per minute MHR. For exercise purposes, divide MHR by 2 for 50% of MHR, or 85 beats per minute, in this example. You'll find many different methods of calculating a preferred target heart rate for different styles of aerobic exercise.

*KISS:* Keep it Simple, Stupid. For moderate aerobic exercise, just do it at a pace that you can easily keep up with for 30–60 minutes. To add some "vigor," walk a bit faster for brief periods until you get a bit out of breath and start to sweat. As you get more fit, it will take more to get out of breath and sweaty. For beginners, best to keep it simple. Don't worry about HIIT, LISS, $VO_2$ max, or MHR. Just get moving! Once you're a pro, read some books and learn more about how all this works.

## 10,000 Steps a Day

The current craze is walking 10,000 steps a day (approximately 5 miles). This originated in the 1970s in Japanese walking clubs and carried over to the United States in the early 2000s (Yuenyongchaiwat, 2016). Under the current usage of the idea, these 10,000 steps are not walked consecutively. Most people walk 4–6,000 steps a day in normal daily activity, leaving a deficit of 4–6,000 steps, requiring one to purposely walk for an extra 30–60 minutes daily.

## Fitbits

I'm not a fan of electronic step trackers. They are notoriously inaccurate. I tried out a couple of old-fashioned mechanical pedometers and two types of Fitbits for a couple months last summer. I found that at a normal walking speed, I took 2,000 steps per mile. Both the mechanical pedometer and the Fitbits were extremely accurate in counting steps *while walking nonstop*.

While wearing a mechanical pedometer, I was seeing about 5,000 steps during my 7 a.m.–5 p.m. workday, with an extra 2,000 steps before and after work. Most of these "steps" were just normal, daily activity—nothing I would count as "moderate aerobic exercise."

When wearing a Fitbit, I saw anywhere from 10,000 to 20,000 steps during my workday! That's a 5,000–15,000-step error. A quick web search shows that this is a very common complaint, and there are some hacks to increase the accuracy such as wearing the Fitbit on your left hand or decreasing the sensitivity. I tried several things but never got the accuracy I was hoping for.

My advice is to ditch the Fitbits and pedometers. Walk an extra 30–60 minutes every day and don't worry about how many steps you've taken. Automated step counters will mislead you into thinking you don't need to exercise with purpose. That said, Fitbits can do some pretty amazing things like track your sleep, heart rate, and even food intake. If you're a techie, you'll have fun with it, but expect it to be quite inaccurate.

***Non-negotiable:*** *Walk, at any speed you can, 30 minutes, 3 times a week.*

# CHAPTER 30

# STRENGTH TRAINING

> **TL;DR:** *Strength training improves your overall metabolism and helps you maintain your weight. A good program only takes 20–30 minutes, 1–3 times a week. Learn the proper movements so you don't waste time or hurt yourself. Don't be a noob.*

As aerobic exercise is for your heart, so strength training is for your muscles. The benefits of strength training reach far beyond your muscles. The terms "resistance" and "strength" training can be used interchangeably for the purpose of this discussion. We can use weights, machines, bands, or our own body to provide resistance for strengthening our muscles. Most people's minds automatically go to pictures of musclemen lifting giant barbells, but there are other ways to do this, as you'll soon see.

Strength training is about more than just getting stronger. Strength training is a proven way to slow down aging and prevent disease. If more people knew exactly *why* we need strength training, there'd be no room in the gym. It doesn't take much time at all! Just 20 minutes a couple times a week is perfectly enough, ideal even. Strength training can be as easy or as hard as you make it.

## Why Do It?

Adults who do not do any kind of strength training will lose 3–8% of their muscle mass every ten years, have a much lower resting metabolism, and greater fat accumulation compared to adults who keep up with a strength-training program. Benefits of a good strength-training program can be summed up as follows (Westcott, 2012):

- Enhances cardiovascular health by reducing resting blood pressure, decreasing LDL cholesterol and triglycerides, and increasing HDL cholesterol.
- Improves physical performance, movement control, walking speed, functional independence, cognitive abilities, and self-esteem.
- Prevents type 2 diabetes by decreasing visceral fat, reducing HbA1c, and improving insulin sensitivity.
- Reduces low back pain and eases discomfort associated with arthritis and fibromyalgia.
- Reverses specific aging factors in skeletal muscles.
- Strengthens bones.

## Convinced? Good!

Now that you understand *why* you need to strength train, we can get started. Just about everyone agrees that all we need is at least two strength training sessions per week, but most people don't have a good strength-training program. Adding this to your routine will pay massive dividends toward your weight loss goals, lifelong weight maintenance, and health.

Like aerobic exercise, strength training has some key elements: strength training also needs to be *intentional, timed, controlled, and meaningful*.

**Intentional:** You don't get to say, "I just hauled in the groceries, that was a real workout!" No. Doesn't count, sorry. You need to intentionally work specific muscle groups (arms, back, chest, core, legs, and shoulders).

**Timed:** You'll need to set aside 15–30 minutes, at least twice a week, to train your muscles.

**Controlled:** You need to have a plan. You should do exercises that work each muscle group and perform 8–12 reps of each exercise in 1–3 sets with a minute or two resting between sets. This is proven advice, not bro-science. You need to learn to do each exercise properly. There are tons of free videos online to watch, or you can get help at the gym. No freelancing! Injuries abound when people don't do this properly.

**Meaningful:** The resistance you use to strengthen your muscles needs to be heavy enough that you feel it. Using too little resistance doesn't do much good, but *too much* is not good either. Over time, you may need to increase the resistance you use.

## Lingo

I've probably used some terms you might not recognize. Sets? Reps? Let me explain. Bodybuilders and gym rats have developed their own language. Here are a few words you need to know:

- *1RM:* One Rep Max. This is the heaviest weight you can possibly lift once.

- *Bro-science:* Things that people at the gym say with no scientific evidence that it works. "Do 4,000 push-ups a day for best results? Sounds like *bro-science* to me."

- *Bulking:* A phase bodybuilders use to gain muscle. "Wow, you ate a whole chicken. Are you *bulking* for a competition?"

- *Cutting:* A phase bodybuilders go through to lose weight. "You look great. Are you *cutting*?"

- *Hypertrophy:* Causing muscles to expand to mammoth proportions using targeted training.

- *Noob:* Short for newbie. A person "new" to the gym scene.

- *Reps:* The number of times you do each movement. "Twenty *reps* of pushups in one set."

- *Sets:* The number of times you do an exercise. "Three *sets* of push-ups."

- *Plates:* Weights used on barbells or dumbbells.

- *PR:* Personal Record. This is your own Olympic gold medal. If you really want to get some street cred at the gym, after your last set of the day, slam down the weights and parade around yelling, "Woooooo! PR, baby, PR! In yo' face, bro!"

---

*Fitness Industry Insider Secret: A team of researchers concluded that a <u>single set</u> of several basic exercises performed <u>twice a week</u> will result in superior strength compared to other more time-consuming programs (Feigenbaum, 1997).*

---

As you get stronger, you'll likely want to start doing more. However, we must realize that not all of us have the time to make a career out of strength training. Performing one set of key exercises is enough to create meaningful change.

## Is All Resistance Training Created Equal?

No. People train for different outcomes (Mangine, 2015). Building large, veiny muscles requires a special type of resistance training, known as *hypertrophy training* (Mangine, 2015). Training to increase endurance requires another (Mangine, 2015). We are going for "strength" here as opposed to becoming the next Mr. Universe or an Olympic swimmer.

| Type of Program | % of 1RM | Repetitions per Set | Sets per Session |
|---|---|---|---|
| Strength | 50–70% | 6–12 | 1–3 |
| Endurance | 40–60% | 13–60 | 2–4 |
| Large Muscles | 60–80% | 6–12 | 4–8 |

1RM, or One Rep Max, is the heaviest weight you can possibly lift.

Strength training to increase one's muscle *tone* is a very rewarding activity. It will make you feel great and not worn out. But as I've said before, getting started is the hardest part! I'll describe it thoroughly later, but in case you're wondering how much weight you'll actually be lifting, here's a quick way to find out.

**Determining your 1RM:** Find a weight that you can easily pick up and put down about 10 times, but not 20 times. You should get tired somewhere in the middle. This will be about 50% of your 1RM.

Don't let the details get you down! This is just a primer into strength training. I'll have you walking and talking like a gym rat soon enough.

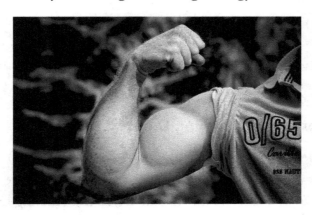

## Will I Lose Weight?

Strength training is not strictly done for weight loss, it's done to make you healthy—but it certainly won't hurt your weight loss efforts (Villareal, 2017). The long-range goal may be weight loss, but many people are under the assumption that strength training will burn fat from targeted areas of the body; this is simply not true, no matter what the beautiful people on TV tell you.

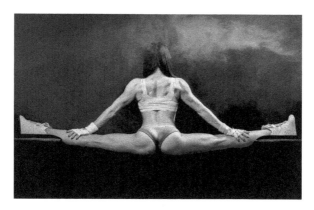

## Different Methods of Strength Training

The next several chapters will discuss specific methods of strength training. While there are countless YouTube videos, books, and programs to check out, I want to go through each one of these methods in detail so you have a reference for each strength training method as it relates to weight maintenance.

We'll be looking at these, arranged from level of effort and experience required:

- Bodyweight exercises
- Resistance bands
- Weight machines
- Weightlifting (free weights)

Each one has its place. My intent is to help you develop a plan you can stick to and not feel like a total noob in the gym.

## How to Spot a Noob in the Gym

I once stayed at a hotel with a nice little gym. While I was walking on the treadmill, a gentleman wearing jeans and a jacket came in and looked around. He spent about five minutes positioning a weight bench in front of a mirror and another five minutes picking dumbbells off the rack. Finally, he brought a very small dumbbell to his bench and started doing bicep curls. He did about 60, then switched arms for 60 more. Then he set the weight on the ground and proceeded to take a nap on the weight bench. *Noob!*

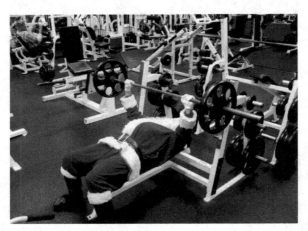

Here are some total noob moves:
- Wear street clothes to work out in.
- Use the machines completely wrong.
- Lift too light or too heavy.
- Bring kids in the gym and let them run around.
- Don't wipe down the equipment after use.
- Try to use *every* machine.
- Work only one muscle group.

- Give advice to everyone.
- Quit in February.

At least after you read the rest of this chapter you won't be a *total* noob. I'm only half joking here—the gym can be a daunting place! It will help if you go in with a plan and can talk intelligently to the staff.

## Muscle Groups

A proper strength-training program will work all the muscle groups:

- Arms
- Back
- Chest
- Core
- Legs
- Shoulders

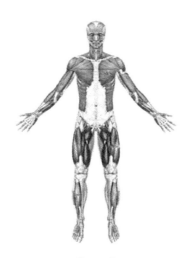

Medlineplus.gov

**Non-negotiable:** *Get started with a strength-training program soon. For now, drop and give me 10.*

# CHAPTER 31

# STRENGTH TRAINING METHOD 1: BODYWEIGHT EXERCISES

**TL;DR:** *Exercise like a prisoner or soldier: push-ups, pull-ups, squats, and planks.*

Bodyweight exercise is a strength training method using only your body's own weight and gravity. There are a couple of basic bodyweight moves that most people can master easily. You'll be doing 8–12 reps for 1–3 sets during each strength training session (Thomas, 2014). A good bodyweight strength training session only takes 15–20 minutes. These exercises are great for men and women. We'll be focusing on four very effective moves:

- Squats
- Push-ups
- Planks
- Pull-ups

Even if your plan is to join a gym or buy some weights, it pays to learn these basic bodyweight moves. You can do them anywhere, even at work. If you master these, you'll have all you need for a good strength-training program. If you are still on the fence about strength training, do these bodyweight exercises for six months and see what you think then. I'll bet you'll be hooked and ready for more.

## Squats

The squat is a lower body exercise that trains the muscles of the legs, back, and core.

Squats are a central movement for most strength-training programs and should never be overlooked. Squats work the largest muscles in your body (quadriceps) as well as help you with balance and flexibility.

Squats are easy to master. The fitness industry likes to complicate things, so they've invented dozens of variations, most of which will just help you hurt yourself. Here are some popular variations you might like to try (from Wikipedia):

- Bodyweight squat: The most basic form.
- Face-the-wall squat: A bodyweight squat done facing a wall, toes against the wall, making balance even more difficult than the overhead squat.
- Hindu squat: A squat done standing on toes, heels raised, instead of flat-footed. This form helps to strengthen the legs, calves, lower back, and thighs.
- Hindu-jumper squat: Similar to a Hindu squat, but with a jump of about six inches after each rep.
- Jump squat: A bodyweight squat where one jumps forcefully off the floor at the top.
- Overhead squat: A bodyweight squat with the hands held over your head so that more balance is required, working your core area more.
- Pistol squat: A bodyweight single-leg squat while the other leg is extended off the floor.
- Prisoner squat: A version of the bodyweight squat where fingers are interlocked behind your head.
- Shrimp squat: A version of the pistol squat where the other

leg is held behind the body with a hand. Sometimes called the flamingo squat.

The only difficult thing about squats is getting up the ambition to do them. Squats are a good workout. You'll feel them the next day! That's good. If you have bad knees, you'll most likely not want to go crazy with squats. Perhaps try wall sits or glute bridges; no exercise is worth injuring yourself over!

To perform a simple squat, stand up straight, hands on hips or out-stretched for balance, and bend at the knees until you are as low as you can go. Straighten up and repeat.

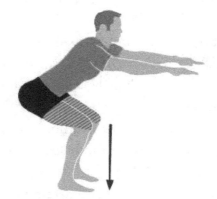

*Marcel Kollmar, CC BY-SA 3.0. (Wikipedia)*

***Pro Tip:*** *The 30-day squat challenge was popularized on social media to "build a better booty." this challenge involves progressively doing more squats every day for a month. Try it!*

## Push-ups

Push-ups are one of the most basic exercises done in nearly every fitness program. Push-ups are ubiquitous to military and prisoner life due to their simplicity, ease of mastery, endless variations, and effectiveness. Push-ups work the core, chest, and arms.

It's easier to show than describe, but you already know what a push-up is.

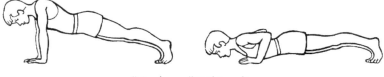

*"Push-up," Wikipedia*

## Variations

Some variations for you to search online and explore later:

- Backhanded push-up
- Clap push-up
- Guillotine push-up
- Hindu push-up
- Knuckle push-up
- Maltese push-up
- Narrow-grip push-up
- One-arm push-up
- Planche push-up
- Single-leg push-up
- Spiderman push-up

The most common push-up position is with hands and feet spaced about shoulder-width apart, but simply varying the distance between hands and between feet creates an entirely new exercise and works slightly different muscles. To keep things interesting, have fun creating your own version of the push-up.

You'll be doing 10–20 reps and 1–3 sets of push-ups in each strength training session.

## Planks

**Front plank:** This is basically a push-up, but instead of moving up and down, you hold the position for 30 seconds to 2 minutes. Planks can be done by resting on the forearms or hands, depending on the level of difficulty desired. Front planks work the muscles of the arms, core, back, and legs.

**Side plank:** These are a bit more difficult, but they're easy to master. Your weight is distributed on one forearm and a foot, working the muscles to the side of the core. When doing side planks, you should switch sides after the desired time has elapsed. Normally 30 seconds to 2 minutes.

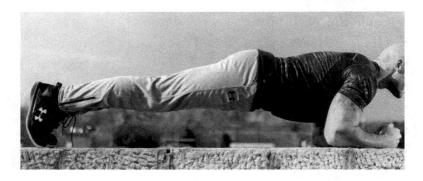

Planks are probably the best core exercise you can do. Plank challenges dominated the internet a couple years ago; people enjoyed posting pictures of themselves planking on various objects to hilarious result.

Planking seems like it would be easy, but give it a try! Try holding your planks for 30 seconds at first and work your way to 2 or more minutes. The world record plank was held for over *10 hours*!

## Pull-ups

Pull-ups are a bit more advanced. This is another exercise that is ever-present in the military and prisons because of their effectiveness and simplicity. Once you've mastered your first pull-up, the hardest one, you are on your way to doing many more. Pull-ups work the muscles of the arms, back, chest, shoulders, and core. You should strive for doing 5–10 reps of pull-ups in 1–3 sets for a good strength workout.

The hardest thing about pull-ups is that you'll need a pull-up bar. You may need help getting a suitable bar installed if you want to do these at home. You can find cheap doorway pull-up bars that can be installed in any home doorway; but be warned, they'll damage the wall if you install it wrong or buy a cheap one.

Every gym in the world has pull-up bars. Every playground has pull-up bars. You'll find places to do pull-ups just about everywhere you look. They can even be done on a tree branch or gazebo rail. My pull-up bar is a piece of pipe secured between two trees in my backyard.

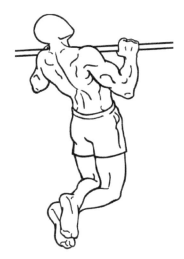

*Everkinetic, CC BY-SA 3.0, Wikipedia*

I'm assuming most readers have not done many pull-ups lately, if ever. The best way to get started with pull-ups is a technique called "negative" pull-ups. This is where you stand on a stool, grip the bar, raise your feet off the stool, and lower yourself to the ground. Once you've done 10–20 of these a day for a couple weeks, you'll most likely be able to do an actual pull-up. It helps to have the stool underneath to use as a "cheat" as you learn to do pull-ups. Pull-ups are quite rewarding. They give you a great workout. And you'll make everyone jealous of your skills.

What about the hand grip? You can either grip the bar overhanded or underhanded (fingers pointing toward you). Some prefer one way over the other, it also pays to alternate the grips periodically to work different sets of muscles.

I highly recommend the use of pull-ups in an advanced bodyweight strength training routine. I fully understand they are difficult to master and hard to find a suitable bar. If you are working out in a gym, there are machines that simulate pull-ups you might like to try.

## That's It

Squats, push-ups, planks, and pull-ups. These are the only four exercises you need for an effective strength-training program of your own. There are others, and you might explore them as you get stronger. Crunches, wall-sits, weighted pull-ups, and countless variations of the "big four." These exercises can be performed by anyone, they can all be done to exactly *your* requirements and capabilities.

*Non-negotiable: Practice doing squats, push-ups, and planks today and tomorrow. Do pull-ups if you have a bar. Design a program for the next couple weeks that uses bodyweight exercises, and stick to it.*

# CHAPTER 32

# STRENGTH TRAINING METHOD 2: RESISTANCE BANDS

**TL;DR:** *Resistance bands might seem lame, but they are very effective, cheap, and easy to use.*

Resistance bands are a cheap and effective method for first-time strength trainers and pros alike. If you can't afford free weights or just don't have the space, resistance bands are perfect. The best thing about resistance bands is that you can easily travel with them and use them anywhere.

I was not convinced you could get a good workout with resistance bands until I bought a set. It turns out they are extremely effective. In fact, exercise physiologists recently studied the effects of using elastic bands for strength training versus traditional weights. They found that bands were just as effective and make a very good strength-training program (Iversen, 2017). It might not look as cool as pumping iron, but who cares?

Resistance bands come in two styles, loops and tubes. They are so cheap you can easily afford to buy a set of each. There are dozens of variations you can do for strength training using resistance bands, and the exercises are comparable to using free weights, according to research. You could easily keep a set in your desk drawer at work and knock out a couple sets when the boss steps out—try that with an Olympic barbell! I have a couple sets; my wife and I both love them. Bottom line: Totally worth it.

## Buying Resistance Bands

They're very affordable, so it's best to buy new and get exactly what you need. The most expensive set of resistance bands on Amazon is like 30 bucks, so don't freak out when you see how many styles, options, and sizes there are when you go look. Get a couple different sets so you're sure to get one that works for you. Most come with instructions, and some even have videos or their website. I'll describe a couple of the most popular here. Please don't overlook these as an integral part of a strength-training program if you're still reluctant to try.

Resistance bands come in two styles:

**Loop bands:** These look like giant rubber bands. These are used for full-body workouts or warm-up stretching. Most sets contain four or five loop bands of various sizes for beginners through advanced users. Some of the nicest sets are around $10 (seriously!). One of my favorite sets I own is the Limm, set of 5, 12" bands for $9.97.

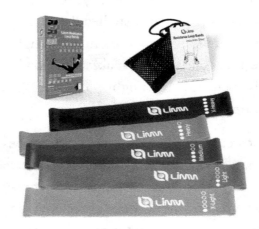

*Amazon.com*

**<u>Tube bands:</u>** This style looks like surgical tubing with pre-attached or removable handles. These are versatile, and they're suitable for a full-body workout. These can be attached to a door for more variety in workouts. Most sets come with different "weights" of bands that can even be stacked to greatly increase the workout force. These run a bit more expensive, but a good set is still under $30. I'm very happy with the set my wife and I use, the *Fitness Insanity* set for $23.97. Comes with five stackable bands, door anchors, ankle straps, and a nice guidebook.

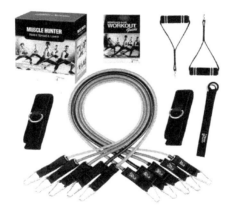

*Amazon.com*

If you're still in a buying mood, get a resistance band workout poster to hang on the wall where you work out. This one from Amazon shows 40 different workouts you can do using resistance bands. It's well worth the $20 it costs to have a quick reference for the proper stances and different movements you can do.

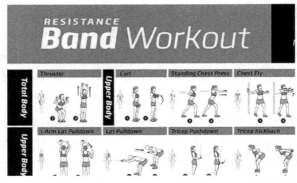

*Amazon.com*

Don't get suckered in by the "booty blasters" and other specialty bands that can cost over $100. These are just gimmicks. Stick with the basic loops and tubes, you (and your credit card) will be much happier, and you'll be getting a product you can use in many different ways for a successful workout.

## Designing a Good Resistance Band Program

Make sure you are working all your muscle groups:

- Arms
- Back
- Chest
- Core
- Legs
- Shoulders

If you find it's difficult to use the bands to work your legs, mix the band exercises with bodyweight squats. I think you'll find you really like using resistance bands if you don't like exercising in general. Just resist the urge to overdo it with too many reps using the lighter bands. Use the heaviest band that you find you can do 8–10 times in a row. If you can do the band exercise 20 or 30 times, you are using too light of a band.

Find one or two exercises that work each body part, and perform the same exercise during each session for at least a couple months. After a while, you might want to switch things up and use some other movements. There's nothing wrong with mixing bodyweight, resistance bands, and even free weights into one workout. Make a game of it, but be consistent.

***Non-negotiable:*** *Get on Amazon or visit Walmart, pick up a set of resistance bands, and try them out.*

# CHAPTER 33

# STRENGTH TRAINING METHOD 3: WEIGHT MACHINES

**TL;DR:** *Learn to use the machines correctly. Go from machine to machine with no rest in between. Do 8–12 reps and 2–3 sets on each machine. Don't look like a noob.*

If you think the gym is daunting, just wait until you enter the machine room. You'll need to join a gym if you want to use machines. Take advantage of the employees; they will show you how to use these machines to ensure you are doing the movements correctly. The machines also usually have a graphic that shows how to use them correctly. Weight machines mostly isolate muscle groups so you can work just one or two muscles at a time. Start with a weight you can comfortably lift 10–12 times, and develop a program that suits you. Keep notes and be consistent. You'll quickly look like you know what you're doing, and you won't hurt yourself.

Joining a gym has many great benefits. You can try out all the different equipment and weights, most have organized classes for beginners. Gyms usually offer aerobics classes, and some even have a pool sauna, snack bar, and store. If you belong to a gym, take advantage of all the weight machines; these cost thousands of dollars each and are too big for home gyms.

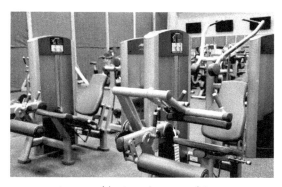

*Leg curl/extension machines*

**Best machines (author's picks):**

- Assisted Pull-up and Dip Machines (arms/shoulders)
- Chest Press Machine (chest)
- Leg Curl Machine (hamstrings)
- Lat Pulldown Machine (chest)
- Seated Row Machine (back)
- Shoulder Press Machine (shoulders)

**Worst machines (author's opinion):** (Do not be tempted to try these machines without special help and lots of experience)

- Hip Abductor/Adductor Machines (spine/knee injuries)
- Lying Leg Press Machine (herniated disks)
- Standing Calf Raise Machine (spine injuries)

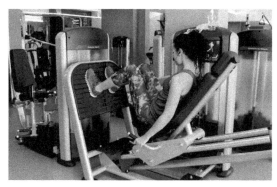

*Lying Leg Press Machine*

Make some notes when you are using weight machines in your gym; it's nearly impossible to remember what weight you used last time since the machines will have to be adjusted every time you use them. Some might argue my selections, but this list will get you off to a good start. A word of caution—some machines are designed for aerobic workouts, like rowing machines or stair climbers. Don't be misled into using these when you are doing resistance exercises.

## Don't Look Like a Noob

When you've worked up the courage to actually go into a gym, here are some pro tips to make your first visit much more enjoyable.

1. Have a machine in mind; make a list and stick to it. Try to use 4–6 machines during your workout.

2. Walk up to the machine and read the card showing proper form.

3. Sit in the seat and get it adjusted just right. There will be several levers to adjust height and positioning. Ask for help if you can't figure it out, some are difficult at first.

4. Once the seat is adjusted, select your desired weight. You'll see a metal pin in a stack of weights with the weight listed beside the holes. Start with a low weight. The worst noob mistake you can make is to lift a set of weights that does not have the pin inserted or is only inserted halfway. The resulting crash will ensure everyone knows your noob status.

5. Spend a minute or two adjusting the weight stack until you find a good weight that you can lift 8–12 times. Make a note of the weight you used. Wipe the machine with your towel, even if you didn't get it sweaty—people will notice.

6. Move on to the next machine.

7. Hit the machines on your list one after the other with little rest between machines.

8. When you've finished one round, go back and do it again as many times as you wish. On your first visit to a gym, one round is plenty. It's better to take notes and get the feel of the place before going in for a proper workout. Next visit, try to do 2–3 sets on each machine.

9. On your way out, help a noob adjust his seat and weight stack.

---

***Fitness Industry Insider Secret:*** *Only a small percentage of people exercise for overall health reasons, and even fewer know how to mix aerobic and strength training effectively (Guess, 2012):*

- *Most people join gyms or start an exercise program for the single purpose of losing weight.*
- *Most gyms advertise in a way that attracts those looking for quick weight loss.*
- *Most people do not understand the connections between exercise and health beyond weight loss.*
- *Most people who exercise do not do any strength training, only cardio.*
- *Most people quit fitness programs because they do not see the weight loss they had hoped for.*

---

***Non-negotiable:*** *Stop by a couple of gyms where you live and see what you think. Ask if they have a free trial membership. If they do, take it.*

# CHAPTER 34

# STRENGTH TRAINING METHOD 4: FREE WEIGHTS

> **TL;DR:** *Free weights (i.e., barbells, dumbbells, and kettlebells) can be used to create an excellent strength-training program. Learn the basic movements and either buy your own or join a gym and use theirs.*

Lifting weights is probably the most rewarding exercise you can do. You target certain sets of muscles that make you look good; biceps and legs, for instance. Bodybuilders and bodybuilding competitions wouldn't exist if it weren't for weightlifting. If you are happy with the bodyweight exercises I showed you earlier, you don't need to lift weights. But dollars to donuts, you'll *want to*.

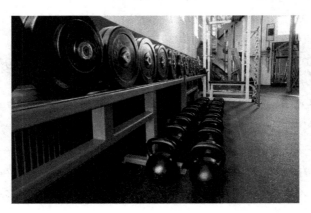

The idea of walking into the free-weight room of a gym makes most noobs want to run and hide. If you go in and just start picking up heavy things and putting them back down, you're just playing. You'll get hurt, and people will point and laugh at you like a noob. If you don't want to take the time to learn the basics of weightlifting by watching videos or reading books, it's best if you join a gym and hire a personal trainer. Explain that you want to be shown a *basic strength-training program* with some supervision for a couple weeks. Personal trainers specialize in this kind of thing. The gym staff will appreciate that you're trying, and they'll be much happier to help you out. Soon everyone will be giving you tips.

Weightlifting seems scary. It would appear that only giant, hulking people lift weights ... and that's usually the case in most gyms. Rarely do you see a small group of soccer moms spotting each other on the bench press. But we all *should* be doing strength training; it's one of the basic tenets of weight maintenance and well-being recommended by nearly every agency that oversees public health. If fewer than 20% of Americans exercise at all, the number of people who do strength training must be something like 5% or less. Weightlifters love their community, and they're happy to welcome new members into their group. But they're just as happy to laugh at noobs.

If you hate the thought of personal trainers and gyms, here's a basic weightlifting program you can set up with little fear of hurting yourself.

## Free Weights

Free-weight exercises can be performed with dumbbells, kettlebells, or barbells. These exercises are easily done at home. Weights are inexpensive, but you can find them for cheap on Craigslist or at a used sporting goods store. To determine the proper weight you need, start with a weight you can easily lift about 12 times, but not 20 times. Usually this will be in the 10-pound to 50-pound weight range for most exercises. If you've never lifted free weights before and are unsure, you can start with weights as small as 5 pounds and slowly add weight as it becomes easier. A good home set-up would look like this:

- 5 dumbbells ranging from 10–50 pounds; or a set of adjustable-weight dumbbells
- 1 barbell with plates (weights) that add up to 150 pounds
- 2 or 3 kettlebells around 10–40 pounds
- 1 weight bench; flat or inclined

A set-up like this would cost about the same as a yearly gym membership. For the DIYer, there are hundreds of videos on YouTube showing proper form. Please watch some before starting.

## Free-Weight Exercises

These exercises are done "almost to failure" meaning that the last couple reps of the last set are *just about* all you can physically do (Nóbrega, 2016). On your last set, you need to have sufficiently tired the muscles being worked so much that more reps are nearly impossible. A 2–3 minute recovery period will allow you to do another set (de Salles, 2009).

*One-armed Dumbbell Rows:* This is a great exercise for your free-weight program. Dumbbell rows work the muscles of the back and shoulders. There is little danger of injury with this exercise, but care should be taken to ensure proper form.

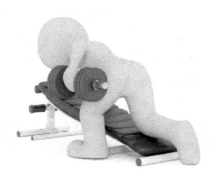

Proper position:

- Stand next to a weight bench.
- Place one knee on the bench.
- Lift a dumbbell off the ground.
- Keep your back straight and abs tight.
- Lift using the muscles of the back.

Routine: Perform 1–3 sets of 8–12 reps with 1–2 minutes of rest between sets. Repeat for each arm.

***Bicep Curls:*** Bicep curls can be done in several ways using either a barbell or dumbbells. Bicep curls work the muscles of the arms: biceps, shoulders, forearms, and wrists.

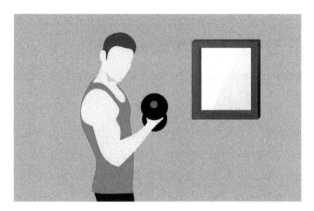

Proper Position:

- Hold a barbell or dumbbell in each hand; stand with your feet slightly apart.
- Start with weights hanging.
- "Curl" both arms upward to shoulder height.
- Slowly lower the dumbbells.

Routine: Perform 8–12 reps in 1–3 sets with 1–3 minutes of rest between sets.

***Triceps Extensions:*** Triceps extensions work the triceps, the muscles at the back of the upper arm. Used in conjunction with bicep curls to give a full-arm strength workout. You can use a single dumbbell, a barbell weight, or a special triceps extension bar.

Proper Position:

- Grasp a dumbbell with both hands. Your feet should be about shoulder width apart.
- Slowly lift the dumbbell over your head until both arms are fully extended.
- The weights of the dumbbell should be resting in the palms of your hands.
- Keep your upper arms close to your head and lower the weights. The upper arms remain stationary, only the forearms move.
- Return the arms to the starting position.

Routine: Perform 8–12 reps in 1–3 sets with 1–3 minutes of rest between sets.

***Weighted Squats:*** Weighted squats or "goblet squats" add a new dimension to bodyweight squats with some added weight to really work the big muscles in the legs, hips, calves, back, and core. Goblet squats can be performed with a single dumbbell, a kettlebell, a barbell plate, a jug of water, a sandbag, or 30 copies of this book.

Proper Position:

- Stand up straight holding a heavy object.
- Keep your feet shoulder-width apart.
- Squat down by bending the knees, go as low as you can, keeping your back straight.
- Return to your standing position.

Routine: Perform a couple reps of bodyweight squats to warm up, then do 8–12 reps for 1–3 sets with 1–2 minutes of rest in between.

The four exercises I've described here will give you a good start and can easily be done at home. If you go to a gym, walk straight to the free weights and start doing these four basic movements, people will think you're a pro. They might even call you "bro," (even if you're a gal).

Start slow and allow several days between weightlifting sessions. Muscles need time to repair. This is actually essential for building muscle. If you overdo it, you won't see the gains you're after. After a couple weeks, you'll find you might want to add more weights. Great. As you develop "muscle memory" of the movements, you'll be more comfortable, and you might want to start branching out to other free weight techniques.

## Lifts You Should *Not* Do

Some free-weight movements are best left to the pros with years of training. No matter how tempting, for the purposes of this exercise program, do not be tempted to do these exercises unless you have a personal trainer and several weight lifting friends who can help you keep good form ("spotters") and save you from getting trapped beneath a weight bar. The following weight lifting techniques are the most dangerous, in my opinion:

- Bench press (shoulder, chest injuries)
- Deadlifts (back/spine injuries)
- Squat racks (lower back/knee/hip injuries)

It's *so easy to get hurt* by lifting heavy things incorrectly that *it's simply not worth taking the chance*. You think you have problems being overweight now, just wait until you slip a disk or overextend a joint. You could be looking at a lifetime of pain killers and surgeries.

But there are some very safe weight lifting exercises that can be done with free weights that have very little risk of injury. These are the ones I want you to focus on.

**"But I don't want big muscles!"**

The strength-training program I've outlined above will give you muscles as nature designed. The big, bulky muscles you see on body-builders come from a completely different type of exercise known as "hypertrophy" training. Hypertrophy training requires lots more time in the gym, lots more lifting, heavier weights, eating specialized meals, and taking many supplements (Schoenfeld, 2010).

## Supplements

Please, please, please stay away from muscle building supplements. These are mostly scams or used by professionals (Kreider, 1999). Do not be tempted to start taking any of these oft-used "muscle building" supplements. You don't need them:

- Arginine
- Beta-alanine
- Beta-hydroxy-beta-methylbutyrate (HMB)
- Betaine
- Branched-chain amino acids (BCAAs)
- Caffeine
- Citrulline
- Creatine
- Dehydroepiandrosterone (DHEA)
- Glutamine
- Iron
- Protein Supplements
- Quercetin
- Ribose
- Sodium bicarbonate

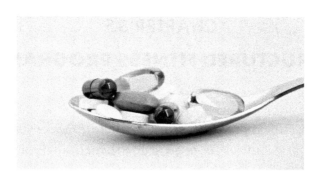

**Fitness Industry Insider Secret:** *Exercise supplements don't increase fitness levels or cure diseases, and they can be dangerous (Starr, 2015).*

Additionally, shy away from pre- and post-workout "recovery" bars and drinks. Completely avoid any type of steroid or testosterone booster, estrogen blocker, or other hormonal biohacks. You will be surrounded by offers "you can't refuse" once you enter the fitness world. You don't need any of it. Real food and exercise go hand in hand.

**Non-negotiable:** *Watch some videos of strength training techniques. Keep an eye out for someone selling used free weights and weightlifting equipment. Consider getting your own free weights for home use if you have the space.*

# CHAPTER 35

## STRUCTURED FITNESS PROGRAMS

> **TL;DR:** *Fitness programs require structure. Make your own program, buy DVDs, or go to an instructor-led course.*

It's hard *not* to notice ads and commercials for exercise programs. They're filled with sexy, rock-hard bodies, music, and ear-to-ear grins. Of course we want to be like those people! But today's exercise programs are as intimidating as gyms and diet plans. Highly charismatic leaders convince us that if we'd only exercise like they do, we'll soon look like them, and life will be great.

> **Fitness Industry Insider Secret:** *A recent study determined that 86% of advertisements for online fitness programs promote "harmful health messages." These messages normalize dysfunctional behaviors and promote fixating on certain body parts (Blackstone, 2018).*

Most of these programs are really good, but only for the right person. It can be fun to buy an exercise program on DVD, app, or stream it to your TV and follow along for a couple weeks to get reenergized in your current program. Lots of people would rather go to an exercise class led by a competent instructor. And other people want nothing to do with structure; they prefer to create their own programs.

Some of the celebrity trainers you see are really good at what they do, which is mostly to motivate people to exercise. Some of the hottest names right now are Jillian Michaels, Shaun T, Gunnar Peterson, and Harley Pasternak. Exercise programs rely on intense marketing, the stuff of late-night infomercials, and Facebook ad campaigns. P90X, for instance has made over $500 million, and the CrossFit brand generates over $4 billion!

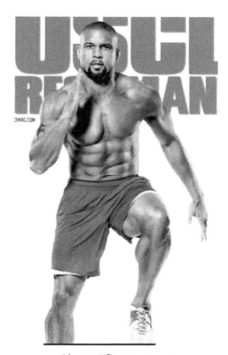

ShaunTfitness.com

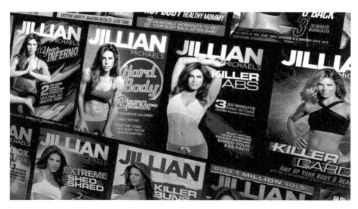

Jillianmichaels.com

The biggest mistake is thinking that if you follow a popular program, you'll quickly shed all of the excess fat you've accumulated. If fast weight loss is your motivation, you'll be disappointed. But if you want to get in better shape and kick your workout up a notch, these programs are for you.

## Types of Exercise Programs

There are three types of exercise programs:

- Self-made, self-monitored
- In-person, studio-based, guided programs (e.g., CrossFit and Zumba)
- At-home, DVD-based, semi-guided programs (e.g., P90X, Insanity)

*Self-made programs* are used by most successful exercisers. With a bit of reading and practice, you can develop your own exercise program based on aerobic and strength training exercises. I recommend everyone do this. You can even incorporate some of the other programs, like Zumba or Insanity, into your personalized routine.

*In-person, studio-based, guided programs* like CrossFit and Zumba, or other more generic aerobics classes, are very popular. These programs are offered at local gyms, workplaces, hospitals, or even libraries. "No one to exercise with" is a common excuse used by non-exercisers. Getting out amongst other exercisers is a great way to meet people and stay motivated to continue an exercise program. If the instructor is knowledgeable and likable, this type of program is very worthwhile. Sometimes it takes some exploring to find the right fit for your personality and goals. Beware of the "bootcamp/summer body" type of programs that pop up locally unless you are familiar with the instructors and programs.

*At-home, DVD-based, semi-guided programs* appeal to many people as well. "No time for the gym" is the number one excuse given by non-exercisers. Busy people love the convenience of self-paced, digital programs and turn to these for their workouts. There are even online subscription-based programs that allow you to exercise with other groups in real-time. The Peloton bicycle program has been extremely popular in the last couple years. While there are no statistics on how long people stick with DVD-based exercise programs, you can bet it's very low. A much better tactic is to develop your own routine and use these guided programs just to break up the monotony if you start to get burned out on your current program.

Here's a quick rundown on some of the top programs in case you've been wondering how they work. As you read through this list, try to take some elements from each that you can use in your own program.

## Top-Selling Commercial Fitness Programs Reviewed

### DVD-Based:

#### *Insanity*

It's called "Insanity" for a reason … it's insane! Not for beginners unless you just want to watch something to motivate you while you do some *sane* exercises. The insanity workouts are led by Shaun T, an intensely insane fitness trainer. His jumps and kicks will leave you breathless just watching.

The good thing about Insanity is that it doesn't require any special equipment, just some room in front of a TV to do 30 minutes of fast-paced cardio and bodyweight exercises. Insanity uses a method known as HIIT, or high-intensity interval training. It's like jumping jacks on steroids. You'll work to maximum capacity for about 40 seconds with 30–40 seconds of rest before doing it again. The basic

Insanity package is a 2-month program that gets increasingly harder as the weeks progress.

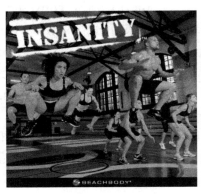

*Amazon.com*

Insanity is based on an exercise technique known as *plyometrics*. Plyometrics was popularized by Soviet Olympians during the 1970s. This technique uses explosive jumps to train the muscles for instant power and maximum elasticity. Plyometrics is used by athletes in sports such as basketball, tennis, track, and volleyball.

Jumping is hard on the knees and joints. If you try Insanity, be sure to follow the initial stretching sequences or you'll injure yourself very quickly. Insanity is a full-body workout that will leave you breathless, perfect for your weekly "vigorous aerobics" requirements.

The 2-month Insanity course is available from Beachbody.com and costs about $150 for the DVD set and instruction books.

I give Insanity a low rating because it's too hard for most people and too expensive.

*2 out of 5 stars.*

## *P90X*

P90X was developed by Tony "The Master of Motivation" Horton. This program is a mixture of strength training and aerobic conditioning. It uses a principal called "muscle confusion" in which different muscle groups are continually being worked throughout the program. For strength training, P90X relies heavily on pull-ups and resistance bands. A partial list of exercises you'll do on P90X include:

- Closed Grip Overhand Pull-up
- Groucho Walk
- Reverse Grip Chin-ups
- Sneaky Lunge
- Speed Squats
- Three-way Lunge
- Wide Front Pull-ups

P90X is DVD-based, so you'll need to buy one of the many packages offered. Some packages just have DVDs, while more advanced packages have pull-up bars, resistance bands, and other exercise equipment.

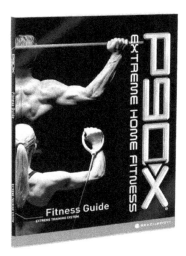

*Amazon.com*

345

An integral part of P90X is the diet plan. It starts off with a low-carb diet that progressively adds more carbs as the weeks go on. P90X is also big on supplements, so you'll be confronted with an endless array of slimming shakes, vitamins, and performance-enhancing formulas.

P90X is available from Beachbody.com and costs anywhere from $100–$600 depending on the plan you choose.

I give P90X a low rating because it's too hard for most people to follow, especially the diet plan. Its heavy use of supplements and exercises performed with twisting moves has great potential for injuries.

*1 out of 5 stars*

## Studio-Based:

### *Zumba*

"Ditch the Workout, Join the Party," is Zumba's calling card. Zumba is an instructor-led aerobic exercise program that has taken the world by storm. Born in Columbia and brought to America in 2001, Zumba boasted over 10,000 studios across the United States by 2007. Now there are something like 100,000 or more!

Zumba is a great workout, sort of like the old aerobics classes of the '80s and '90s, but with a more party-like atmosphere and a total Latin-music vibe. The Zumba company is a force to behold, they've expanded from simple classes to:

- Zumba®
- Zumba® Step
- Zumba® Toning
- Aqua Zumba®
- Zumba Sentao™

- Zumba® Gold
- Zumba® Gold-Toning
- Zumba® Kids
- Zumba® Kids Jr.
- Zumbini™
- Zumba In The Circuit™

If organized classes are your thing, check out Zumba. They offer classes for every fitness level, low-impact, high-impact, and even strength training. More likely than not, there's a Zumba class available near you. There's even a full DVD selection for home-exercisers.

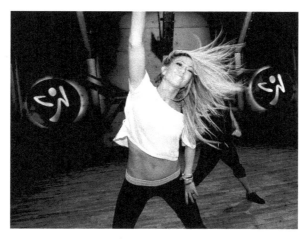

*Amazon.com*

The only drawback to Zumba is the cost. At $5–$20 per class, you could rack up some hefty dues. But if you do it wisely, just go every now and then. Done once a week or a couple times a week, it might be the perfect venue for people who need organization and lots of companions.

*5 out of 5 stars for guided programs.*

### CrossFit

CrossFit has followed a similar trajectory as Zumba, starting in the early 2000s. They've grown to offering classes in over 13,000 locations (called "boxes") in 2019. CrossFit is an instructor-led program that incorporates elements of both aerobic and strength training. CrossFit appeals mainly to athletic people who enjoy competition and hard workouts.

CrossFit is a bit expensive at around $150 a month, and classes are usually held in barebones locations like garages, warehouses, or outside, so you won't have access to a full gym in most cases.

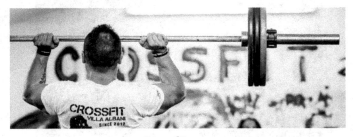

*Crossfit.com*

If Zumba is for people looking to lose weight, CrossFit is for people looking to get strong. Critiques of CrossFit are that the instructors are often not well-trained for the intense, injury-prone workouts they lead, and injuries are common. But that's also part of the appeal of CrossFit. If you like a no-holds-barred, all-out *beast mode* workout, check out CrossFit.

*3 out of 5 stars.* Too difficult for most people and expensive.

## Internet/App-Based:

### *Bodyrock.tv*

Bodyrock.tv seems to be a big seller, but the creators have to know they are promoting an unhealthy brand. Perhaps this program appeals to waif-like runway models or people with body-image issues.

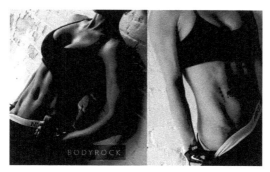

*Bodyrock.tv*

They do have an impressive online store where they sell cool things like pink barbells and weighted vests alongside books and meal plans. Bodyrock.tv recommends a super-low-carb diet. I'm really surprised they haven't jumped on the "keto" bandwagon yet.

Bodyrock.tv uses a combination of weights and aerobics for maximum weight loss. They use DVDs and live internet courses with numerous packages priced according to the plan you choose. The website is hard to navigate, and many of the links didn't work when I tried them. They are well-known for offering free videos of their workout programs, but I could not access any of them. To me, the website seemed more about selling DVDs and fitness gear than offering a robust workout program.

If super-skinny models are your thing, check them out.

*1 out of 5 stars.* Pure marketing. Based on hype, advertising, and unhealthy body image obsession.

> **Fitness Industry Insider Secret:** *Fitness program instructors are more likely to have eating disorders than the general public (Bratland, 2015).*

### My Fitness by Jillian Michaels

Jillian Michaels is most well-known as the hard-ass coach on *The Biggest Loser*. She's now widely accepted as a fitness expert. You see her everywhere on talk shows and in commercials. Jillian recently started My Fitness, an app-based program that seems to be very well-thought-out and has something for everyone.

Jillian also released her latest book, *6 Keys*, this year, and it's getting lots of great reviews. Here's a deal for you: visit her website, jillianmichaels.com, and you can get three months of her My Fitness program for free if you buy the book.

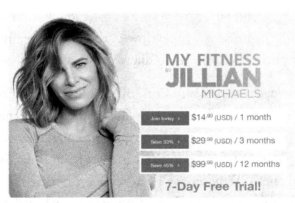

*JillianMichaels.com*

If you like Jillian Michaels, you'll love My Fitness by Jillian Michaels. If you're not a fan, you'll find that her workouts are a bit "canned" and don't offer much in the way of variety, but that could quickly change if the program gets lots of subscribers.

Go check out her website if this sounds interesting. She gives away a free seven-day trial for the asking.

*5 out of 5 stars.* It's a relatively new program, so expect bugs. Jillian has enough experience to guide most people, and she understands the difference between "health" and "fat loss."

### *iBodyFit*

iBodyFit has been around since 2006 and has won about every award possible in the fitness world. While I am a little bit disappointed that their website uses images that may encourage body dysmorphia, this is the best internet-based plan out there and only gets better. Prices range from about $50–$150 a month depending on the plan you choose. At the upper end, you'll have access to a live trainer who will help you develop a personalized eating and exercise program based on your goals. At the lower end, you'll have access to hundreds of exercise videos, personalized support, and feedback.

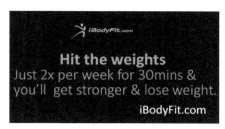

*iBodyFit.com*

The iBodyFit website has lots of free content and a decent blog, so go check them out. They have a great reputation in the fitness industry and offer something for everyone.

*4.5 out of 5 stars.* Good value, great product. Marked down for gratuitous use of extra-skinny models in their ads.

**Non-negotiable:** *Create an exercise program; it doesn't have to be insane. The best program is one that you will adhere to for many years.*

# CONCLUSION TO PART 4

Physical fitness needs to become part of your life. Like brushing your teeth and taking a shower, exercise needs to become part of your daily routine. Physical fitness also needs some structure if you are to keep at it. This can be as simple as plotting out a simple routine that's done at home or in the gym—think walking, bodyweight exercises, and more. Or you can sign up for an instructor-led program and attend classes several nights a week. DVD and internet or app-based programs have also been really popular. With the rise of the smartphone, having some apps to help you exercise is an awesome idea.

Your aerobic fitness and strength are what will get you through life unscathed. Your body is an incredible thing. Treat it right and it will reward you in ways you never thought possible. Exercise shouldn't be looked at as a chore to dread, but rather something that you get to do. Just like eating right, sleeping well, and living a stress-free life, these are rewards, not punishments. Don't become complacent.

# EPILOGUE

So, there you have it folks. Everything I know about the topic of dieting. I hope you learned something. Here are some things *I* learned:

- The Diet and Fitness Industries are in worse shape than I ever imagined.

- Most commercial diet programs are terrible. They rely on ultra-processed foods and miss most of the elements that *could* make a diet work.

- Viral marketing of fad diets has messed up everyone's perception of weight loss.

- Most overweight people have no idea how to lose weight or exercise correctly.

- Losing weight requires a lot more motivation, planning, education, and technology than I realized.

- It's nearly impossible to lose weight without a plan. "Watching what I eat" is not a *weight loss* plan that will work. Over 90% of dieters use that plan.

- "Watching what I eat" is a fine *weight maintenance* plan.

- Exercising and giving up ultra-processed food are mandatory for sustained weight loss.

- Sleep and stress are possibly more important than food and exercise.

- Most people, even super-elite athletes and bodybuilders, are unhappy with how they look.

I wrote this book in a way that should appeal to doctors and nutritionists as well as people in need of losing weight. I'd like to see doctors giving this book out to all their overweight patients. Please recommend this book to your doctor. If anyone needs help ordering this book in quantity for a steep discount, let me know.

It was fun writing this book. It helped me to learn where I need to focus my efforts in staying a successful weight loss maintainer. It's a small club, it would be nice to get some company! Come visit me at my blog, www.thediethack.com, and let me know how you're doing.

# APPENDIX: THE MINNESOTA STARVATION EXPERIMENT

The topic of calories continually evokes heated debate in dieting circles. One camp says calories don't matter; the other says calories are everything. Somewhere in the middle lies the truth. No one can argue that calories from *refined* sugar, oil, or wheat offer the same nutritional value as the equivalent number of calories from fruit, vegetables, and whole grains. Perhaps to an engineer, but not to a nutritionist. And certainly not to our body and our gut microbes.

Counting calories is the gold-standard for weight loss. One need not meticulously count grams of fat or carbohydrates on a low-calorie diet if wholesome food is consumed, just counting calories is enough. How many calories a person requires to maintain, gain, or lose weight is dependent on several factors such as the metabolism of the body at rest and calories burned through activity. Further, this calculation also varies with the subject's lean body mass, health, metabolic rate, gut flora, inflammation, and genetics. The food itself is also a factor. Some food digests easier, and some food causes a thermal effect, which causes a small boost in metabolism (Howell, 2017).

## Experimental Starvation in Man

To show the power of calories, I want to share an experiment conducted during World War II on the effects of starvation. In this experiment, 34 healthy men volunteered to be starved for six months so that scientists could better understand what happens to humans when deprived of food. This research was needed to better serve victims of concentration camps, prisoners of war, and people in famine-stricken countries.

I obtained a photocopy of the original 48-page report that was produced by Dr. Ancel Keys, lead researcher for this experiment. This paper was a preliminary briefing for the war department on the first phase of a two-phase project. It shows the raw data of the first phase, unmuddled by interpretation and editing. The first phase of the experiment examined starvation, the second phase was related to rehabilitation. This report and its follow-up on rehabilitation were later transformed into a two-volume text that is 1,385 pages in length and contains over 2,000 referenced citations. The full report can be purchased on Amazon for $1,199 in textbook format, sold as *The Biology of Human Starvation. Volumes 1 and 2* (Keys, 1950).

I am a total geek for old research papers. Government reports are even better, especially when stamped, "Approved for Public Release." This one was written on a manual typewriter, covered in coffee stains, and found in the two-prong manila folder in which it had resided for the past 74 years.

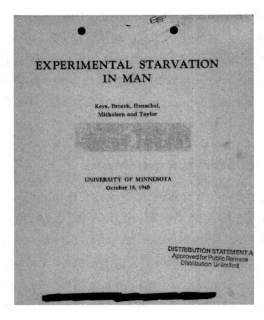

## The Experiment

The first phase of the experiment was designed to study the effects of starvation, specifically:

1. Changes of basic physiological functions.
2. Changes in the psychological condition.
3. Metabolic adaptations to starvation.
4. The order in which physical performance deteriorates.
5. How rapidly does occupational work capacity deteriorate?
6. What tests might be used to measure nutritional state and performance potential?
7. Can starvation effects be predicted or estimated?

## The Subjects

Thirty-four healthy normal-weight men aged 20–33 years. Heights ranged from 5'5" to 6'3". Weights ranged from 135 to 182 pounds. These subjects were conscientious objectors, that is they refused to join the military for religious or moral reasons. Instead, they were placed in civil service jobs. They all volunteered willingly in the hopes that their sacrifice would save lives. The subjects were treated kindly and fairly, although I doubt a similar experiment would be allowed under today's regulatory landscape regarding protection of human rights.

## The Study Design

- During a three-month standardization period, the subjects were fed regular meals containing 3,000–3,400 calories per day while engaging in regular fitness activities, walking, and doing daily work that was not physically demanding.

- During the six-month starvation period, the subjects were fed two meals per day with a daily calorie intake of about 1,700 calories. During this time, the subjects were to attempt to keep up with as much physical activity as possible and maintain social contact with others.

- Throughout the study, the subjects were given many medical and psychological tests to determine the extent of damage occurring from starvation.

## Results

- During the three-month standardization period, some subjects gained weight, some lost weight.
- During the six-month starvation period, all subjects lost from 1.13 to 2.69 pounds per week.
- The subjects lost an average of 37 pounds, or 24% of initial weight.
- The weight loss was linear and greatly determined by calorie intake.
- Final weights varied mostly due to rates of edema (swelling) and inflammation.
- Basal metabolism (calories burned at rest) dropped almost 40% on average.
- Strength, work ability, and mental functions declined.

## The Control Diet

The control diet was used for 90 days at the beginning of the experiment to "standardize" the subjects prior to entering the starvation phase. By eating this set menu, fatter participants became leaner, and leaner men gained weight. The most weight *lost* was 12.5 pounds, and the most *gained* was 8.5 pounds. The average among the 34 subjects was a 4-pound loss in weight.

The control diet was designed to provide 3,000–3,400 calories per day using three different menus. This "standardization" diet looks to be very healthy and representative of how people ate in the 1940s. Note the absence of ultra-processed food and a heavy intake of fresh fruit and vegetables. Missing is soda pop, candy bars, and fried food that is now so popular. They were drinking over a quart of milk daily. I dare say that most overweight people would lose weight if they followed this same eating pattern today.

Representative diets during standardization period.
Caloric values calculated from standard dietary tables.

| Date January 24, 1945 | | January 30, 1945 | | February 8, 1945 | |
|---|---|---|---|---|---|
| Food served | Wt. per person (gms.) | Food served | Wt. per person (gms.) | Food served | Wt. per person (gms.) |
| Tomato juice | 100 | Grapefruit juice | 100 | Vegetable juice | 100 |
| Corn Flakes | 30 | Bran Flakes | 30 | Bran Flakes | 30 |
| Sugar | 10 | Bread | 150 | Jam | 70 |
| Butter | 30 | Butter | 30 | Bread | 150 |
| Bread (white) | 150 | Sugar | 10 | Butter | 30 |
| Milk | 540 | Jam | 70 | Sugar | 10 |
| Soda crackers | 6 | Milk | 540 | Milk | 720 |
| Split-pea soup | 125 | Vegetable soup | 110 | Soda cracker | 8 |
| Hamburger | 40 | Crackers | 8 | Cream of corn | |
| Gravy | 75 | Macaroni and | | soup | 110 |
| Potatoes | 120 | cheese | 200 | Ground beef | 65 |
| Wax beans | 100 | Scrambled eggs | 60 | Gravy | 75 |
| French Dressing | 15 | Bacon | 20 | Potatoes | 210 |
| Rice pudding | 75 | Cabbage | 75 | Green beans | 100 |
| Swiss steak | 50 | Sponge cake | 30 | Apricots | 45 |
| Gravy | 75 | Orange sauce | 30 | Lettuce | 15 |
| Squash | 100 | Beef roast | 60 | Apple Betty | 100 |
| Pickles | 20 | Parsnips | 100 | Pork chops | 60 |
| Apple pie | 125 | Potatoes (mashed) | 200 | Peas | 100 |
| | | Tomatoes (fresh) | 75 | Apple sauce | 100 |
| | | Mayonnaise | 10 | Gingercake | 60 |
| | | Gravy | 75 | Sweet potatoes | 170 |
| | | Ice cream | 75 | | |
| | | Vanilla wafer | 5 | | |
| Total Protein 131 gms. | | 89 gms. | | 90 gms. | |
| Total Fat 128 gms. | | 146 gms. | | 114 gms. | |
| Total Calories 3410 | | 3056 | | 3032 | |

## The Starvation Diet

While officially called a "semi-starvation" diet in the report, the plan was designed to mimic the effects of starvation. I had never before considered 1,700 calories to be anywhere near a "starvation" level of eating. I would have guessed a much lower number, like 800 calories or less. It truly shook me to the core that these men were left so emaciated after eating a well-balanced diet consisting of 1,700 calories per day. To visualize this emaciation, here are some before-and-after pictures included in the original report.

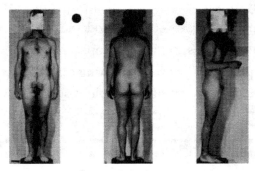

*Subject #20. Initial Weight 143 lbs.*

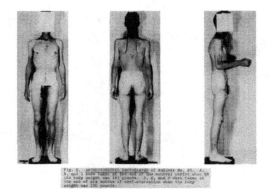

*Subject #20. Final Weight 106 lbs.*

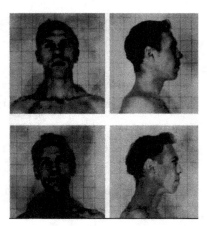

*Subject #29. Facial Features Before and After.*

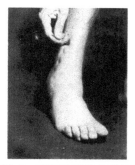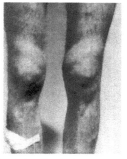

Fig. 13. PHOTOGRAPHS TAKEN AT SIX MONTHS of semi-starvation showing extensive ankle edema in subject No. 170 and swelling of the knee due to fluid in the joint in subject No. 20.

*Swelling and Edema*

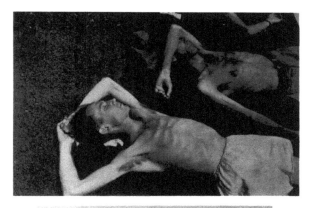

Fig. 7. RELAXATION, FOURTH MONTH OF SEMI-STARVATION. Developing emaciation is evident in a casual glance at a group while sunbathing.

*Weight loss effects after 4 months*

## Starvation Food

The starvation diet menus were surprisingly well-rounded and quite like low-fat weight loss diets used today. I examined the calorie counts by using FitDay's calorie tracking tools and found the calorie counts to be within 10% accuracy.

Here are the "semi-starvation diet" breakfast selections. The subjects were only allowed to eat twice a day. These menus were rotated throughout the experiment:

Complete menus for the semi-starvation period.

Breakfast

| Menu No. 1 Food served | Wt. gms. | Menu No. 2 Food served | Wt. gms. | Menu No. 3 Food served | Wt. gms. |
|---|---|---|---|---|---|
| Farina | 200 | Oatmeal | 190 | Pancakes | 100 |
| (27 gms. dry unenriched farina) | | (27 gms. dry oat-meal) | | (45 gms. gra-ham flour | |
| Jam | 20 | Jam | 20 | 50 gms. skim milk | |
| Milk | 40 | Milk | 40 | 1.2 gms. egg | |
| Sugar | 10 | Sugar | 10 | 2.8 gms. sugar | |
| Fried potatoes | 150 | Fried potatoes | 200 | 0.9 gms. lard) | |
| Jello with dried apples | 100 | Gingerbread | 50 | Syrup | 50 |
| Bread | | Bread | 180 | Jam | 20 |
| (whole wheat) | 180 | (whole wheat) | | Applesauce | 70 |
| | | | | Cornbread | 110 |
| | | | | Bread | 180 |
| | | | | (whole wheat) | |

And the dinners:

Supper

| Food served | Wt. gms. | Food served | Wt. gms. | Food served | Wt. gms. |
|---|---|---|---|---|---|
| Fish chowder | 200 | Bean and pea soup | 185 | Potato soup | 250 |
| (102 gms. potatoes | | (5 gms. dried peas | | (100 gms. po-tatoes | |
| 11 gms. onions | | 16 gms. dried beans | | 10 gms. onions | |
| 11 gms. celery | | | | 30 gms. skim milk | |
| 7 gms. fish | | 15 gms. fresh ham) | | 5 gms. whole wheat bread | |
| 20 gms. milk | | Macaroni and cheese | 255 | 25 gms. beef) | |
| 7 gms. butter | | (130 gms. wet macaroni | | Stew | 285 |
| 2 gms. flour) | | 12 gms. lard | | (90 gms. tur-nips | |
| Spaghetti and meat balls | 200 | 108 gms. skim milk | | 20 gms. carrots | |
| (100 gms. wet spa-ghetti | | 2 gms. flour | | 35 gms. green beans | |
| 20 gms. beef | | 35 gms. American cheese) | | 5 gms. lard | |
| 7 gms. oatmeal | | Rutabagas | 40 | 10 gms. onions) | |
| 5 gms. onions | | Steamed potatoes | 100 | Steamed potatoes | 205 |
| 60 gms. tomatoes) | | Lettuce salad | 100 | | |
| Steamed potatoes | 150 | (80 gms. lettuce | | | |
| Peas and carrots | 55 | 10 gms. vinegar | | | |
| (38 gms. peas | | 10 gms. sugar) | | | |
| 17 gms. carrots) | | | | | |
| Cabbage salad | 120 | | | | |
| (100 gms. cabbage | | | | | |
| 10 gms. sugar | | | | | |
| 10 gms. vinegar) | | | | | |

Here is my analysis of Menu No. 1 using the FitDay calorie tracker:

## *Breakfast:*

| Food Name | Amount | Unit | Cals | Fat (g) | Carbs (g) | Prot (g) |
|---|---|---|---|---|---|---|
| Cereals, farina, enriched, dry | 27 | grams | 100 | 0.1 | 21.1 | 2.9 |
| Jams and preserves | 20 | grams | 56 | 0.0 | 13.8 | 0.1 |
| Milk, whole | 40 | grams | 24 | 1.3 | 1.8 | 1.3 |
| Sugar | 10 | grams | 39 | 0.0 | 10.0 | 0.0 |
| Potatoes, red, flesh and skin, baked | 150 | grams | 134 | 0.2 | 29.4 | 3.4 |
| Gelatin desserts, KRAFT, JELL-O Brand Sugar Free Low Calorie... | 100 | grams | 8 | 0.0 | 0.0 | 1.4 |
| Bread, whole wheat | 180 | grams | 477 | 6.5 | 85.0 | 19.8 |

*Breakfast totals: 838 calories, 8.1g fat, 161g carbs, 28.9g protein*

## *Dinner:*

| Food Name | Amount | Unit | Cals | Fat (g) | Carbs (g) | Prot (g) |
|---|---|---|---|---|---|---|
| Potatoes, white, flesh and skin, baked | 150 | grams | 141 | 0.2 | 31.6 | 3.2 |
| Onions, sweet, raw | 11 | grams | 4 | 0.0 | 0.8 | 0.1 |
| Celery, raw | 11 | grams | 2 | 0.0 | 0.3 | 0.1 |
| Fish, raw | 7 | grams | 6 | 0.1 | 0.0 | 1.2 |
| Milk, whole | 20 | grams | 12 | 0.7 | 0.9 | 0.6 |
| Butter | 7 | grams | 50 | 5.7 | 0.0 | 0.1 |
| Flour, white | 2 | grams | 7 | 0.0 | 1.5 | 0.2 |
| Spaghetti, cooked | 100 | grams | 157 | 0.9 | 30.7 | 5.8 |
| Ground beef, raw | 20 | grams | 51 | 4.0 | 0.0 | 3.4 |
| Cereals, QUAKER, Quick Oats, Dry | 7 | grams | 26 | 0.5 | 4.8 | 1.0 |
| Onions, sweet, raw | 5 | grams | 2 | 0.0 | 0.4 | 0.0 |
| Tomatoes, raw | 60 | grams | 11 | 0.1 | 2.4 | 0.5 |
| Potatoes, red, flesh and skin, raw | 150 | grams | 105 | 0.2 | 23.9 | 2.8 |
| Peas, green, raw | 38 | grams | 31 | 0.2 | 5.5 | 2.1 |
| Carrots, raw | 17 | grams | 7 | 0.0 | 1.6 | 0.2 |
| Cabbage, green, raw | 100 | grams | 25 | 0.1 | 5.8 | 1.3 |
| Sugar, raw | 10 | grams | 38 | 0.0 | 9.7 | 0.0 |
| Vinegar | 10 | grams | 2 | 0.0 | 0.1 | 0.0 |

*Dinner totals: 674 calories, 12.8g fat, 120g carbs, 22.5g protein*

Menu No. 1 totals (FitDay Estimate): 1,512 calories, 20.9g fat, 281g carbs, 51.4g protein

Menu No. 1 totals (Original Estimate): 1,680 calories, 10.2g fat, 344.5g carbs, 52.6g protein

## Why the discrepancy?

Calories are an estimate at best. Perhaps standardized calorie charts have changed over the last 75 years. I'm sure that other calorie trackers would result in even more differences. At any rate, the semi-starvation diet is very close to what the researchers designed when measured by today's techniques. At only 10% off, it's well within the standards for calories counting (Jumpertz, 2013).

## Other Measurements of the Starvation Diet

Further analyzed with the FitDay counter, we can see the ratio of fat, protein, and carbs. The starvation diet contains an impressive 24 grams of fiber.

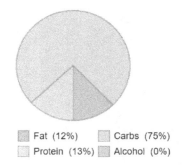

|  | Grams | Calories | %-Cals |
|---|---|---|---|
| **Calories** |  | 1,512 |  |
| **Fat** | 20.9 | 186 | 12 % |
| Saturated | 8.2 | 73 | 5 % |
| Polyunsaturated | 3.9 | 34 | 2 % |
| Monounsaturated | 5.5 | 49 | 3 % |
| **Carbohydrate** | 281.0 | 1,125 | 75 % |
| Dietary Fiber | 24.4 |  |  |
| **Protein** | 51.4 | 199 | 13 % |
| **Alcohol** | 0.0 | 0 | 0 % |

Fat (12%)  Carbs (75%)
Protein (13%)  Alcohol (0%)

Nutrient wise, not the best, but I've seen worse profiles for modern weight loss diets:

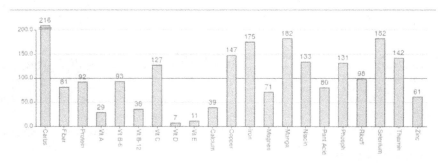

## Experimental Tweaks

During the experiment, Dr. Keys wanted to control the weight being lost by each man, so he altered the diets slightly each week depending on the number of pounds lost. By knowing exactly what each person had eaten, it was possible to add or subtract some food to dial in the desired weight loss.

Though the menus were set, each man received a slightly different amount of bread and potatoes to achieve the desired effect of weight loss. If a subject lost too much, he was given a few extra slices of bread or extra potatoes. If he did not lose enough, he was given less bread or potatoes. Everything else was held constant.

This fine-tuning worked well until the latter months of the experiment. As the men's health deteriorated, they began to accumulate fluid (edema and swelling). This gave the impression of weight gain when looking at the scale.

During the six-month starvation experiment, the monthly averages for food intake based on tweaks and personalized adjustments came out to:

- Month 1 – 1,834 calories
- Month 2 – 1,822 calories
- Month 3 – 1,766 calories
- Month 4 – 1,661 calories
- Month 5 – 1,695 calories
- Month 6 – 1,764 calories

To create sustained weight loss, the calories had to be reduced as time went on. Toward the end of the experiment, the men's weights stabilized and they were given a bit more food to prevent muscle wasting.

## Formulaic Weight Loss

Dr. Keys' method of adding and subtracting bread and potatoes worked so well that he was able to develop a formula for predicting weight loss. Hammered out on a manual typewriter and punched with two holes in 1945, the math looks exactly like this:

Mathematically, the general curve required for weight versus time is represented by a parabola with vertical axis and zero slope at 24 weeks. The equation is: $W_x = W_f + K (24-t)^2$, where $W_f$ is final weight, t is time in weeks and $W_x$ is weight at time t. If $W_0$ is initial weight and G is the desired total per cent of weight loss, then the equation can be written: $W_x = W_0 (100-G)/100 + K (24-t)^2$. For each case the constant K is obtained: $576 K = W_0 (G)/100$. The foregoing method was used to obtain the prediction curves for each man, such as shown in Figures 2, 3, 4 and 5.

The formula might look complicated, but the math works. Restrict calories, and it's just a matter of time until the desired weight is lost. Here's a chart showing how effective this method is (my annotations added):

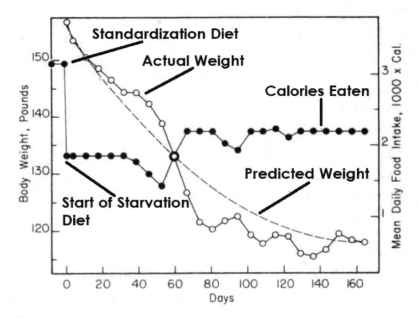

*Keys' Figure 4. Body weight and food intake. Subject 29 (explanatory notes added by author).*

## The Human Side of Weight Loss

While the math works, humans aren't keen on starving. The researchers noted that morale plummeted during the last two months of the experiment. The subjects showed progressive apathy and depression. The education program faltered, and social relations dwindled. The subjects became increasingly upset at mealtime when they would get fewer rations than others due to weight fluctuations. Several men had periods of "serious emotional stress" that responded to counseling, however one subject was removed in the second month for undisclosed "psychological reasons."

Physically, the men noted an alarming "creaking" of the joints. Toward the end, they appeared "lifeless and staring." Hair was dull and unkempt. There was a tremendous atrophy of the supraspinatus muscle, a muscle that keeps the shoulders from slumping. Several military observers noted that the men looked exactly like people liberated from German concentration camps.

The men's complaints were logged throughout the project:

- Excessive appetite and hunger
- Tiredness and fatigue
- Muscle soreness
- Apathy
- General irritability
- Inability to concentrate
- Depression
- Dizziness
- Lack of ambition
- Moodiness
- Sensitivity to noise
- Muscle cramps
- Coldness

- Feeling "old" (described as low libido, weak, depressed, no ambition)
- Clothes not fitting well
- Need for more sleep
- Hunger pains
- Vivid dreams

Surprisingly, there were few complaints of gastric issues, constipation, or diarrhea. The 24 grams of daily fiber were important in this regard.

In the starvation experiment, much attention was given to keeping the men fully engaged by providing nutrition education, keeping diaries, filling out questionnaires, participating in scheduled and informal interviews, and having constant contact between staff and subjects.

## Surprises

Throughout the report, Dr. Keys mentioned several surprise findings:

- Dental health remained surprisingly normal.
- Vitamin deficiencies were very meager.
- The morale of the subjects remained surprisingly high the first few months.
- Speed tests (tapping speed, body reaction time) were surprisingly unaffected by starvation.
- Inflammation was a constant confounder for accurately measuring weight.
- The heart was consistently decreased in size.
- Average heart rate dropped from 55 to 36 beats per minute ("startling" the researchers).
- The "creaking" of joints was shocking and surprising to both researchers and subjects.

I was surprised by several things as well. I was surprised how much muscle was lost and how much fat remained. This figure illustrates the relative amounts of muscle and fat that were lost over the six-month starvation diet:

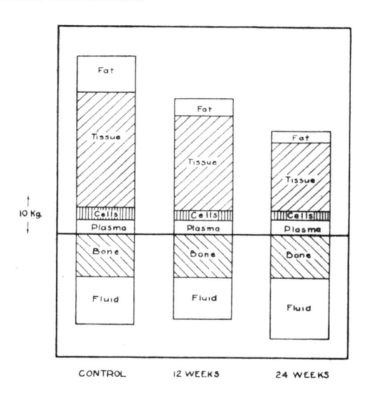

From the report, this diagram indicates that the men lost an average of 41% of their lean body mass (LBM) by the end of the experiment. At the halfway point (12 weeks), they'd lost about 20% of LBM. LBM was lost at a rate of about 8% per month. Perhaps this was the result of such low protein intakes during the starvation period. However, using the men's ages and weights their recommended (lower) level of protein intake based on today's standards would be approximately 50–60 grams per day. The starvation diets contained an average of 49g/day, hardly a massive deficit.

Regarding body fat, the men lost about 45% of their body fat at 12 weeks and 68% by the end of the study. They started at an average of 13% body fat. At 12 weeks they were measured at 7% body fat, and 5% at the end of the experiment in week 24. I was surprised that they retained even 5% in light of the serious muscle wasting that was evident. But I guess that just reinforces that the body will hang on to some fat no matter what. To be muscular and very low in body fat is non-typical.

**What Ifs?**

- What if the study had included obese subjects as well?

- What if a different diet was used (e.g. low-carb, high-protein, carnivore, potato hack, meal-replacement shakes)?

- What if they had gone on for a year?

- What if this was done today, would results be the same?

- What if a person tried to follow the diets used for weight loss?

## Ancel Keys

Ancel Keys was a world-renowned nutrition researcher and physiologist. His experiments on starvation have never been replicated, and generations of scientists rely on his work. Besides studying the effects of starvation during World War II, Keys also invented K-rations, the MRE (Meal, ready-to-eat) of the day. K-rations contained 3,200 calories and according to Keys, "had a piece of hard sausage, dry biscuits, a block of chocolate, a stick of chewing gum, matches, and a couple of cigarettes, all in a waterproof package to fit in a uniform pocket" (Keys, 1990).

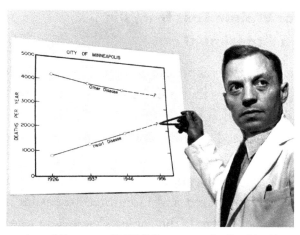

*Ancel Keys, ca 1957 (Minnesota Daily, 2018)*

After the war, Keys spent the rest of his career studying the effects of diet on heart disease and overall health. His works shaped a lifetime of nutritional advice on dietary fat, cholesterol, and heart disease (Keys, 1957). Though his work is often criticized (Minnesota Daily, 2016), much of this criticism is baseless (Minger, 2011). He noted differences in fermentable versus nonfermentable fiber in the treatment of high cholesterol, but the science of gut health was non-existent at the time, and his findings went nowhere (Keys, 1961). He was an early proponent of using the Body Mass Index (BMI) to predict obesity (Keys, 1972).

In later life, Keys became an author and promoted a diet he called "The Mediterranean Diet" (Keys, 1975). Keys died in 2004 at age 100 after spending the last 28 years of his life living in Southern Italy (Brody, 2004).

## Lessons for Weight Loss from the Starvation Experiment

The raw data from this report can be applied to weight loss diets of today. Weight loss diets that use the Intensive Weight Loss Intervention model described in other parts of *The Diet Hack* are almost guaranteed to succeed (Hollis, 2008). This model uses a closely guided program and tracks calories very closely while providing structure, support, and education. In the starvation experiment, every bite was carefully measured and monitored to ensure no cheating or miscalculations occurred. The subjects were kept engaged in the planning and rationale of the experiment. The subjects had high morale throughout most of the experiment.

### Results versus Calories

This experiment uniquely highlights that *results* trump *calories* when trying to lose weight. During the 24-week starvation diet, Keys and his research team carefully compared expected results with actual results and adjusted food rations (calories) to raise or lower the subject's weight with remarkable precision. Modern dieters should take note! I've talked with many dieters who could not lose weight eating at a specific calorie level. When we examined their diet by meticulously tracking food intake with a calorie-tracking app, we found they were overestimating calories by several hundred per day. In a real-world situation, accurately counting calories is extremely difficult. Careful use of calorie calculators will help to ensure your results meet your expectations.

### Biggest Loser Effect

I was quite surprised that a daily intake of 1,700 calories resulted in such rapid decline in the physical and mental fitness of the subjects. This experiment helped to shape my views on weight loss diets and my advice that weight loss diets should not be taken lightly nor used by people who are not truly overweight in an unhealthy sense. Weight loss through calorie restriction is hard on a body and results in metabolic changes that make keeping the weight off very hard. The 40% reduction in resting energy metabolism seen in this experiment is a very real danger for dieters who attempt to lose too fast or cut calories too far. Recently deemed "The Biggest Loser Effect," this reduction in metabolic rate can take years to recover from (Fothergill, 2016).

## Mental Effects

Dieting also takes a mental toll that few can afford. As with professional bodybuilders before a competition, the starvation subjects continually obsessed about food. In a real-world setting without constant supervision, this obsession will occasionally lead to sporadic binges and feelings of guilt (French, 1994).

## Water Weight

Calorie restriction is a proven method for weight loss, but when fat stores are low, the weight lost is mostly from lean body mass and hidden by an increase in inflammation (Williams, 2015). Weight loss stalls and plateaus plague diet plans and are the subject of many weight loss forum threads. Invariably someone will mention "water weight" but still the tendency is to restrict calories further to "break" the stall. Perhaps the better tweak would be to add 200–300 calories instead of reducing.

## Muscle Loss

This paper also made me realize that a weight loss diet is an extreme protocol and not to be taken lightly. Cutting calories to a level where fat is lost and muscle is preserved is the holy grail of dieting. Many methods promise this result; one known as the Protein Sparing Modified Fast is quite popular in some dieting circles but relies on taking many supplements and has a complicated set of instructions that few have the gumption to follow. Just Google, "How to lose fat without losing muscle" and you'll see the extent of interest in this phenomenon. Your head will spin when you start clicking the links. A proven technique encourages obese dieters to perform regular physical activity, especially strength training, and to eat protein at 1.25 to 1.6 times the recommended RDA (Cava, 2017) (Phillips, 2016). In bodybuilding circles, the standard advice is to eat 1 gram of protein per pound of bodyweight, which is more than twice the recommended amount.

## Calorie Limits

I think the key to proper weight loss dieting is to expect some loss of muscle mass during your active fat loss phase. You should never cut calories so low that your body suffers. And you should eat plenty of protein. The chart I developed in Part 2 reflects levels of calories and protein that should result in minimal muscle loss during dieting.

| Current Body Weight | Calories Needed for Weight Loss (Assuming a BMI over 27) | Protein Needed to Prevent Lean Body Mass Loss (1g/kg) |
|---|---|---|
| 250–300 pounds | 2,200–2,500 calories | 113–136 grams |
| 200–250 | 2,000–2,200 | 90–113 |
| 180–200 | 1,900–2,200 | 81–90 |
| 160–180 | 1,600–1,900 | 72–81 |
| 150 or less | 1,500–1,800 | 68–72 |

The food you eat should be highly nutritious and minimally processed to preserve lean body mass. Inflammation will hide weight loss, and the Western diet is highly inflammatory to most overweight people. The calories need to be carefully tracked and monitored. You cannot "eyeball" 2,000 calories to any degree that's useful for weight loss (Archer, 2018). Remember, "Watching what I eat" is not a valid weight loss program. You must know precisely how much you are eating to lose weight at a formulaic rate. Studies that compare estimated calorie values against actual measurements show disparities of more than 37% among dieters (Brown, 2016).

## The Dreaded Stall

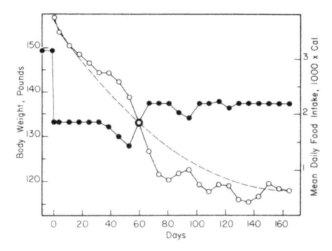

*Keys' Figure 4. Body weight and food intake. Subject 29.*

Take note of the calories eaten by Subject 29 as shown in Keys' Figure 4. He started the starvation period at 1,700 calories per day. Between days 30 and 40, Subject 29 experienced a "plateau" or weight stall, as commonly seen by weight loss dieters. Keys reduced the man's calorie allowance by 100 calories per week for three weeks, and the plateau was broken. In fact, this subject started losing weight rapidly after the stall. Keys then increased the man's calorie intake by about 800 calories to slow the rapid weight loss seen while eating below 1,500 calories per day. Several more stalls were seen at the 80- and 120-day marks. These were also broken by lowering calories slightly the week following a stall in weight loss. As the man's weight increased and decreased, calories were slowly raised and lowered by 100 or so per week and the weight loss continued its downward trend as predicted. Subject 29 lost nearly 30 pounds over 24 weeks, most of this time he was eating approximately 2,100 calories per day. This carefully controlled feeding study speaks volumes to the effects of carefully tracking calorie intake, adjusting as necessary, and the short-lived nature of weight loss plateaus when calories are carefully considered.

## Accountability

Accountability is huge. Imagine how the starvation experiment would have worked if the 34 subjects were instructed to eat 1,500 calories worth of self-monitored food per day and come in for a weekly weigh-in. I discussed an experiment in Section 3 of *The Diet Hack* in which 75 overweight people were intensively monitored and lost weight but upon cessation of support, they all regained at a linear rate (Ross, 2018). This is the human condition. To eat freely and feel good. Unfortunately, that just can't be the case for most people if we are to maintain a healthy weight.

To this end, there must be a level of accountability inserted into the well-designed weight loss diet. Many commercial weight loss programs know this, which is why they provide support. Books are interesting to read but cannot provide support unless the author has set up some system such as a forum or website where support can be obtained. Several community-based forums exist where people can develop their own accountability systems, but most people don't understand the importance of accountability in weight loss and miss this step completely.

## Conclusion

I'd heard stories about this experiment for many years. Several books have been written about the ordeals of the subjects, but mostly from a human-interest point of view, and with many inaccuracies as I am now learning. I think by reviewing the raw data and seeing the initial reactions of Dr. Keys, you gain more insight than by simply reading the 1,300-page final report. The final report undoubtedly contains personal bias and politically correct assumptions. Dieters today could take some lessons from the 1945 starvation experiment:

- Accurately count and track calories for best results.
- Become engaged in the weight loss program.
- Keep a log of measurements for future analysis.
- Ensure social support is available to keep your morale high.
- Spend some time in selecting the best-quality nutritious food for your diet.
- Eat plenty of fiber.
- Muscle loss occurs on most diets.
- Fat is very stubborn.
- Tweak food intake according to expectations.

I hope you found this essay on the Minnesota Starvation Experiments useful.

Yours in health,

Tim Steele
2019

# ABOUT THE AUTHOR

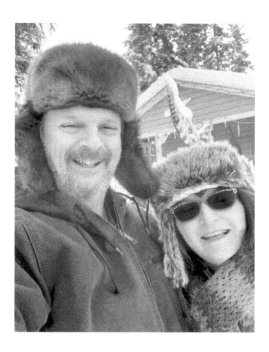

Tim Steele is author of the best-selling book *The Potato Hack: Weight Loss Simplified*. Tim's work is predicated on the idea that human health is based on gut health, which food can either work for or against. Using knowledge he's gained through years of working with various health-related industries and his own health challenges, he offers intentional, actionable formulas for reaching optimum health and shedding weight—for good. Tim holds a Master of Science degree in biotechnology. His company, Steele Biotech, provides regulatory oversight for pharmaceutical and supplement manufacturers and the fledgling cannabis industry. He enjoys traveling, gardening, beekeeping and spending time with family. Tim and his wife Jackie reside in North Pole, Alaska.

# BEFORE YOU GO...

Liked what you read? Please leave this book a review on Amazon, then check out my blog, www.thediethack.com for more information and to chat with others on a similar health journey. If you have any questions about my books, you can contact me directly through my blog. I'm always happy to hear what readers think and help you achieve your maximum potential.

Yours in health,

Tim Steele

# REFERENCES

Agamennone, Valeria, Cyrille AM Krul, Ger Rijkers, and Remco Kort. "A practical guide for probiotics applied to the case of antibiotic-associated diarrhea in The Netherlands." *BMC Gastroenterology* 18, no. 1 (2018): 103.

Aguayo-Patrón, Sandra, and Ana Calderón de la Barca. "Old fashioned vs. ultra-processed-based current diets: possible implication in the increased susceptibility to type 1 diabetes and celiac disease in childhood." *Foods* 6, no. 11 (2017): 100.

Albaugh, Vance L., and Naji N. Abumrad. "Surgical treatment of obesity." *F1000Research* 7 (2018).

Allen, Joseph G., Sara Gale, R. Thomas Zoeller, John D. Spengler, Linda Birnbaum, and Eileen McNeely. "PBDE flame retardants, thyroid disease, and menopausal status in US women." *Environmental Health* 15, no. 1 (2016): 60.

Andersen, J. C. "Stretching before and after exercise: effect on muscle soreness and injury risk." *Journal of Athletic Training* 40, no. 3 (2005): 218.

Andersen, Ross E., Kelly D. Brownell, Glen D. Morgan, and Susan J. Bartlett. "Weight loss, psychological, and nutritional patterns in competitive female bodybuilders." *Eating Disorders* 6, no. 2 (1998): 159–167.

Andersen, Ross E., Susan J. Barlett, Glen D. Morgan, and Kelly D. Brownell. "Weight loss, psychological, and nutritional patterns in competitive male body builders." *International Journal of Eating Disorders* 18, no. 1 (1995): 49–57.

Anderson, James W., Pat Baird, Richard H. Davis, Stefanie Ferreri, Mary Knudtson, Ashraf Koraym, Valerie Waters, and Christine L. Williams. "Health benefits of dietary fiber." *Nutrition Reviews* 67, no. 4 (2009): 188–205.

Anderson, Kristin L. "A review of the prevention and medical management of childhood obesity." *Child and Adolescent Psychiatric Clinics of North America* (2017).

Araújo, Joana, Jianwen Cai, and June Stevens. "Prevalence of Optimal Metabolic Health in American Adults: National Health and Nutrition Examination Survey 2009–2016." *Metabolic Syndrome and Related Disorders* (2018).

Archer, Edward, Carl J. Lavie, and James O. Hill. "The Failure to Measure Dietary Intake Engendered a Fictional Discourse on Diet-Disease Relations." *Frontiers in Nutrition* 5 (2018).

Arora, Teresa, Hoda Gad, Omar M. Omar, Sopna Choudhury, Odette Chagoury, Javaid Sheikh, and Shahrad Taheri. "The associations among objectively estimated sleep and obesity indicators in elementary schoolchildren." *Sleep Medicine* 47 (2018): 25–31.

Astrup, Arne, and Mads F. Hjorth. "Low-fat or low carb for weight loss? It depends on your glucose metabolism." *EBioMedicine* 22 (2017): 20–21.

Atkinson Jr, Richard, Gail Butterfield, William Dietz, John Fernstrom, Arthur Frank, Barbara Hansen, Steven Heymsfield, Robin Kanarek, Mary Mays, and Barbara Moore. "Weight Management: State of the Science and Opportunities for Military Programs." *National Academy of Sciences* (2003).

Baxter, Nielson T., Alexander W. Schmidt, Arvind Venkataraman, Kwi S. Kim, Clive Waldron, and Thomas M. Schmidt. "Dynamics of Human Gut Microbiota and Short-Chain Fatty Acids in Response to Dietary Interventions with Three Fermentable Fibers." *mBio* 10, no. 1 (2019): e02566-18.

Benjamin, Emelia J. "Heart disease and stroke statistics—2017 update: a report from the American Heart Association." *Circulation* 135, no. 10 (2017): e146.

Berlowitz, Dan R., Capri G. Foy, Lewis E. Kazis, Linda P. Bolin, Molly B. Conroy, Peter Fitzpatrick, Tanya R. Gure et al. "Effect of intensive blood-pressure treatment on patient-reported outcomes." *New England Journal of Medicine* 377, no. 8 (2017): 733–744.

Blackstone, Sarah R., and Lynn K. Herrmann. "Extreme body messages: themes from Facebook posts in extreme fitness and nutrition online support groups." *mHealth* 4 (2018).

Blair, Steven N., Harold W. Kohl, Carolyn E. Barlow, Ralph S. Paffenbarger, Larry W. Gibbons, and Caroline A. Macera. "Changes in physical fitness and all-cause mortality: a prospective study of healthy and unhealthy men." *Jama* 273, no. 14 (1995): 1093–1098.

Bliss, Edward S., and Eliza Whiteside. "The gut-brain axis, the human gut microbiota and their integration in the development of obesity." *Frontiers in Physiology* 9 (2018).

Bond, Dale S., Suzanne Phelan, Tricia M. Leahey, James O. Hill, and Rena R. Wing. "Weight-loss maintenance in successful weight losers: surgical vs. non-surgical methods." *International Journal of Obesity* 33, no. 1 (2009): 173.

Booth, Frank W., Christian K. Roberts, and Matthew J. Laye. "Lack of exercise is a major cause of chronic diseases." *Comprehensive Physiology* 2, no. 2 (2012): 1143.

Botchlett, Rachel, Shih-Lung Woo, Mengyang Liu, Ya Pei, Xin Guo, Honggui Li, and Chaodong Wu. "Nutritional approaches for managing obesity-associated metabolic diseases." *Journal of Endocrinology* (2017): JOE-16.

Boutcher, Stephen H. "High-intensity intermittent exercise and fat loss." *Journal of Obesity* (2010).

Brandsma, Eelke, Niels J. Kloosterhuis, Mirjam Koster, Daphne C. Dekker, Marion JJ Gijbels, Saskia van der Velden, Melany Ríos-Morales et al. "A proinflammatory gut microbiota increases systemic inflammation and accelerates atherosclerosis." *Circulation Research* 124, no. 1 (2019): 94–100.

Brantley, P. J., L. J. Appel, J. Hollis, V. J. Stevens, J. Ard, C. M. Champagne, P. J. Elmer et al. "Weight Loss Maintenance (WLM): design and rationale of a multi-center trial to sustain weight loss." *Clinical Trials (London, England)* 5, no. 5 (2008): 546.

Bratland-Sanda, Solfrid, Merethe Pauline Nilsson, and Jorunn Sundgot-Borgen. "Disordered eating behavior among group fitness instructors: a health-threatening secret?" *Journal of Eating Disorders* 3, no. 1 (2015): 22.

Bray, George A., Steven R. Smith, Lilian DeJonge, Russell de Souza, Jennifer Rood, Catherine M. Champagne, Nancy Laranjo et al. "Effect of diet composition on energy expenditure during weight loss: the POUNDS LOST Study." *International Journal of Obesity* 36, no. 3 (2012): 448.

Brody, Jane E. "Dr. Ancel Keys, 100, Promoter of Mediterranean Diet, Dies" (2004). *The New York Times.*

Brown, Ruth E., Karissa L. Canning, Michael Fung, Dishay Jiandani, Michael C. Riddell, Alison K. Macpherson, and Jennifer L. Kuk. "Calorie estimation in adults differing in body weight class and weight loss status." *Medicine and Science in Sports and Exercise* 48, no. 3 (2016): 521.

Buresh, Robert, and Kris Berg. "Exercise for the management of type 2 diabetes mellitus: factors to consider with current guidelines." *The Journal of Sports Medicine and Physical Fitness* 58, no. 4 (2018): 510–524.

Butler, Merlin G., Austen McGuire, and Ann M. Manzardo. "Clinically relevant known and candidate genes for obesity and their overlap with human infertility and reproduction." *Journal of Assisted Reproduction and Genetics* 32, no. 4 (2015): 495–508.

Cabré, Eduard, and Eugeni Domènech. "Impact of environmental and dietary factors on the course of inflammatory bowel disease." *World Journal of Gastroenterology: WJG* 18, no. 29 (2012): 3814.

Cai, Gui-Hong, Jenny Theorell-Haglöw, Christer Janson, Magnus Svartengren, Sölve Elmståhl, Lars Lind, and Eva Lindberg. "Insomnia symptoms and sleep duration and their combined effects in relation to associations with obesity and central obesity." *Sleep Medicine* 46 (2018): 81–87.

Calbet, Jose AL, Jesús G. Ponce-González, Jaime de La Calle-Herrero, Ismael Perez-Suarez, Marcos Martin-Rincon, Alfredo Santana, David Morales-Alamo, and Hans-Christer Holmberg. "Exercise preserves lean mass and performance during severe energy deficit: the role of exercise volume and dietary protein content." *Frontiers in Physiology* 8 (2017): 483.

Cava, Edda et al. "Preserving Healthy Muscle during Weight Loss" *Advances in Nutrition (Bethesda, Md.)* vol. 8,3 511–519. 5 May. (2017), doi:10.3945/an.116.014506

CDC. "CDC: 1 in 3 antibiotic prescriptions unnecessary." Atlanta: CDC Newsroom (2016).

Centers for Disease Control. "Attempts to Lose Weight Among Adults in the United States, 2013–2016." Retrieved from www.cdc.gov (2018).

Ceria-Ulep, Clementina D., Alice M. Tse, and Reimund C. Serafica. "Defining exercise in contrast to physical activity." *Issues in Mental Health Nursing* 32, no. 7 (2011): 476–478.

Chadid, Susan, Martha R. Singer, Bernard E. Kreger, M. Loring Bradlee, and Lynn L. Moore. "Midlife weight gain is a risk factor for obesity-related cancer." *British Journal of Cancer* (2018): 1.

Champagne, Catherine M., Stephanie T. Broyles, Laura D. Moran, Katherine C. Cash, Erma J. Levy, Pao-Hwa Lin, Bryan C. Batch et al. "Dietary intakes associated with successful weight loss and maintenance during the Weight Loss Maintenance trial." *Journal of the American Dietetic Association* 111, no. 12 (2011): 1826–1835.

Chaput, Jean-Philippe, Vicky Drapeau, Marion Hetherington, Simone Lemieux, Véronique Provencher, and Angelo Tremblay. "Psychobiological effects observed in obese men experiencing body weight loss plateau." *Depression and Anxiety* 24, no. 7 (2007): 518–521.

Chassaing, Benoit, Tom Van de Wiele, Jana De Bodt, Massimo Marzorati, and Andrew T. Gewirtz. "Dietary emulsifiers directly alter human microbiota composition and gene expression ex vivo potentiating intestinal inflammation." *Gut* (2017).

Chaudhry, Hammad S., and Steve S. Bhimji. *Cushing Syndrome.* (2017).

Chemycal. "France set to ban titanium dioxide nanoparticles from food products, EFSA is still re-evaluating." Retrieved from www.chemycal.com (2018).

Choi, Candace "No accounting for these tastes: Artificial flavors a mystery." Retrieved from www.medicalxpress.com (2018).

Ciorba, Matthew A. "A gastroenterologist's guide to probiotics." *Clinical Gastroenterology and Hepatology* 10, no. 9 (2012): 960–968.

Clearinghouse, N. D. D. I. "Digestive Diseases Statistics for the United States." Bethesda, MD: *National Institutes of Health* (2013).

Cook, Chad M., Courtney N. McCormick, Mandi Knowles, and Valerie N. Kaden. "A Commercially Available Portion-Controlled Diet Program Is More Effective for Weight Loss than a Self-Directed Diet: Results from a Randomized Clinical Trial." *Frontiers in Nutrition* 4 (2017): 55.

Cook, Laura E., Bethany J. Finger, Mark P. Green, and Andrew J. Pask. "Exposure to atrazine during puberty reduces sperm viability, increases weight gain and alters the expression of key metabolic genes in the liver of male mice." *Reproduction, Fertility and Development* (2019).

Cooper, Christopher B., Eric V. Neufeld, Brett A. Dolezal, and Jennifer L. Martin. "Sleep deprivation and obesity in adults: a brief narrative review." *BMJ Open Sport & Exercise Medicine* 4, no. 1 (2018): e000392.

Costa, Caroline Santos, Bianca Del-Ponte, Maria Cecília Formoso Assunção, and Iná Silva Santos. "Consumption of ultra-processed foods and body fat during childhood and adolescence: A systematic review." *Public Health Nutrition* 21, no. 1 (2018): 148–159.

Courtemanche, Charles, Rusty Tchernis, and Benjamin Ukert. "The effect of smoking on obesity: Evidence from a randomized trial." *Journal of Health Economics* 57 (2018): 31–44.

Da Costa Louzada, Maria Laura, Camila Zancheta Ricardo, Euridice Martinez Steele, Renata Bertazzi Levy, Geoffrey Cannon, and Carlos Augusto Monteiro. "The share of ultra-processed foods determines the overall nutritional quality of diets in Brazil." *Public Health Nutrition* 21, no. 1 (2018): 94–102.

Davis, Cindy D. "The gut microbiome and its role in obesity." *Nutrition Today* 51, no. 4 (2016): 167.

Davy, Brenda M., Elizabeth A. Dennis, A. Laura Dengo, Kelly L. Wilson, and Kevin P. Davy. "Water consumption reduces energy intake at a breakfast meal in obese older adults." *Journal of the American Dietetic Association* 108, no. 7 (2008): 1236–1239.

De Coster, Sam, and Nicolas van Larebeke. "Endocrine-disrupting chemicals: associated disorders and mechanisms of action." *Journal of Environmental and Public Health* (2012).

de Salles, Belmiro Freitas, Roberto Simao, Fabrício Miranda, Jefferson da Silva Novaes, Adriana Lemos, and Jeffrey M. Willardson. "Rest interval between sets in strength training." *Sports Medicine* 39, no. 9 (2009): 765–777.

Dennis, Elizabeth A., Ana Laura Dengo, Dana L. Comber, Kyle D. Flack, Jyoti Savla, Kevin P. Davy, and Brenda M. Davy. "Water consumption increases weight loss during a hypocaloric diet intervention in middle-aged and older adults." *Obesity* 18, no. 2 (2010): 300–307.

Department of Health and Human Services. "Key Recommendations: Components of Healthy Eating Patterns." Retrieved from www.health.gov/dietaryguidelines (2015).

Devoto, F., L. Zapparoli, R. Bonandrini, M. Berlingeri, A. Ferrulli, L. Luzi, G. Banfi, and E. Paulesu. "Hungry brains: A meta-analytical review of brain activation imaging studies on food perception and appetite in obese individuals." *Neuroscience & Biobehavioral Reviews* (2018).

Diether, Natalie E., and Benjamin P. Willing. "Microbial Fermentation of Dietary Protein: An Important Factor in Diet–Microbe–Host Interaction." *Microorganisms* 7, no. 1 (2019): 19.

Dirlewanger, M., V. Di Vetta, E. Guenat, P. Battilana, G. Seematter, P. Schneiter, E. Jequier, and L. Tappy. "Effects of short-term carbohydrate or fat overfeeding on energy expenditure and plasma leptin concentrations in healthy female subjects." *International Journal of Obesity* 24, no. 11 (2000): 1413.

Domecq, Juan Pablo, Gabriela Prutsky, Aaron Leppin, M. Bassam Sonbol, Osama Altayar, Chaitanya Undavalli, Zhen Wang et al. "Drugs commonly associated with weight change: a systematic review and meta-analysis." *The Journal of Clinical Endocrinology & Metabolism* 100, no. 2 (2015): 363–370.

Dreher, Mark. "Whole Fruits and Fruit Fiber Emerging Health Effects." *Nutrients* 10, no. 12 (2018): 1833.

Duffey, Kiyah J., and Barry M. Popkin. "High-fructose corn syrup: is this what's for dinner?" *The American Journal of Clinical Nutrition* 88, no. 6 (2008): 1722S–1732S.

Duncan, Glen E. "The 'fit but fat' concept revisited: population-based estimates using NHANES." *International Journal of Behavioral Nutrition and Physical Activity* 7, no. 1 (2010): 47.

Dwyer, Johanna, Paul Coates, and Michael Smith. "Dietary supplements: regulatory challenges and research resources." *Nutrients* 10, no. 1 (2018): 41.

El Aidy, Sahar, Timothy G. Dinan, and John F. Cryan. "Gut microbiota: the conductor in the orchestra of immune–neuroendocrine communication." *Clinical Therapeutics* 37, no. 5 (2015): 954–967.

Espeland, Mark A., W. Jack Rejeski, Delia S. West, George A. Bray, Jeanne M. Clark, Anne L. Peters, Haiying Chen, Karen C. Johnson, Edward S. Horton, and Helen P. Hazuda. "Intensive Weight Loss Intervention in Individuals Ages 65 Years or Older: Results from the Look AHEAD Type 2 Diabetes Trial." *Journal of the American Geriatrics Society* 61, no. 6 (2013): 912.

Fan, Sicun, Fred Breidt, Robert Price, and Ilenys Pérez-Díaz. "Survival and Growth of Probiotic Lactic Acid Bacteria in Refrigerated Pickle Products." *Journal of Food Science* 82, no. 1 (2017): 167–173.

FDA. "FDA Removes 7 Synthetic Flavoring Substances from Food Additives List." Retrieved from www.fda.gov (2018).

FDA(2). "CFR Title 21, Section 1, Subpart B, paragraph 101.22." Retrieved from www.accessdata.fda.gov (2018).

FDA(3). "Listing of Color Additives Exempt From Certification; Mica-Based Pearlescent Pigments." Federal Register. Retrieved from www.federalregister.gov (2015).

Feigenbaum, Matthew S., and Michael L. Pollock. "Strength training: rationale for current guidelines for adult fitness programs." *The Physician and Sportsmedicine* 25, no. 2 (1997): 44–64.

Fildes, Alison, Judith Charlton, Caroline Rudisill, Peter Littlejohns, A. Toby Prevost, and Martin C. Gulliford. "Probability of an obese person attaining normal body weight: cohort study using electronic health records." *American Journal of Public Health* 105, no. 9 (2015): e54–e59.

Fisher, Gordon, Andrew W. Brown, Michelle M. Bohan Brown, Amy Alcorn, Corey Noles, Leah Winwood, Holly Resuehr, Brandon George, Madeline M. Jeansonne, and David B. Allison. "High intensity interval-vs moderate intensity-training for improving cardiometabolic health in overweight or obese males: a randomized controlled trial." *PloS One* 10, no. 10 (2015): e0138853.

Foraster, Maria, Ikenna C. Eze, Danielle Vienneau, Emmanuel Schaffner, Ayoung Jeong, Harris Héritier, Franziska Rudzik et al. "Long-term exposure to transportation noise and its association with adiposity markers and development of obesity." *Environment International* 121 (2018): 879–889.

Foster-Schubert, Karen E., Catherine M. Alfano, Catherine R. Duggan, Liren Xiao, Kristin L. Campbell, Angela Kong, Carolyn E. Bain, Ching-Yun Wang, George L. Blackburn, and Anne McTiernan. "Effect of diet and exercise, alone or combined, on weight and body composition in overweight-to-obese postmenopausal women." *Obesity* 20, no. 8 (2012): 1628–1638.

Fothergill, Erin, Juen Guo, Lilian Howard, Jennifer C. Kerns, Nicolas D. Knuth, Robert Brychta, Kong Y. Chen et al. "Persistent metabolic adaptation 6 years after 'The Biggest Loser' competition." *Obesity* 24, no. 8 (2016): 1612–1619.

Freeman, A.M. and Pennings, N., "Insulin resistance." In StatPearls [Internet]. *StatPearls Publishing.* (2018).

French, Simone A., and Robert W. Jeffery. "Consequences of dieting to lose weight: effects on physical and mental health." *Health Psychology* 13, no. 3 (1994): 195.

Fritsch, Jane. "95% Regain Lost Weight. Or Do They?" *NY Times* (1999).

Gadiraju, Taraka V., Yash Patel, J. Michael Gaziano, and Luc Djoussé. "Fried food consumption and cardiovascular health: A review of current evidence." *Nutrients* 7, no. 10 (2015): 8424–8430.

Galgani, Jose E., Cedric Moro, and Eric Ravussin. "Metabolic flexibility and insulin resistance." *American Journal of Physiology-Endocrinology and Metabolism* 295, no. 5 (2008): E1009–E1017.

Geiker, Nina Rica Wium, Arne Astrup, Mads Fiil Hjorth, A. Sjödin, L. Pijls, and C. Rob Markus. "Does stress influence sleep patterns, food intake, weight gain, abdominal obesity and weight loss interventions and vice versa?" *Obesity Reviews* 19, no. 1 (2018): 81–97.

Geisler, Corinna, Carla M. Prado, and Manfred J. Müller. "Inadequacy of body weight-based recommendations for individual protein intake—lessons from body composition analysis." *Nutrients* 9, no. 1 (2016): 23.

Gerrior, Shirley, Wenyen Juan, and Basiotis Peter. "An easy approach to calculating estimated energy requirements." *Preventing Chronic Disease* 3, no. 4 (2006).

Ghany, Abdel. "Safe food additives: A review." *Journal of Biological and Chemical Research.* (2015).

Gibson, A. A., R. V. Seimon, J. Franklin, T. P. Markovic, N. M. Byrne, E. Manson, I. D. Caterson, and Amanda Sainsbury. "Fast versus slow weight loss: Development process and rationale behind the dietary interventions for the TEMPO Diet Trial." *Obesity Science & Practice* 2, no. 2 (2016): 162–173.

Gillois, Kévin, Mathilde Lévêque, Vassilia Théodorou, Hervé Robert, and Muriel Mercier-Bonin. "Mucus: An Underestimated Gut Target for Environmental Pollutants and Food Additives." *Microorganisms* 6, no. 2 (2018): 53.

Gomes, João Pedro, Abdulla Watad, and Yehuda Shoenfeld. "Nicotine and autoimmunity: The lotus' flower in tobacco." *Pharmacological Research* (2017).

Gotthardt, Juliet D., Jessica L. Verpeut, Bryn L. Yeomans, Jennifer A. Yang, Ali Yasrebi, Troy A. Roepke, and Nicholas T. Bello. "Intermittent fasting promotes fat loss with lean mass retention, increased hypothalamic norepinephrine content, and increased neuropeptide Y gene expression in diet-induced obese male mice." *Endocrinology* 157, no. 2 (2016): 679–691.

Grandl, Gerald, Leon Straub, Carla Rudigier, Myrtha Arnold, Stephan Wueest, Daniel Konrad, and Christian Wolfrum. "Short-term feeding of a ketogenic diet induces more severe hepatic insulin resistance than an obesogenic high-fat diet." *The Journal of Physiology* 596, no. 19 (2018): 4597–4609.

Guess, Nicola. "A qualitative investigation of attitudes towards aerobic and resistance exercise amongst overweight and obese individuals." *BMC Research Notes* 5, no. 1 (2012): 191.

Hall, Kevin D. "Did the Food Environment Cause the Obesity Epidemic?" *Obesity* 26, no. 1 (2018): 11–13.

Hall, Kevin D., and Scott Kahan. "Maintenance of lost weight and long-term management of obesity." *Medical Clinics* 102, no. 1 (2018): 183–197.

Halson, Shona L. "Sleep in elite athletes and nutritional interventions to enhance sleep." *Sports Medicine* 44, no. 1 (2014): 13–23.

Hamdy, Osama, Mhd Wael Tasabehji, Taha Elseaidy, Shaheen Tomah, Sahar Ashrafzadeh, and Adham Mottalib. "Fat Versus Carbohydrate-Based Energy-Restricted Diets for Weight Loss in Patients With Type 2 Diabetes." *Current Diabetes Reports* 18, no. 12 (2018): 128.

Haskins, Ron. "The school lunch lobby." Retrieved from www.educationnext. org (2005).

Hayek, Nabil. "Chocolate, gut microbiota, and human health." *Frontiers in Pharmacology* 4 (2013): 11.

Headland, Michelle Louise, Peter Marshall Clifton, and Jennifer Beatrice Keogh. "Effect of intermittent compared to continuous energy restriction on weight loss and weight maintenance after 12 months in healthy overweight or obese adults." *International Journal of Obesity* (2018): 1.

Healthday. "A slam dunk: late-night tweets harm NBA players' performance." Retrieved from www. medicalxpress.com (2018).

Hensrud, Donald. *The Mayo Clinic Diet.* (2017).

Herrmann, Stephen D., Erik A. Willis, Jeffery J. Honas, Jaehoon Lee, Richard A. Washburn, and Joseph E. Donnelly. "Do changes in energy intake and non-exercise physical activity affect exercise-induced weight loss? Midwest Exercise Trial-2." *Obesity (Silver Spring, Md.)* 23, no. 8 (2015): 1539.

Hewagalamulage, S. D., T. K. Lee, I. J. Clarke, and B. A. Henry. "Stress, cortisol, and obesity: a role for cortisol responsiveness in identifying individuals prone to obesity." *Domestic Animal Endocrinology* 56 (2016): S112–S120.

Heymsfield, Steven B., MC Cristina Gonzalez, Wei Shen, Leanne Redman, and Diana Thomas. "Weight loss composition is one-fourth fat-free mass: a critical review and critique of this widely cited rule." *Obesity Reviews* 15, no. 4 (2014): 310–321.

HHS. "USDA Dietary Guidelines for Americans, 2010" Retrieved from www. nhlbi.nih.gov (2010).

HHS(2). "HHS/USDA Dietary Guidelines for Americans: 2005." Retrieved from www.nhlbi.nih.gov (2005).

Hicks, L.A., et al., "US Outpatient Antibiotic Prescribing Variation According to Geography, Patient Population, and Provider Specialty in 2011." *Clinical Infectious Diseases* 60, no. 9 (2015): 1308–16.

Hirshkowitz, Max, Kaitlyn Whiton, Steven M. Albert, Cathy Alessi, Oliviero Bruni, Lydia DonCarlos, Nancy Hazen et al. "National Sleep Foundation's sleep time duration recommendations: methodology and results summary." *Sleep Health* 1, no. 1 (2015): 40–43.

Højgaard, Betina, Dorte Gyrd-Hansen, Kim Rose Olsen, Jes Søgaard, and Thorkild IA Sørensen. "Waist circumference and body mass index as predictors of health care costs." *PLoS One* 3, no. 7 (2008): e2619.

Hollis, Jack F., Christina M. Gullion, Victor J. Stevens, Phillip J. Brantley, Lawrence J. Appel, Jamy D. Ard, Catherine M. Champagne et al. "Weight loss during the intensive intervention phase of the weight-loss maintenance trial." *American Journal of Preventive Medicine* 35, no. 2 (2008): 118–126.

Homayoni Rad, Aziz, Elnaz Vaghef Mehrabany, Beitullah Alipoor, and Leila Vaghef Mehrabany. "The comparison of food and supplement as probiotic delivery vehicles." *Critical Reviews in Food Science and Nutrition* 56, no. 6 (2016): 896–909.

Horne, James. "Too weighty a link between short sleep and obesity?" *Sleep* 31, no. 5 (2008): 595.

Howell, Scott, and Richard Kones. "'Calories in, calories out' and macronutrient intake: the hope, hype, and science of calories." *American Journal of Physiology-Endocrinology and Metabolism* 313, no. 5 (2017): E608–E612.

Hruby, Adela, JoAnn E. Manson, Lu Qi, Vasanti S. Malik, Eric B. Rimm, Qi Sun, Walter C. Willett, and Frank B. Hu. "Determinants and consequences of obesity." *American Journal of Public Health* 106, no. 9 (2016): 1656–1662.

Hu, Tian, Katherine T. Mills, Lu Yao, Kathryn Demanelis, Mohamed Eloustaz, William S. Yancy Jr, Tanika N. Kelly, Jiang He, and Lydia A. Bazzano. "Effects of low-carbohydrate diets versus low-fat diets on metabolic risk factors: a meta-analysis of randomized controlled clinical trials." *American Journal of Epidemiology* 176, no. suppl_7 (2012): S44–S54.

Ingargiola, Michael J., Saba Motakef, Michael T. Chung, Henry C. Vasconez, and Gordon H. Sasaki. "Cryolipolysis for fat reduction and body contouring: safety and efficacy of current treatment paradigms." *Plastic and Reconstructive Surgery* 135, no. 6 (2015): 1581.

INRA-France. "Food additive E171: First findings of oral exposure to titanium dioxide nanoparticles." ScienceDaily. www.sciencedaily.com/releases/2017/01/170124124355.htm (accessed November 28, 2018).

Iversen, Vegard M., Paul Jarle Mork, Ottar Vasseljen, Ronny Bergquist, and Marius S. Fimland. "Multiple-joint exercises using elastic resistance bands vs. conventional resistance-training equipment: A cross-over study." *European Journal of Sport Science* 17, no. 8 (2017): 973–982.

Jalonick, Mary Clare. "Pizza is a vegetable? Congress says yes." Retrieved from www.nbcnews.com (2011).

Jarde, Alexander, Anne-Mary Lewis-Mikhael, Paul Moayyedi, Jennifer C. Stearns, Stephen M. Collins, Joseph Beyene, and Sarah D. McDonald. "Pregnancy outcomes in women taking probiotics or prebiotics: a systematic review and meta-analysis," *BMC Pregnancy and Childbirth* 18, no. 1 (2018): 14.

Jaslow, Ryan. "CDC: 80 percent of American adults don't get recommended exercise." *CBC News*. May 3, 2013.

Jenkins, A. B., T. P. Markovic, A. Fleury, and L. V. Campbell. "Carbohydrate intake and short-term regulation of leptin in humans." *Diabetologia* 40, no. 3 (1997): 348–351.

Jéquier, Eric, and George A. Bray. "Low-fat diets are preferred." *The American Journal of Medicine* 113, no. 9 (2002): 41–46.

Johannsen, Darcy L., Nicolas D. Knuth, Robert Huizenga, Jennifer C. Rood, Eric Ravussin, and Kevin D. Hall. "Metabolic slowing with massive weight loss despite preservation of fat-free mass." *The Journal of Clinical Endocrinology & Metabolism* 97, no. 7 (2012): 2489–2496.

Johnston, Bradley C., Steve Kanters, Kristofer Bandayrel, Ping Wu, Faysal Naji, Reed A. Siemieniuk, Geoff DC Ball et al. "Comparison of weight loss among named diet programs in overweight and obese adults: a meta-analysis." *Jama* 312, no. 9 (2014): 923–933.

Jovanović, Boris. "Critical review of public health regulations of titanium dioxide, a human food additive." *Integrated Environmental Assessment and Management* 11, no. 1 (2015): 10–20.

Jumpertz, Reiner, Colleen A. Venti, Duc Son Le, Jennifer Michaels, Shannon Parrington, Jonathan Krakoff, and Susanne Votruba. "Food label accuracy of common snack foods." *Obesity* 21, no. 1 (2013): 164–169.

Kaur, Jaspinder. "A comprehensive review on metabolic syndrome." *Cardiology research and practice* (2014).

Kearney, John. "Food consumption trends and drivers." *Philosophical Transactions of the Royal Society B: Biological Sciences* 365, no. 1554 (2010): 2793–2807.

Keys, A., and M. Keys. "How to eat well and stay well the Mediterranean way." (1975).

Keys, Ancel. "Recollections of pioneers in nutrition: from starvation to cholesterol." *Journal of the American College of Nutrition* 9, no. 4 (1990): 288–291.

Keys, Ancel, Flaminio Fidanza, Martti J. Karvonen, Noboru Kimura, and Henry L. Taylor. "Indices of relative weight and obesity." *Journal of Chronic Diseases* 25, no. 6–7 (1972): 329–343.

Keys, Ancel, Francisco Grande, and Joseph T. Anderson. "Fiber and pectin in the diet and serum cholesterol concentration in man." *Proceedings of the Society for Experimental Biology and Medicine* 106, no. 3 (1961): 555–558.

Keys, Ancel, J. Brozek, Austin Henschel, O. Michelsen, H. Longstreet Taylor, E. Simonson, A. S. Skinner, and SM WELLS. "The biology of human starvation. Volumes 1 and 2." *The Biology of Human Starvation. Volumes 1 and 2.* (1950).

Keys, Ancel, Joseph T. Anderson, and Francisco Grande. "Prediction of serum-cholesterol responses of man to changes in fats in the diet." *Lancet* 273 (1957): 959–966.

Koleva, M., A. Nacheva, and M. Boev. "Somatotype and disease prevalence in adults." *Reviews on Environmental Health* 17, no. 1 (2002): 65–84.

Koliaki, Chrysi, Theodoros Spinos, Marianna Spinou, Maria-Eugenia Brinia, Dimitra Mitsopoulou, and Nicholas Katsilambros. "Defining the Optimal Dietary Approach for Safe, Effective and Sustainable Weight Loss in Overweight and Obese Adults." *In Healthcare*, vol. 6, no. 3, p. 73. Multidisciplinary Digital Publishing Institute (2018).

Kopf, Julianne C., Mallory J. Suhr, Jennifer Clarke, Seong-il Eyun, Jean-Jack M. Riethoven, Amanda E. Ramer-Tait, and Devin J. Rose. "Role of whole grains versus fruits and vegetables in reducing subclinical inflammation and promoting gastrointestinal health in individuals affected by overweight and obesity: A randomized controlled trial." *Nutrition Journal* 17, no. 1 (2018): 72.

Kreider, Richard B. "Dietary supplements and the promotion of muscle growth with resistance exercise." *Sports Medicine* 27, no. 2 (1999): 97–110.

Kresser, Chris. "Are You Undereating? Here Are 6 Common Signs and Symptoms." Retrieved from www.chriskresser.com (2018).

Kreuter, Roxane, Miriam Wankell, Golo Ahlenstiel, and Lionel Hebbard. "The role of obesity in inflammatory bowel disease." *Biochimica et Biophysica Acta (BBA)-Molecular Basis of Disease* (2018).

Krishnaswami, Ashok, Rohini Ashok, Stephen Sidney, Michael Okimura, Beth Kramer, Lindsey Hogan, Michael Sorel, Sheri Pruitt, and Wayne Smith. "Real-World Effectiveness of a Medically Supervised Weight Management Program in a Large Integrated Health Care Delivery System: Five-Year Outcomes." *The Permanente Journal* 22 (2018).

LaLanne, Jack. *Live Young Forever: 12 Steps to Optimum Health, Fitness and Longevity.* (2009).

Le Bourvellec, Carine, Sylvie Bureau, Catherine MGC Renard, Daniel Plenet, Hélène Gautier, Line Touloumet, Thierry Girard, and Sylvaine Simon. "Cultivar and year rather than agricultural practices affect primary and secondary metabolites in apple fruit." *PloS One* 10, no. 11 (2015): e0141916.

Lee, Hayan, Sunho Kim, and Donghee Kim. "Effects of exercise with or without light exposure on sleep quality and hormone reponses." *Journal of Exercise Nutrition & Biochemistry* 18, no. 3 (2014): 293.

Lee, Megan. "Five types of food to increase your psychological well-being." Retrieved from www.theconversation.com (2018).

Leidy, Heather J., Peter M. Clifton, Arne Astrup, Thomas P. Wycherley, Margriet S. Westerterp-Plantenga, Natalie D. Luscombe-Marsh, Stephen C. Woods, and Richard D. Mattes. "The role of protein in weight loss and maintenance–." *The American Journal of Clinical Nutrition* 101, no. 6 (2015): 1320S–1329S.

Lemstra, Mark, Yelena Bird, Chijioke Nwankwo, Marla Rogers, and John Moraros. "Weight loss intervention adherence and factors promoting adherence: a meta-analysis." *Patient Preference and Adherence* 10 (2016): 1547.

Levy, David T., Ron Borland, Eric N. Lindblom, Maciej L. Goniewicz, Rafael Meza, Theodore R. Holford, Zhe Yuan et al. "Potential deaths averted in USA by replacing cigarettes with e-cigarettes." *Tobacco Control* 27, no. 1 (2018): 18–25.

Li, Jingmei, Keith Humphreys, Louise Eriksson, Kamila Czene, Jianjun Liu, and Per Hall. "Effects of childhood body size on breast cancer tumour characteristics." *Breast Cancer Research* 12, no. 2 (2010): R23.

Li, Junyou. "Current status and prospects for in-feed antibiotics in the different stages of pork production—A review." *Asian-Australasian Journal of Animal Sciences* 30, no. 12 (2017): 1667.

Lichtenstein, Alice H., Lawrence J. Appel, Michael Brands, Mercedes Carnethon, Stephen Daniels, Harold A. Franch, Barry Franklin et al. "Diet and lifestyle recommendations revision 2006: a scientific statement from the American Heart Association Nutrition Committee." *Circulation* 114, no. 1 (2006): 82–96.

Liu, Ann G., Nikki A. Ford, Frank B. Hu, Kathleen M. Zelman, Dariush Mozaffarian, and Penny M. Kris-Etherton. "A healthy approach to dietary fats: understanding the science and taking action to reduce consumer confusion." *Nutrition Journal* 16, no. 1 (2017): 53.

Liu, Yanghui, D. C. Lee, Yehua Li, Weicheng Zhu, Riquan Zhang, Xuemei Sui, Carl J. Lavie, and Steven N. Blair. "Associations of Resistance Exercise with Cardiovascular Disease Morbidity and Mortality." *Medicine and Science in Sports and Exercise* (2018).

Liu (2), Yuying, Jane Alookaran, and J. Rhoads. "Probiotics in Autoimmune and Inflammatory Disorders." *Nutrients* 10, no. 10 (2018): 1537.

Lock, Jaclyn Y., Taylor L. Carlson, Chia-Ming Wang, Albert Chen, and Rebecca L. Carrier. "Acute exposure to commonly ingested emulsifiers alters intestinal mucus structure and transport properties." *Scientific Reports* 8, no. 1 (2018): 10008.

Longo, Valter D., and Mark P. Mattson. "Fasting: molecular mechanisms and clinical applications." *Cell Metabolism* 19, no. 2 (2014): 181–192.

Longo, Valter D., and Satchidananda Panda. "Fasting, circadian rhythms, and time-restricted feeding in healthy lifespan." *Cell Metabolism* 23, no. 6 (2016): 1048–1059.

Loprinzi, Paul, Ellen Smit, Hyo Lee, Carlos Crespo, Ross Andersen, and Steven N. Blair. "The 'fit but fat' paradigm addressed using accelerometer-determined physical activity data." *North American Journal of Medical Sciences* 6, no. 7 (2014): 295.

Lowe, Michael R., and C. Alix Timko. "Dieting: really harmful, merely ineffective or actually helpful?" *British Journal of Nutrition* 92, no. S1 (2004): S19–S22.

MacCormack, Jennifer K., and Kristen A. Lindquist. "Feeling hangry? When hunger is conceptualized as emotion." *Emotion* (2018).

Macfarlane, S. M. G. T., G. T. Macfarlane, and JH T. Cummings. "Prebiotics in the gastrointestinal tract." *Alimentary Pharmacology & Therapeutics* 24, no. 5 (2006): 701–714.

MacFarquhar, Jennifer K., Danielle L. Broussard, Paul Melstrom, Richard Hutchinson, Amy Wolkin, Colleen Martin, Raymond F. Burk et al. "Acute selenium toxicity associated with a dietary supplement." *Archives of Internal Medicine* 170, no. 3 (2010): 256–261.

MacLean, Paul S., Audrey Bergouignan, Marc-Andre Cornier, and Matthew R. Jackman. "Biology's response to dieting: the impetus for weight regain." *American Journal of Physiology-Regulatory, Integrative and Comparative Physiology* 301, no. 3 (2011): R581–R600.

Mangine, Gerald T., Jay R. Hoffman, Adam M. Gonzalez, Jeremy R. Townsend, Adam J. Wells, Adam R. Jajtner, Kyle S. Beyer et al. "The effect of training volume and intensity on improvements in muscular strength and size in resistance-trained men." *Physiological Reports* 3, no. 8 (2015).

Mann, Steven, Christopher Beedie, and Alfonso Jimenez. "Differential effects of aerobic exercise, resistance training and combined exercise modalities on cholesterol and the lipid profile: review, synthesis and recommendations." *Sports Medicine* 44, no. 2 (2014): 211–221.

Mann, Traci, A. Janet Tomiyama, Erika Westling, Ann-Marie Lew, Barbra Samuels, and Jason Chatman. "Medicare's search for effective obesity treatments: diets are not the answer." *American Psychologist* 62, no. 3 (2007): 220.

Markowiak, Paulina, and Katarzyna Śliżewska. "Effects of probiotics, prebiotics, and synbiotics on human health." *Nutrients* 9, no. 9 (2017): 1021.

Maugeri, Andrea, Jose Medina-Inojosa, Sarka Kunzova, Antonella Agodi, Martina Barchitta, Ondrej Sochor, Francisco Lopez-Jimenez, Yonas Geda, and Manlio Vinciguerra. "Sleep Duration and Excessive Daytime Sleepiness Are Associated with Obesity Independent of Diet and Physical Activity." *Nutrients* 10, no. 9 (2018): 1219.

Maynard, Andrew. "Dunkin' Donuts ditches titanium dioxide – but is it actually harmful?" Retrieved from www.phys.org (2015).

Mayo Clinic. "Are high-protein diets safe for weight loss?" Retrieved from www.mayoclinic.org (2018).

McAllister, Emily J., Nikhil V. Dhurandhar, Scott W. Keith, Louis J. Aronne, Jamie Barger, Monica Baskin, Ruth M. Benca et al. "Ten putative contributors to the obesity epidemic." *Critical Reviews in Food Science and Nutrition* 49, no. 10 (2009): 868–913.

McGraw, Phil. *The 20/20 Diet.* (2015).

McLaughlin, Elizabeth, Jane Ellen Smith, Kelsey Serier, Jamie Smith, Dominique Santistevan, and Jeremiah Simmons. "What does self-reported 'dieting' mean? Evidence from a daily diary study of behavior." *Appetite.* (2018).

Mead, M. Nathaniel. "Benefits of sunlight: a bright spot for human health." *Environmental Health Perspectives* 116, no. 4 (2008): A160.

MedicalXpress. "More than skin deep: cosmetic surgery industry booming." Retrieved from www.medicalxpress.com (2018).

Melanson, E. L. "The effect of exercise on non-exercise physical activity and sedentary behavior in adults." *Obesity Reviews* 18 (2017): 40–49.

Mickel, Kelly. "Alison Sweeney's Stay-Slim Secrets for Reaching Fitness Goals." Retrieved from www.fitnessmagazine.com (2018).

Mincer, Dana L., and Ishwarlal Jialal. "Hashimoto Thyroiditis." In StatPearls [Internet]. *StatPearls Publishing*, 2018.

Minger, Denise. "The Truth About Ancel Keys: We've All Got It Wrong" (2011). Blog of Denise Minger, retrieved 9 January 2019.

Minnesota Daily, "Nutritionist Ancel Keys, once the pride of UMN research, presents a fat problem for modern science" (2016).

Montesi, Luca, Marwan El Ghoch, Lucia Brodosi, Simona Calugi, Giulio Marchesini, and Riccardo Dalle Grave. "Long-term weight loss maintenance for obesity: a multidisciplinary approach." *Diabetes, Metabolic Syndrome and Obesity: Targets and Therapy* 9 (2016): 37.

Moore, June. "Nutrition apps provide weight stability for industrial hygiene warriors." *American Journal of Industrial Hygiene* 66, no. 6 (2019): 10.

Morin, Jean-Pascal, Luis F. Rodríguez-Durán, Kioko Guzmán-Ramos, Claudia Perez-Cruz, Guillaume Ferreira, Sofia Diaz-Cintra, and Gustavo Pacheco-López. "Palatable hyper-caloric foods impact on neuronal plasticity." *Frontiers in Behavioral Neuroscience* 11 (2017): 19.

Morris, Anne M., and Debra K. Katzman. "The impact of the media on eating disorders in children and adolescents." *Paediatrics & Child Health* 8, no. 5 (2003): 287–289.

Myles, Ian A. "Fast food fever: reviewing the impacts of the Western diet on immunity." *Nutrition Journal* 13, no. 1 (2014): 61.

Nackers, Lisa M., Kathryn R. Middleton, Pamela J. Dubyak, Michael J. Daniels, Stephen D. Anton, and Michael G. Perri. "Effects of prescribing 1,000 versus 1,500 kilocalories per day in the behavioral treatment of obesity: a randomized trial." *Obesity* 21, no. 12 (2013): 2481–2487.

National Institutes of Health. "Are you at a healthy weight?" www.nhlbi.nih.gov (2018).

National Weight Control Registry. "Success Stories." Accessed March 5, 2019. http://www.nwcr.ws/stories.htm.

Ness-Abramof, Rosane, and Caroline M. Apovian. "Drug-induced weight gain." *Drugs of Today* 41, no. 8 (2005): 547.

NIH. "Sleep Deprivation and Deficiency." Retrieved from www. nhlbi.nih.gov (2018).

Nóbrega, Sanmy R., and Cleiton A. Libardi. "Is resistance training to muscular failure necessary?" *Frontiers in Physiology* 7 (2016): 10.

Oja, Pekka, and Sylvia Titze. "Physical activity recommendations for public health: development and policy context." *EPMA Journal* 2, no. 3 (2011): 253–259.

Ortega, Francisco B., Xuemei Sui, Carl J. Lavie, and Steven N. Blair. "Body mass index, the most widely used but also widely criticized index: would a criterion standard measure of total body fat be a better predictor of cardiovascular disease mortality?" In *Mayo Clinic Proceedings*, vol. 91, no. 4, pp. 443–455. Elsevier, (2016).

Orvanová, Eva. "Somatotypes of weight lifters." *Journal of Sports Sciences* 8, no. 2 (1990): 119–137.

Pai, Aditi. "Weight Watchers acquires weight loss selfie startup Weilos." *Mobihealthnews.* (2015).

Paoli, Antonio, A. Rubini, J. S. Volek, and K. A. Grimaldi. "Beyond weight loss: a review of the therapeutic uses of very-low-carbohydrate (ketogenic) diets." *European Journal of Clinical Nutrition* 67, no. 8 (2013): 789.

Patel, Harsh, Hassan Alkhawam, Raef Madanieh, Niel Shah, Constantine E. Kosmas, and Timothy J. Vittorio. "Aerobic vs anaerobic exercise training effects on the cardiovascular system." *World Journal of Cardiology* 9, no. 2 (2017): 134.

Patterson, Ruth E., Gail A. Laughlin, Andrea Z. LaCroix, Sheri J. Hartman, Loki Natarajan, Carolyn M. Senger, María Elena Martínez et al. "Intermittent fasting and human metabolic health." *Journal of the Academy of Nutrition and Dietetics* 115, no. 8 (2015): 1203–1212.

Pawluk, April. "CRISPR: No Sign of Slowing Down." *Cell* 174, no. 5 (2018): 1041.

Phillips, Stuart M. "A brief review of higher dietary protein diets in weight loss: a focus on athletes." *Sports Medicine* 44, no. 2 (2014): 149–153.

Phillips, Stuart M., Stéphanie Chevalier, and Heather J. Leidy. "Protein 'requirements' beyond the RDA: implications for optimizing health." *Applied Physiology, Nutrition, and Metabolism* 41, no. 5 (2016): 565–572.

Pinho, Maria Gabriela M., Joreintje D. Mackenbach, Hélène Charreire, Jean-Michel Oppert, Helga Bardos, Harry Rutter, Sofie Compernolle, Joline WJ Beulens, Johannes Brug, and Jeroen Lakerveld. "Spatial access to restaurants and grocery stores in relation to frequency of home cooking." *International Journal of Behavioral Nutrition and Physical Activity* 15, no. 1 (2018): 6.

Poti, Jennifer M., Bianca Braga, and Bo Qin. "Ultra-processed Food Intake and Obesity: What Really Matters for Health—Processing or Nutrient Content?." *Current Obesity Reports* 6, no. 4 (2017): 420–431.

Poulimeneas, Dimitrios, Mary Yannakoulia, Costas Anastasiou, and Nikolaos Scarmeas. "Weight Loss Maintenance: Have We Missed the Brain?" *Brain Sciences* 8, no. 9 (2018): 174.

Pulido-Arjona, Leonardo, Jorge Enrique Correa-Bautista, Cesar Agostinis-Sobrinho, Jorge Mota, Rute Santos, María Correa-Rodríguez, Antonio Garcia-Hermoso, and Robinson Ramírez-Vélez. "Role of sleep duration and sleep-related problems in the metabolic syndrome among children and adolescents." *Italian Journal of Pediatrics* 44, no. 1 (2018): 9.

Qiu, Feifei, Chun-Ling Liang, Huazhen Liu, Yu-Qun Zeng, Shaozhen Hou, Song Huang, Xiaoping Lai, and Zhenhua Dai. "Impacts of cigarette smoking on immune responsiveness: Up and down or upside down?" *Oncotarget* 8, no. 1 (2017): 268.

Quigley, Eamonn MM. "Leaky gut–concept or clinical entity?." *Current Opinion in Gastroenterology* 32, no. 2 (2016): 74–79.

Quigley, Eamonn MM. "Prebiotics and probiotics in digestive health." *Clinical Gastroenterology and Hepatology* (2019).

Rask-Andersen, Mathias, Torgny Karlsson, Weronica Ek, Asa Johansson. "Genome-wide association study of body fat distribution identifies adiposity loci and sex-specific genetic effects." *Nature Communications* 10, 339 (2019): 1.

Requena, Teresa, M. Carmen Martínez-Cuesta, and Carmen Peláez. "Diet and microbiota linked in health and disease." *Food & Function* 9, no. 2 (2018): 688–704.

Riebl, Shaun K., and Brenda M. Davy. "The hydration equation: Update on water balance and cognitive performance." *ACSM's Health & Fitness Journal* 17, no. 6 (2013): 21.

Rockford Press. *The DASH Diet for Weight Loss*. (2014).

Rodgers, Blake, Kate Kirley, and Anne Mounsey. "Prescribing an antibiotic? Pair it with probiotics." *The Journal of Family Practice* 62, no. 3 (2013): 148.

Rodriguez, Julie, Sophie Hiel, and Nathalie M. Delzenne. "Metformin: old friend, new ways of action–implication of the gut microbiome?" *Current Opinion in Clinical Nutrition & Metabolic Care* 21, no. 4 (2018): 294–301.

Ross, Kathryn M., Peihua Qiu, Lu You, and Rena R. Wing. "Characterizing the Pattern of Weight Loss and Regain in Adults Enrolled in a 12-Week Internet-Based Weight Management Program." *Obesity* 26, no. 2 (2018): 318–323.

Sarica, Kemal. "Obesity and stones." *Current Opinion in Urology* 29, no. 1 (2019): 27–32.

Scheffler, Frederika, Sanja Kilian, Bonga Chiliza, Laila Asmal, Lebogang Phahladira, Stefan du Plessis, Martin Kidd et al. "Effects of cannabis use on body mass, fasting glucose and lipids during the first 12 months of treatment in schizophrenia spectrum disorders." *Schizophrenia Research* (2018).

Schoenfeld, Brad J. "The mechanisms of muscle hypertrophy and their application to resistance training." *The Journal of Strength & Conditioning Research* 24, no. 10 (2010): 2857–2872.

Schulte, Maureen MB, Jui-he Tsai, and Kelle H. Moley. "Obesity and PCOS: the effect of metabolic derangements on endometrial receptivity at the time of implantation." *Reproductive Sciences* 22, no. 1 (2015): 6–14.

Schüz, Benjamin, Natalie Schüz, and Stuart G. Ferguson. "It's the power of food: individual differences in food cue responsiveness and snacking in everyday life." *International Journal of Behavioral Nutrition and Physical Activity* 12, no. 1 (2015): 149.

Schwarz, Neil A., B. Rhett Rigby, Paul La Bounty, Brian Shelmadine, and Rodney G. Bowden. "A review of weight control strategies and their effects on the regulation of hormonal balance." *Journal of Nutrition and Metabolism* (2011).

Simon, Jean-Christophe, Julian R. Marchesi, Christophe Mougel, and Marc-André Selosse. "Host-microbiota interactions: from holobiont theory to analysis." *Microbiome* 7, no. 1 (2019): 5.

Singh, Vishal, Beng San Yeoh, Benoit Chassaing, Xia Xiao, Piu Saha, Rodrigo Aguilera Olvera, John D. Lapek Jr et al. "Dysregulated microbial fermentation of soluble fiber induces cholestatic liver cancer." *Cell* 175, no. 3 (2018): 679–694.

Sinha, Rajita, and Ania M. Jastreboff. "Stress as a common risk factor for obesity and addiction." *Biological Psychiatry* 73, no. 9 (2013): 827–835.

Sisson, Mark. *The Primal Blueprint: Reprogram your genes for effortless weight loss, vibrant health, and boundless energy.* (2013).

Skocaj, Matej, Metka Filipic, Jana Petkovic, and Sasa Novak. "Titanium dioxide in our everyday life; is it safe?" *Radiology and Oncology* 45, no. 4 (2011): 227–247.

Slaght, Jana, Martin Sénéchal, Travis J. Hrubeniuk, Andrea Mayo, and D. R. Bouchard. "Walking cadence to exercise at moderate intensity for adults: a systematic review." *Journal of Sports Medicine* (2017).

Sleep Foundation. "The Relationship Between Sleep and Industrial Accidents." Retrieved from www.sleepfoundation.org (2018).

Smith, Reuben L., Maarten R. Soeters, Rob CI Wüst, and Riekelt H. Houtkooper. "Metabolic flexibility as an adaptation to energy resources and requirements in health and disease." *Endocrine Reviews* 39, no. 4 (2018): 489–517.

Soeliman, Fatemeh Azizi, and Leila Azadbakht. "Weight loss maintenance: A review on dietary related strategies." *Journal of Research in Medical Sciences: The Official Journal of Isfahan University of Medical Sciences* 19, no. 3 (2014): 268.

Spring, Bonnie, Christine Pellegrini, H. G. McFadden, Angela Fidler Pfammatter, Tammy K. Stump, Juned Siddique, Abby C. King, and Donald Hedeker. "Multicomponent mHealth Intervention for Large, Sustained Change in Multiple Diet and Activity Risk Behaviors: The Make Better Choices 2 Randomized Controlled Trial." *Journal of Medical Internet Research* 20, no. 6 (2018): e10528.

Stahlhut, Richard W., John Peterson Myers, Julia A. Taylor, Angel Nadal, Jonathan A. Dyer, and Frederick S. vom Saal. "Experimental BPA Exposure and Glucose-Stimulated Insulin Response in Adult Men and Women." *Journal of the Endocrine Society* 2, no. 10 (2018): 1173–1187.

Starr, Ranjani R. "Too little, too late: ineffective regulation of dietary supplements in the United States." *American Journal of Public Health* 105, no. 3 (2015): 478–485.

Steele, Eurídice Martínez, Barry M. Popkin, Boyd Swinburn, and Carlos A. Monteiro. "The share of ultra-processed foods and the overall nutritional quality of diets in the US: evidence from a nationally representative cross-sectional study." *Population Health Metrics* 15, no. 1 (2017): 6.

Steele, Eurídice Martinez, and Carlos A. Monteiro. "Association between dietary share of ultra-processed foods and urinary concentrations of phytoestrogens in the US." *Nutrients* 9, no. 3 (2017): 209.

Steele, Eurídice Martínez, Larissa Galastri Baraldi, Maria Laura da Costa Louzada, Jean-Claude Moubarac, Dariush Mozaffarian, and Carlos Augusto Monteiro. "Ultra-processed foods and added sugars in the US diet: evidence from a nationally representative cross-sectional study." *BMJ Open* 6, no. 3 (2016): e009892.

Steele, Tim. "Life begins at forty–hybridomas: ageing technology holds promise for future drug discoveries." *GABI Journal-Generics and Biosimilars Initiative Journal* 5, no. 1 (2016): 21–26.

Stein, Michael D., and Peter D. Friedmann. "Disturbed sleep and its relationship to alcohol use." *Substance Abuse* 26, no. 1 (2006): 1–13.

Stockman, Mary-Catherine, Dylan Thomas, Jacquelyn Burke, and Caroline M. Apovian. "Intermittent Fasting: Is the Wait Worth the Weight?" *Current Obesity Reports* 7 (2018): 172–185.

Stott-Miller, Marni, Marian L. Neuhouser, and Janet L. Stanford. "Consumption of deep-fried foods and risk of prostate cancer." *The Prostate* 73, no. 9 (2013): 960–969.

Stratakis, Constantine A., and Sosipatros A. Boikos. "Genetics of adrenal tumors associated with Cushing's syndrome: a new classification for bilateral adrenocortical hyperplasias." *Nature Reviews Endocrinology* 3, no. 11 (2007): 748.

Sun, M., W. Feng, F. Wang, P. Li, Z. Li, M. Li, G. Tse, J. Vlaanderen, R. Vermeulen, and L. A. Tse. "Meta-analysis on shift work and risks of specific obesity types." *Obesity Reviews* 19, no. 1 (2018): 28–40.

Suter, Paolo M., and Angelo Tremblay. "Is alcohol consumption a risk factor for weight gain and obesity?" *Critical Reviews in Clinical Laboratory Sciences* 42, no. 3 (2005): 197–227.

Sutherland, Elizabeth. "Healing metabolism: a naturopathic medicine perspective on achieving weight loss and long-term balance." *The Permanente Journal* 9, no. 3 (2005): 16.

Swift, Damon L., Neil M. Johannsen, Carl J. Lavie, Conrad P. Earnest, and Timothy S. Church. "The role of exercise and physical activity in weight loss and maintenance." *Progress in Cardiovascular Diseases* 56, no. 4 (2014): 441–447.

Syed-Abdul, Majid M., Qiong Hu, Miriam Jacome-Sosa, Jaume Padilla, Camila Manrique-Acevedo, Colette Heimowitz, and Elizabeth J. Parks. "Effect of carbohydrate restriction-induced weight loss on aortic pulse wave velocity in overweight men and women." *Applied Physiology, Nutrition, and Metabolism* (2018).

Tang, Jason, Charles Abraham, Colin Greaves, and Tom Yates. "Self-directed interventions to promote weight loss: a systematic review of reviews." *Journal of Medical Internet Research* 16, no. 2 (2014).

The Heart Foundation. "The Top 10 Excuses for Not Exercising (and Solutions!)." Retrieved from www.theheartfoundation.org (2018).

Thomas, Diana M., Corby K. Martin, Leanne M. Redman, Steven B. Heymsfield, Steven Lettieri, James A. Levine, Claude Bouchard, and Dale A. Schoeller. "Effect of dietary adherence on the body weight plateau: a mathematical model incorporating intermittent compliance with energy intake prescription." *The American Journal of Clinical Nutrition* 100, no. 3 (2014): 787–795.

Thomas, Michael H., and Steve P. Burns. "Increasing lean mass and strength: A comparison of high frequency strength training to lower frequency strength training." *International Journal of Exercise Science* 9, no. 2 (2016): 159.

Thomas, Sunil, Jacques Izard, Emily Walsh, Kristen Batich, Pakawat Chongsathidkiet, Gerard Clarke, David A. Sela et al. "The host microbiome regulates and maintains human health: a primer and perspective for non-microbiologists." *Cancer Research* 77, no. 8 (2017): 1783–1812.

Tokuhara, Daisuke, Yosuke Kurashima, Mariko Kamioka, Toshinori Nakayama, Peter Ernst, and Hiroshi Kiyono. "A comprehensive understanding of the gut mucosal immune system in allergic inflammation." *Allergology International* (2019).

Tox Town. "Endocrine disruptors. What are they?" Retrieved from www.toxtown.nlm.nih.gov (2018).

Traversy, Gregory, and Jean-Philippe Chaput. "Alcohol consumption and obesity: an update." *Current Obesity Reports* 4, no. 1 (2015): 122–130.

Trexler, Eric T., Abbie E. Smith-Ryan, and Layne E. Norton. "Metabolic adaptation to weight loss: implications for the athlete." *Journal of the International Society of Sports Nutrition* 11, no. 1 (2014): 7.

Tsai, Yu-Ling, Tzu-Lung Lin, Chih-Jung Chang, Tsung-Ru Wu, Wei-Fan Lai, Chia-Chen Lu, and Hsin-Chih Lai. "Probiotics, prebiotics and amelioration of diseases." *Journal of Biomedical Science* 26, no. 1 (2019): 3.

Turk, Melanie Warziski, Kyeongra Yang, Marilyn Hravnak, Susan M. Sereika, Linda J. Ewing, and Lora E. Burke. "Randomized clinical trials of weight-loss maintenance: A review." *The Journal of Cardiovascular Nursing* 24, no. 1 (2009): 58.

University of Zurich. "Titanium dioxide nanoparticles can exacerbate colitis." ScienceDaily. www.sciencedaily.com/releases/2017/07/170719100521.htm (accessed November 28, 2018).

Upadhyay, Jagriti, Olivia Farr, Nikolaos Perakakis, Wael Ghaly, and Christos Mantzoros. "Obesity as a disease." *Medical Clinics of North America* (2017).

Vakil, Rachit M., Zoobia W. Chaudhry, Ruchi S. Doshi, Jeanne M. Clark, and Kimberly A. Gudzune. "Commercial Programs' Online Weight-Loss Claims Compared to Results from Randomized Controlled Trials." *Obesity* 25, no. 11 (2017): 1885–1893.

van den Boer, Janet HW, Jentina Kranendonk, Anne van de Wiel, Edith JM Feskens, Anouk Geelen, and Monica Mars. "Self-reported eating rate is associated with weight status in a Dutch population: a validation study and a cross-sectional study." *International Journal of Behavioral Nutrition and Physical Activity* 14, no. 1 (2017): 121.

Vaz, Louise Elaine, Kenneth P. Kleinman, Marsha A. Raebel, James D. Nordin, Matthew D. Lakoma, M. Maya Dutta-Linn, and Jonathan A. Finkelstein. "Recent trends in outpatient antibiotic use in children." *Pediatrics* (2014): peds-2013.

Venkata, Rekhadevi Perumalla, and Rajagopal Subramanyam. "Evaluation of the deleterious health effects of consumption of repeatedly heated vegetable oil." *Toxicology Reports* 3 (2016): 636–643.

Viennois, Emilie, and Benoit Chassaing. "First victim, later aggressor: How the intestinal microbiota drives the pro-inflammatory effects of dietary emulsifiers." *Gut Microbes* 66, no. 8 (2018): 1–4.

Villareal, Dennis T., Lina Aguirre, A. Burke Gurney, Debra L. Waters, David R. Sinacore, Elizabeth Colombo, Reina Armamento-Villareal, and Clifford Qualls. "Aerobic or resistance exercise, or both, in dieting obese older adults." *New England Journal of Medicine* 376, no. 20 (2017): 1943–1955.

Ville, Annette P., Melvin B. Heyman, Rosalinda Medrano, and Janet M. Wojcicki. "Early antibiotic exposure and risk of childhood obesity in Latinos." *Childhood Obesity* 13, no. 3 (2017): 231–235.

Vuong, Ann M., Kimberly Yolton, Kendra L. Poston, Changchun Xie, Glenys M. Webster, Andreas Sjödin, Joseph M. Braun, Kim N. Dietrich, Bruce P. Lanphear, and Aimin Chen. "Childhood polybrominated diphenyl ether (PBDE) exposure and executive function in children in the HOME Study." *International Journal of Hygiene and Environmental Health* 221, no. 1 (2018): 87–94.

Wajchenberg, Bernardo Leo. "Subcutaneous and visceral adipose tissue: their relation to the metabolic syndrome." *Endocrine Reviews* 21, no. 6 (2000): 697–738.

Wang, Lu, I-Min Lee, JoAnn E. Manson, Julie E. Buring, and Howard D. Sesso. "Alcohol consumption, weight gain, and risk of becoming overweight in middle-aged and older women." *Archives of Internal Medicine* 170, no. 5 (2010): 453–461.

Warburton, Darren ER, Crystal Whitney Nicol, and Shannon SD Bredin. "Health benefits of physical activity: the evidence." *Canadian Medical Association Journal* 174, no. 6 (2006): 801–809.

Warner, Melanie. "Why the Food Industry Loves Michelle Obama." Retrieved from www.cbsnews.com (2010).

Weiss, Edward P., Richard C. Jordan, Ethel M. Frese, Stewart G. Albert, and Dennis T. Villareal. "Effects of weight loss on lean mass, strength, bone, and aerobic capacity." *Medicine and Science in Sports and Exercise* 49, no. 1 (2017): 206.

Wells, Kaitlyn. "6 ways to beat pricey gym memberships." Retrieved from www.marketwatch.com (2015).

Westcott, Wayne L. "Resistance training is medicine: effects of strength training on health." *Current Sports Medicine Reports* 11, no. 4 (2012): 209–216.

Widysanto, Allen, and Abdolreza Saadabadi. "Nicotine Addiction." In StatPearls [Internet]. *StatPearls Publishing*, 2018.

Wikipedia. "Grocery Manufacturers Association," Wikipedia, The Free Encyclopedia, https://en.wikipedia.org/w/index.php?title=Grocery_Manufacturers_Association&oldid=850064780 (accessed November 29, 2018).

Williams, R. L., L. G. Wood, C. E. Collins, and R. Callister. "Effectiveness of weight loss interventions–is there a difference between men and women: a systematic review." *Obesity Reviews* 16, no. 2 (2015): 171–186.

Willmer, Mikaela, and Martin Salzmann-Erikson. "'The only chance of a normal weight life': A qualitative analysis of online forum discussions about bariatric surgery." *PloS One* 13, no. 10 (2018): e0206066.

Wing, Rena R., and Suzanne Phelan. "Long-term weight loss maintenance–." *The American Journal of Clinical Nutrition* 82, no. 1 (2005): 222S–225S.

Wolpert, Stuart. "Dieting does not work, UCLA researchers report." Retrieved from newsroom.ucla.edu (2007).

World Health Organization. "Recommended population levels of physical activity for health." *Global Recommendations on Physical Activity for Health* (2010): 15–34.

Wylie-Rosett, Judith, Karin Aebersold, Beth Conlon, Carmen R. Isasi, and Natania W. Ostrovsky. "Health effects of low-carbohydrate diets: where should new research go?" *Current Diabetes Reports* 13, no. 2 (2013): 271–278.

Yannakoulia, Mary, Dimitrios Poulimeneas, Eirini Mamalaki, and Costas A. Anastasiou. "Dietary modifications for weight loss and weight loss maintenance." *Metabolism* (2019).

Yau, Yvonne HC, and Marc N. Potenza. "Stress and eating behaviors." *Minerva Endocrinologica* 38, no. 3 (2013): 255.

Yildiz, Bulent O., Marc A. Suchard, Ma-Li Wong, Samuel M. McCann, and Julio Licinio. "Alterations in the dynamics of circulating ghrelin, adiponectin, and leptin in human obesity." *Proceedings of the National Academy of Sciences* 101, no. 28 (2004): 10434–10439.

Yoo, Ji Youn, and Sung Soo Kim. "Probiotics and prebiotics: Present status and future perspectives on metabolic disorders." *Nutrients* 8, no. 3 (2016): 173.

Yuenyongchaiwat, Kornanong. "Effects of 10,000 steps a day on physical and mental health in overweight participants in a community setting: a preliminary study." *Brazilian Journal of Physical Therapy* AHEAD (2016): 0–0.

Zaleski, Amanda L., Beth A. Taylor, and Paul D. Thompson. "Coenzyme Q10 as Treatment for Statin-Associated Muscle Symptoms—A Good Idea, but...." *Advances in Nutrition* 9, no. 4 (2018): 519S–523S.

Zinöcker, Marit, and Inge Lindseth. "The Western Diet–Microbiome-Host Interaction and Its Role in Metabolic Disease." *Nutrients* 10, no. 3 (2018).

Zomosky, Lisa. "3 Weight Loss Services Your Plan May Cover." May 19, 2015. https://blogs.webmd.com/public-health/20150519/3-weight-loss-services-your-plan-may-cover.

Zou, Maggie L., Paul J. Moughan, Ajay Awati, and Geoffrey Livesey. "Accuracy of the Atwater factors and related food energy conversion factors with low-fat, high-fiber diets when energy intake is reduced spontaneously." *The American Journal of Clinical Nutrition* 86, no. 6 (2007): 1649–1656.

CPSIA information can be obtained
at www.ICGtesting.com
Printed in the USA
LVHW050720290820
664472LV00013B/1543